After Freud Left

After Freud Left

A Century of Psychoanalysis in America

EDITED BY JOHN BURNHAM

The University of Chicago Press
Chicago and London

The University of Chicago Press, Chicago 60637
The University of Chicago Press, Ltd., London
© 2012 by The University of Chicago
All rights reserved. Published 2012.
Paperback edition 2014
Printed in the United States of America

23 22 21 20 19 18 17 16 15 14   2 3 4 5 6

ISBN-13: 978-0-226-08137-3 (cloth)
ISBN-13: 978-0-226-21186-2 (paper)
ISBN-13: 978-0-226-08139-7 (ebook)
10.7208/chicago/9780226081397.001.0001

Library of Congress Cataloging-in-Publication Data

After Freud left: a century of psychoanalysis in America / edited by John Burnham
    pages; cm
  Includes bibliographical references and index.
  ISBN 978-0-226-08137-3 (cloth: alkaline paper)—ISBN 0-226-08137-0 (cloth: alkaline paper)   1. Psychoanalysis—United States—History.
2. Psychiatry—United States—History—20th century.   3. Freud, Sigmund, 1856-1939—Influence.   4. Psychoanalysts—United States.   I. Burnham, John C. (John Chynoweth), 1929–
   RC503.A38 2012
   616.89'17—dc23
                                                            2011050712

♾ This paper meets the requirements of ANSI/NISO Z39.48-1992 (Permanence of Paper).

CONTENTS

Introduction / 1

PART I : 1909 TO THE 1940S: FREUD AND THE PSYCHOANALYTIC MOVEMENT CROSS THE ATLANTIC

Introduction to Part I: Transnationalizing / 25

SONU SHAMDASANI
ONE / Psychotherapy, 1909: Notes on a Vintage / 31

RICHARD SKUES
TWO / Clark Revisited: Reappraising Freud in America / 49

ERNST FALZEDER
THREE / "A Fat Wad of Dirty Pieces of Paper": Freud on America, Freud in America, Freud and America / 85

GEORGE MAKARI
FOUR / *Mitteleuropa* on the Hudson: On the Struggle for American Psychoanalysis after the *Anschluß* / 111

HALE USAK-SAHIN
FIVE / Another Dimension of the Émigré Experience: From Central Europe to the United States via Turkey / 125

PART II : AFTER WORLD WAR II: THE FATE OF FREUD'S LEGACY IN AMERICAN CULTURE

Introduction to Part II: A Shift in Perspective / 157

DOROTHY ROSS
SIX / Freud and the Vicissitudes of Modernism in the United States, 1940–1980 / 163

LOUIS MENAND
SEVEN / Freud, Anxiety, and the Cold War / 189

ELIZABETH LUNBECK
EIGHT / Heinz Kohut's Americanization of Freud / 209

JEAN-CHRISTOPHE AGNEW
NINE / The Walking Man and the Talking Cure / 233

Conclusion / 247
Acknowledgments / 255
Chronological Guide to Events / 257
List of Contributors / 261
Index / 263

INTRODUCTION

From August 29 to September 21, 1909, Sigmund Freud, the Viennese neurologist who devised psychoanalysis, visited the United States, where he gave five lectures at Clark University. That visit is still mentioned in college-level American history textbooks as a symbol of sociocultural changes that began early in the twentieth century and left the United States transformed for all of the decades afterward.[1] Freud, accurately or inaccurately, became the emblem particularly of that complex historical process that scholars have often referred to as the "psychologization" of America. Moreover, his work went beyond psychotherapy into interactions—not always favorable—with all of the major cultural movements of the twentieth century. In this book, leading historians of psychoanalysis and of American culture reflect on what happened to Freud's legacy in the United States during the ten decades after Freud departed from North America. They write with awareness of the persistent attractiveness of the subject of psychoanalysis for both lay and technical audiences. They also write in the knowledge that psychoanalysis has always been controversial, whether considered in the narrow sense of a particular type of psychotherapy or as the associated system of understanding the world, society, and humans as Freud portrayed them.

    1. In U.S. history textbooks, authors began after World War II to recognize that psychoanalysis was of major significance as part of both intellectual and social history. Freud's 1909 visit began to become a convenient symbol around 1970, as more detailed discussions of psychoanalytic ideas, and indeed intellectual and cultural history material in general, diminished in proportion in the content of most texts. See, for example, a transitional work, the textbook that was more widely used than most, or any, John D. Hicks, George E. Mowry, and Robert E. Burke, *The American Nation*, 5th ed. (Boston: Houghton Mifflin, 1971), 512–14, in which there was a whole section on Sigmund Freud, including the small-group photo of the psychoanalysts participating in the Clark conference described below by Richard Skues.

A centennial offers a special opportunity to reflect on a landmark event in history. Usually such reflections confirm historical memory or serve other human purposes.[2] The centennial of Freud's visit invites new perspectives that the passage of a century will have created. The authors of this book take a fresh look at the visit itself and launch an examination of the transnational movement of Freud's ideas to the United States. The essayists also address the dynamic relationship between psychoanalysis and psychoanalytic thinking, on the one hand, and a changing American culture, on the other.[3] Taken together, these essays suggest a variety of new parameters in the histories of psychoanalysis and of American society and culture, at first in 1909 and then in the decades after Freud left.

Freud's American legacy has to some extent been neglected, even implicitly suppressed, for a generation. There has been a flood of scholarship on the biography of Freud and on the European or world history of psychoanalysis. Much of this scholarship focused, directly or indirectly, on non-historical, anachronistic questions about the contemporary validity of psychoanalytic psychology and psychotherapy. These controversies of the late twentieth century have had the effect of obscuring the extent to which earlier intellectuals and public figures in the United States had accepted psychoanalytic ideas and practice as a fresh and vibrant, if contested, part of their world. Except for a general history published in 1995 by Nathan G. Hale Jr. and some specialized research, such as that on psychoanalysis in films or on the history of local figures and organizations, recent historians have produced relatively little on the past cultural transfer and proliferation of psychoanalytic thinking in the United States, where, everyone agrees, Freud's thinking had far greater intellectual and social impact than it did elsewhere on the planet.[4]

---

2. Leon Hoffman, "One Hundred Years after Sigmund Freud's Lectures in America: Towards an Integration of Psychoanalytic Theories and Techniques within Psychiatry," *History of Psychiatry* 21 (2010): 455–70, for example, used this particular centenary as an occasion to assess the place of psychoanalytic practice and theory in current psychiatry. Or for another example, see Alexandra Sacks and George Makari, "Freud in the New World," *American Journal of Psychiatry* 166 (2009): 662–63.

3. The authors of this book implicitly follow the commonsensical integration of intellectual history into cultural history and general history as described by the writers in "The Current State of Intellectual History: A Forum," *Historically Speaking: The Bulletin of The Historical Society*, September 2009, 14–24.

4. Nathan G. Hale Jr., *The Rise and Crisis of Psychoanalysis in the United States: Freud and the Americans, 1917–1985* (New York: Oxford University Press, 1995). Compare *Transnational Psychiatries: Social and Cultural Histories of Psychiatry in Comparative Perspective, c. 1800–2000*, ed. Waltraud Ernst and Thomas Mueller (Newcastle upon Tyne: Cambridge Scholars Publishing, 2010).

With so few reminders from immediately preceding scholars, even well-informed people of the early twenty-first century may be surprised by evidence of how powerfully psychoanalysis and psychoanalytic thinking directly affected American culture fifty years earlier. The essays below display how the best scholars today take seriously the evidence that the impact of Freud's ideas in the United States, for good or for ill, was indeed a major historical event of the twentieth century.

A Rise-and-Fall Narrative, with a Mid-Twentieth-Century Peak

By chance, the invited reflections in this volume, taken together, comprise a narrative of a historical phenomenon with a beginning, a rise to a peak, and a decline. In 1909, hardly any Americans had heard of Freud's writings, not even his publications about his innovations in psychotherapeutic technique. By the mid-twentieth century, Freud's ideas had become a conspicuous—indeed, unavoidable—part of the American cultural landscape. Another half century later, Freud's name was still familiar, but American cultural leaders had many new ways of looking at the world, and only infrequently did they make detailed, direct references to any of Freud's ideas. The authors in this book therefore offer reflections on how Freud's contentions, originating in Europe, gained such remarkable visibility in the United States in the middle of the twentieth century and then how his legacy declined in importance or became relatively invisible at the end of the century.

If there was a high point and then a decline, there had to be a beginning. Earlier historians explored Freud's visit in 1909 and then the critical transfer of psychoanalytic ideas and their carriers and carrier institutions in the 1930s and 1940s, often portraying events in America as local or subsidiary to what happened in Europe.

In the first decades after Freud ended his three-and-a-half-week visit in 1909, up until World War II, psychoanalysis, historians found, spread into the United States mainly through two routes, medicine and the intellectual and cultural avant-garde.[5] As our essays will show, the migration of European analysts and other intellectuals to the United States in the in-

---

5. Nathan G. Hale Jr., *Freud and the Americans: The Beginnings of Psychoanalysis in the United States, 1876–1917* (New York: Oxford University Press, 1971); Hale, *The Rise and Crisis of Psychoanalysis*; John C. Burnham, *Psychoanalysis and American Medicine, 1894–1918: Medicine, Science, and Culture* (New York: International Universities Press, 1967); John C. Burnham, "From Avant-Garde to Specialism," *Journal of the History of the Behavioral Sciences* 15 (1979): 128–34; George Makari, *Revolution in Mind: The Creation of Psychoanalysis* (New York: HarperCollins, 2008).

terwar period then added a set of strong interactions. The leading analytic practitioners were often very sensitive to what in Europe might be called philosophical questions—not only the mind-body problem and the problems of human nature, but questions of education, social distributions, literature, and the arts. Indeed, as a group, psychoanalysts were remarkably interdisciplinary in background. It is no wonder that, arguably, theory could overshadow practice in the professional, disciplined psychoanalysis that flourished so conspicuously in the United States after 1938. And it is no wonder that psychoanalysts had direct intellectual interactions as well as professional contact with leading thinkers and artists. At the high point of both the popularization and prestige of psychoanalysis in the United States in the 1940s–1960s, it was difficult to separate the core psychoanalytic movement from the pervasive cultural impact. A highly disciplined group of analysts, advocating what became known as "American ego psychology," set the technical standard for psychoanalytic practice.[6] At the same time, intellectuals and the wider public found Freudian ideas omnipresent in the culture.

Some partisan latter-day scholars have denied that psychoanalytic ideas were ever important in the United States or anywhere else.[7] Historians and other scholars, however, had already established the existence of the high point of interest in psychoanalysis in the United States in the mid-century decades.[8] Not the least of their evidence was the fact that, for generations, an astonishing number of leading figures among the powerful intellectual and policy elites underwent a personal psychoanalysis—the most notorious, perhaps, being eminent Hollywood figures and others in the world of entertainment and the media.[9] In the technical field of psychiatry, analysts effectively took most of the leadership positions, and their influence continuously spread into medicine and beyond. Indeed, by the World War II

6. *The Hartmann Era*, ed. Martin S. Bergmann (New York: Other Press, 2000).

7. The basis for writing off psychoanalysis is usually that Freud was wrong and therefore is not important in the history of ideas. This is a viewpoint the Canadian philosopher Todd Dufresne suggests in his offhand comment, quoted in his book of interviews, Todd Dufresne, *Against Freud: Critics Talk Back* (Stanford, CA: Stanford University Press, 2007), 146: "Frankly, in very few fields is the level of scholarship so slipshod. . . . [A]nalysts and their patients generally make for such lousy intellectuals . . . intellectuals themselves have produced so many lousy books on psychoanalysis."

8. See especially Hale, *The Rise and Crisis of Psychoanalysis*.

9. See, for example, Stephen Farber and Marc Green, *Hollywood on the Couch: A Candid Look at the Overheated Love Affair Between Psychiatrists and Moviemakers* (New York: William Morrow, 1993); Krin Gabbard and Glen O. Gabbard, *Psychiatry and the Cinema* (Chicago: University of Chicago Press, 1987).

period, even professional psychologists were, however reluctantly, recognizing Freudian teachings and therapies.[10] At the same time, psychoanalysis became fundamental to other kinds of social scientists, beginning especially in the 1930s. One need only review scholarly writings produced in the 1950s era to see the remarkable extent to which intellectuals in anthropology and kindred disciplines, not to mention literature and the arts, explicitly and repeatedly invoked psychoanalytic thinking in their work.[11]

In addition, there are good eyewitness reports from cultural figures of the mid-century period. They confirm that Freudian ideas constituted a major element in American culture at that time. Not only did witnesses agree that the impact of psychoanalytic thinking was significantly greater in the United States than anywhere else; they projected that impact in the United States to the whole world. In 1957, an important historian from New York, Benjamin Nelson, in introducing a centennial volume marking Freud's birth in 1856, raised the question, "Will the Twentieth Century go down in history as the *Freudian Century?*" Nelson compared Freud to major intellectuals of the nineteenth century and to such giants of his own day as Dewey, Sartre, Spengler, and Toynbee, who all "seem shades of yesteryear, without power to express our present experience of the condition of men or the designs of history. Too few years are left in the present [twentieth] Century to exhaust the dimensions of [Freud's] message or to approximate the substance of his hopes."[12]

Such rhetoric, however well informed, seems in the twenty-first century overblown or partisan, and it probably was. Yet other thoughtful cultural observers of fifty years ago also testified with remarkable unanimity that psychoanalytic thinking was conspicuous and momentous in American culture and life in those times. For example, in 1959, Stanford sociologist Richard LaPiere was ardently condemning "Freudianism" and the cultural changes that he and other social commentators associated with it. Yet LaPiere still concluded that in the United States "the growing popularity of Freudianism as an explanation of and justification for human conduct . . . is a change of paramount significance; for Freudianism provides a

---

10. The classic work is David Shakow and David Rapaport, *The Influence of Freud on American Psychology* (New York: International Universities Press, 1964).

11. See, for example, Edward J. K. Gitre, "Importing Freud: First-Wave Psychoanalysis, Interwar Social Sciences, and the Interdisciplinary Foundations of an American Social Theory," *Journal of the History of the Behavioral Sciences* 46 (2010): 239–62.

12. Benjamin Nelson, "Preface," in *Freud and the Twentieth Century*, ed. Benjamin Nelson (New York: Meridian Books, 1957), 9–10.

unique idea of the nature of man, of his potentialities, and of his relations to society."[13] Altogether, evidence of the importance of Freud's legacy in the 1940s–1960s is overwhelming.

This high point ended only in the wake of the cultural events of the 1960s and the simultaneous resurgence of material, non-psychological ideas and new psychopharmaceutical resources for mental illnesses. In the years 1965 to 1975, as psychoactive drugs became well established in psychiatry proper, the new somaticism, along with waves of new psychotherapies, began to marginalize psychoanalytic practitioners in both medicine and society. The Freudian psychoanalytic movement, for so long consisting of the insiders and leaders, suffered from both direct attacks and from simply being sidelined.[14]

Historians are still working to understand how and why Freudian ideas lost their direct influence in the closing decades of the twentieth century. Institutionalized, formal clinical psychoanalysis fragmented and to a substantial extent became socially, or at least economically, inconsequential. Teachers by the twenty-first century were finding that their students had trouble even conceptualizing that people might have unconscious motives and psychological conflicts. It is true that educated Americans still knew Freud's name. They still understood cartoons that showed the stereotyped situation of the patient on the couch being treated by a "psychiatrist." As late as the decades around the turn of the twenty-first century, Sigmund Freud was still newsworthy. In some areas of literary and humanistic studies and among significant numbers of psychotherapists, psychoanalysis was still central or at least deeply influential. But compared to mid-century, by the 1990s the age of Freud had been fading away for some time.

It is true that psychoanalytic ideas labeled as such did tend to disappear also as they became absorbed into the culture. Neo-Freudians had all along emphasized the social environmental sources of personal and social misery and dysfunction. Then in the 1970s and 1980s, leaders in countercultural movements invoked partial ideas from psychoanalysis but seldom accepted Freud's whole schema. In these important transformations, much got lost. Innovators still used Freudian ideas, but only selectively. In new guises, influenced by reworkings of Freud in Europe and feeding into postmodern theories, Freud remained a thinker to be reckoned with—but no longer in a central role in intellectuals' discussions.

13. Richard LaPiere, *The Freudian Ethic* (New York: Duell, Sloan and Pierce, 1959), viii.
14. See especially Paul E. Stepansky, *Psychoanalysis at the Margins* (New York: Other Press, 2009). Another version of the story is in T. M. Luhrmann, *Of Two Minds: The Growing Disorder in American Psychiatry* (New York: Alfred A. Knopf, 2001).

Many historical writers have also been struck by the ways in which additional events coming from outside of psychoanalysis contributed to the loss of momentum and decline of the psychoanalytic movement. At the end of the twentieth century, financial factors did great damage to psychoanalytic psychotherapy when insurance support for treatment evaporated, particularly in the era of managed care.[15] Among intellectuals, such movements as cognitive psychology competed successfully with approaches based on unconscious conflicts. Fresh definitions of criminal and deviant behavior substituted moralism as well as psychoactive drugs for psychoanalytic understanding. The new outpatient practice for seriously ill patients as well as those suffering less disability consisted of prescribing pills, not offering systematic mental healing. New medications and the worship of conscious choice belonged in a world that had decreasing use for psychoanalytic practice and thinking. In the end, the declension of psychoanalysis could appear inevitable. This narrative of the rise and retreat of a constellation of ideas could in fact be framed in terms of classic tragedy.

Phases in Historians' Writings on Psychoanalysis in America

Understanding how historians framed the subject and then neglected it is therefore necessary to appreciate the contributions made in the essays in this book. Historical writing about psychoanalysis in the United States has followed a course closely parallel to that of Freud's overt cultural visibility, and scholarship on Freudianism has also gone through phases. Most of the time, historical writing has focused on Europe. In the dominant Eurocentric narrative, what happened in the United States was a late and derivative phenomenon. Often, too, the history of psychoanalysis has been used for biographical interest or for advocacy of one point of view or another. Two traditions therefore developed in Freud scholarship. One, following the classic model of the history of scientific discovery, consisted of sympathetic biographical accounts of Freud and his followers as they developed psychoanalytic ideas. For many years this literature provided the only historical accounts. They were accounts in which writers often confused Freud the thinker with Freud the symbolic figure and cast all developments in the history of psychoanalysis as historical progress.

Late in the twentieth century, in reaction to the explicit and implicit adulation inherent in such narratives, another group of intellectuals used biographical and historical accounts to argue against both the current and

---

15. One recent summary is in Luhrmann, *Of Two Minds*, chap. 6.

past validity of Freud's teachings. He had, they contended, put over on the world a personal, delusionary system that produced many bad social effects. Moreover, further to justify their attacks on psychoanalytic thinking, they ultimately began to point out that, in fact, by the late twentieth century, psychoanalytic theory and treatment were being abandoned by most psychiatrists and also by their patients.

Freudian partisans responded, and in the closing decades of the twentieth century a number of scholars engaged in what became known as "the Freud Wars." Historian Eli Zaretsky as late as 2008 commented on the profound irony of the contentiousness and anachronism in the general histories of psychoanalysis written in previous decades: "Freud became a historical figure to those who respected and even revered him, while to his enemies he remains a vital, intensely cathected [emotion-arousing] contemporary."[16] It was in the context of these wars, when historical accounts were overtly composed for partisan purposes, that the number of historical works on psychoanalytic thinking in the United States diminished markedly.

Both sides in the Freud wars tended to use biography—of Freud or of those who carried and developed his ideas. The arguments thus tended to be ad hominem—about the person, not about the ideas. Altogether, biography to a remarkable extent drowned out the history of Freud's thought.

In the history of psychoanalysis generally, and not just in the United States, it became clear after the turn of the twenty-first century that a new group of scholars, mostly younger, but some older, were rebelling against the partisanship and contentiousness of the Freud Wars and were bringing a fresh perspective to the history of psychoanalytic ideas and the psychoanalytic movement. I have referred to this movement as "the New Freud Studies," to counter the traditional "Freud Studies"—although the New Freud Studies were important because they tended to go beyond Freud himself.[17] Some of those "New Freud" scholars have contributed to this volume, helping to bring attention once again to the major phenomenon of the impact of Freud's tenets, but this time they are dealing with the impact such conceptualization had on American society and culture.

16. Eli Zaretsky, "Freud in the Twenty-First Century," in *Freud at 150: 21st-Century Essays on a Man of Genius*, ed. Joseph P. Merlino et al. (Lanham, MD: Rowman & Littlefield, 2008), 158.
17. John C. Burnham, "The 'New Freud Studies': A Historiographical Shift," *Journal of the Historical Society* 6 (2006): 213–33. Another discussion of recent historiography is Jacob Cornelis Bos, *Authorized Knowledge: A Study of the History of Psychoanalysis from a Discourse Point of View* (Utrecht: Febo druk bv, 1997), chap. 6. The virtuoso survey of the literature on Freud is Ernst Falzeder, "Is There Still an Unknown Freud? A Note on the Publications of Freud's Texts and on Unpublished Documents," *Psychoanalysis and History* 9 (2007): 201–32.

The New Freud Studies are distinctive not just because recent authors have left behind the hagiography and polemics of the Freud Wars, although they have done that. In the New Freud Studies, scholars insist on broad, inclusive narratives and analyses in which culture interacted with psychoanalytic advocates and opponents. In particular, leading current scholars who seek balance and perspective recognize in many nuanced ways the cultural historical contexts from which psychoanalytic ideas emerged and the changing cultures into which they penetrated. As George Makari, for example, shows in his new general history of psychoanalysis, nineteenth-century science and philosophy and the changing cultures of Vienna and Zurich all fed into the stream in which scholars can trace the history of psychoanalysis.[18] That broad cultural context also marks the essays presented in this book. The authors, coming from different points of departure, implicitly share the assumption expressed in the title of a sociologist's book from the 1930s: "ideas have consequences."

The fact that the authors in the second part of the book begin with the cultural context reveals inadvertently another reason why scholars in recent decades have not attended to the impact of Freud. American intellectual historians have been preoccupied with the political stances of leading thinkers in the mid-twentieth century and after, and much less than earlier with great ideas about human beings and broad historical context. Therefore, scholars have given relatively little attention to psychoanalysis in the United States or to other subjects dealing with non-political high culture, preferring instead, especially when studying the Cold War decades, to focus on sociopolitical writings. The record in fact shows a strong tendency of cultural historians of 1975–95 not to deal with Freud and psychoanalysis, much less in the United States.[19] As eyewitness historian George Cotkin remarked in 1996 about some of his sometime contemporaries, "Cultural studies is unrelenting in its political agenda."[20] The total result has been an extended dearth of publications about intellect, culture, and psychoanaly-

18. Makari, *Revolution in Mind*.
19. A search for example of the *Intellectual History Newsletter* beginning in 1976 provides dramatic confirmation up at least to 1998–99 and even after that. Or see such specialty books as *The "Other" New York Jewish Intellectuals*, ed. Carole S. Kessner (New York: New York University Press, 1994), or other monographs and textbooks alike from the last two or three decades of the century. Non-impressionistic evidence is available from the *Journal of the History of the Behavioral Sciences*: between 1980 and 2000, there was an average of exactly one article a year on psychoanalysis, but only one was on the history of psychoanalysis in the United States.
20. George Cotkin, in *Intellectual History Newsletter*, 1996, 12. A casual perusal of intellectual and cultural history textbooks and survey works confirms, with only a few exceptions, the validity of Cotkin's comment at least concerning any material that would include mentions of psychoanalytic ideas.

sis in America, especially concerning events in the mid-century years. The authors in this book are therefore introducing ideas and viewpoints that are not necessarily familiar to current readers.

Psychoanalytic Thinking in the Culture

For the history of psychoanalysis in the United States specifically, two basic, parallel narratives stand out. One narrative tells of the small group of practitioners of psychoanalysis that came into existence in the years after Freud's visit and how that group grew. Not only did members set up formal organizations around their shared beliefs and practices, but they constituted a community. Over many years, as the community expanded, members diverged on questions of theory and technique that grew out of differences among European analysts as well as local circumstances. Eventually, by the 1970s and 1980s, formal American psychoanalysis had divided into innumerable factions. Yet most practitioners retained the name and identity of psychoanalyst.[21]

Because any well-developed type of psychotherapy like psychoanalysis was and is a technical procedure, much of the discussion about "orthodox" psychoanalysis, over the whole twentieth century, was about techniques. At two critical points in the twentieth century, psychoanalytic techniques and explanations won respect and adoption because many American physicians believed that the Freudian approach was working. The first was in the earliest phase, when the technique was effective with a number of patients whose neuroses had seriously disabled them—and who had not theretofore responded to treatment. The second critical instance, which will be noted again below, came during World War II, when Freudian explanations fitted the problem of "battle fatigue" in a way that convinced numerous practitioners working in the field that psychoanalysis was superior to other approaches.[22] The spread of psychoanalysis therefore on one level falls into the category of the transfer of a technique, albeit a technique that rested on extensive intellectual scaffolding.

Other historians have created the second type of narrative history of psychoanalysis in America. Freud's teachings had an aspect that was related to mental healing but was different. In doing psychotherapy, Freud devised a theory of psychopathology. The psychopathology was, on the one

---

21. Hale, *The Rise and Crisis of Psychoanalysis in the United States*. A recent detailed, carefully documented historical analysis is Stepansky, *Psychoanalysis at the Margins*.
22. This was generally acknowledged at the time, as Hale, *The Rise and Crisis of Psychoanalysis*, 205, picked up.

hand, the rational justification for the technique. But on the other hand, psychopathology led directly to a normal psychology. One could not discuss abnormal psychology without stipulating how the abnormal deviated from the normal. At that point, Freud's explorations eventuated in a new theory of human nature, complete with desires, inhibitions, and hidden motives—all set in a mechanistic association psychology with which educated Americans were already familiar. The psychological mechanisms that Freud and his followers devised were easy to understand and assimilate. Rationalization, projection, displacement, even defense (or warding-off) represented behaviors that were often familiar in everyday life, but usually not theretofore named as mechanical events in a deterministic scientific theory of behavior.

From even before 1920, then, some Americans recognized that Freud spoke to a number of very basic human questions and historical themes. Cultural historians of the twentieth century eventually generated a formidable scholarly literature on the cultural history of psychoanalysis, a significant part in the form of doctoral dissertations.[23] In these specific and restricted studies, many thoughtful writers examined the influence of psychoanalytic thinking in a wide variety of intellectual and disciplinary areas, including psychology, social sciences, religion, literature, film, and journalism. Taken together, these fragments of evidence show that the impact of Freud's ideas in the United States was powerful and remarkable across all of the divisions of learning in a society of growing specialization and disciplinarity. It was in the course of this penetration, use, and diffusion that what were recognizably Freud's teachings became used and misused, integrated with other ideas, distorted into other agendas, and also studied seriously.

The context in which Americans confronted psychoanalytic ideas and thinking involved more than intellectuals and their educated and often socially influential cohorts. At the beginning of the twentieth century, industrialism and urbanization were attaining their maximum momentum in the United States. By the 1950s, American society was becoming a postindustrial, service-industry society. The consumer culture that marked privileged classes earlier came to characterize the whole society, in which commercial forces often used Freudian formulations to manipulate values and also—for example, in advertising—actual spending.

At the same time, throughout the century, the means of communicating ideas on both the popular and technical levels were changing. The audi-

---

23. A good example is Frances Arick Kolb, "The Reaction of American Protestants to Psychoanalysis" (Ph.D. diss., Washington University, 1972).

ences also were changing. Just before Freud's visit, about 10 percent of the population attended high school, which was largely preparatory school, for almost that same percentage of the population went on to college. In such a society, the technical and intellectual elite communities were relatively well defined, and the ideas of cultural lag and classic trickle-down popularization of the thinking of intellectuals were more generally accurate than some later historians would like to admit. By the beginning of the second half of the twentieth century, however, high school graduation was general, and soon more than half of the population had significant post-secondary education. It was members of a greatly expanded American public who were exposed to large doses of Freudian thinking, for example, through the child-rearing advice of Benjamin Spock, whose famous book, first issued in 1945, sold more than twenty million copies.[24] In addition, the effects of changes in the media with the coming of television in the middle of the twentieth century would be easy to underestimate.

In the midst of this rapidly shifting social context, Americans often used Freudian formulations to explain or rationalize changes that were already under way. The most notorious instances were the "sexual revolution" of the early twentieth century and then a second sexual revolution in the age of "the pill" and feminism of the 1960s and after. Many commentators inaccurately or wistfully blamed Freud's teachings for each one. The age of narcissism, as Elizabeth Lunbeck will recount, produced similar interactions and rationales. As one generation gave way to another, many social commentators continued to see the effects of Freud's ideas or of what any given writer believed at that time was a Freudian idea.

In the extensive, indeed, venerable secondary literature, scholars inquired repeatedly about the ways in which psychoanalytic ideas meshed with American culture, a culture that most leading intellectuals of the time believed was distinctive. Already by 1956, the time of the centenary celebrations of Freud's birth, there was a standard idea of special ways in which Americans understood Freud's ideas. In one centenary essay, a shrewd observer of American psychoanalysis, the Chicago economist Walter Weisskopf, identified "two pillars of the Freudian system, its concept of the unconscious and its metapsychology." Freud's "naturalism and biologism did largely accord with American thinking," Weisskopf noted, but "a shift took place, away from the emphasis on individual biological drives, to socially-

---

24. A. Michael Sulman, "The Humanization of the American Child: Benjamin Spock as a Popularizer of Psychoanalytic Thought," *Journal of the History of the Behavioral Sciences* 9 (1973): 258–65.

acquired traits as prime movers of human behavior. . . . Freudian irrationalism, dualism, and pessimism are incompatible with the American optimistic belief in the rational, progressive perfectibility of man and society." Such thinkers as Weisskopf were therefore already identifying a distinctive pattern of Americanizing Freudian thought to deemphasize the gloomy portrait of a harsh civilization in conflict with badly contained drives. Despite people's inner conflicts, Weisskopf concluded, the American way was to hope "that a harmonious integration within the personality and within society is possible."[25]

It is not the intention of the authors of the papers that appear below to duplicate or try to replace such narratives. Nevertheless, our authors do look at the record again and ask: What kinds of revision do these narratives of therapy, worldview, and cultural trends demand? And how can a later generation better understand what happened in a history that overwhelming evidence shows was very important?

Modifying the Narrative and Revising the History

To the standard narrative and literature, the essayists writing below now add two major elements. First, they underline more deeply that the fate of Freud's legacy in the United States was intertwined with other major historical events and streams in the history of American culture. When something new appeared in the culture, psychoanalysis could become part of it. Second, the authors offer substantial revisions to the historical account that over the years had become familiar, and perhaps in recent decades, forgotten.

The essays appear in two parts, arranged very roughly in chronological order. Part I starts with 1909 and the first decades of the story. These authors—Sonu Shamdasani, Richard Skues, Ernst Falzeder, George Makari, and Hale Usak-Sahin—focus primarily on conscious carriers of psychoanalytic ideas in medicine and psychology through the 1940s. It does indeed turn out that, after their work, the standard narrative will no longer look the same as it did.

In 1909, American experts were active in an international psychotherapy movement. Leaders in this movement were trying to standardize terms

---

25. Walter A. Weisskopf, "The 'Socialization' of Psychoanalysis in Contemporary America," in *Psychoanalysis and the Future: A Centenary Commemoration of the Birth of Sigmund Freud*, ed. Benjamin Nelson (New York: National Psychological Association for Psychoanalysis, 1957), 53. Or similarly, *Psychoanalysis and Contemporary American Civilization*, ed. Hendrik M. Ruitenbeek (New York: Dell, 1964).

and methods, but they also were attempting to claim a dominant place for their own particular techniques. Freud's psychoanalysis was only one of the competing techniques and did not stand out from the others. No one in medicine or applied psychology in 1909 could have predicted that psychoanalysis would become a world-changing movement. Nor, at that time, did the Clark University meeting stand out as an important event.

Sonu Shamdasani, in a unique review of the publications of 1909, shows how mistaken Freudocentric writers have been who suggest that Freud's colleagues by that time had recognized the special characteristics and implications of psychoanalysis. By using only the statements of psychologists and psychotherapists from that year, to let us see the times through their eyes, Shamdasani evokes a landscape that makes Freud's rise to prominence after 1909 all the more remarkable, indeed, almost inexplicable. Shamdasani has produced, in fact, a good dose of historical perspective that changes the way we shall view Freud's place in the world—precisely because he shows how it appeared in the eyes of interested Americans in 1909.

G. Stanley Hall, the host of the Clark University meeting, was almost alone in promoting Freud as an important figure. His efforts did pay off, but only slowly, and effects of the visit did not materialize until well after Freud had departed. Freud himself, however, was stimulated by composing the lectures to extend the program of psychoanalysis for the first time far beyond just advocating the technique. His lectures, with this new program and agenda, appeared the next year in English in the United States, making psychoanalysis in a broad context substantially well known among elites in that country. At the same time, Freud's advocate, Ernest Jones, began an aggressive campaign in North America to spread knowledge about psychoanalysis. Meanwhile, Freud, back in Europe, broke from the general psychotherapy movement and launched his own formal movement, the psychoanalytic movement.

To uncover this fresh narrative sequence, Richard Skues applies a historical microscope to the iconic 1909 Clark conference and lectures. What he finds goes even further than previous scholars have ventured in showing how casually Freud approached his trip and how local and in some ways unimportant the Clark meetings were. But then Skues shows how unintentional circumstances intervened. It was accidental that Freud in those lectures and for that audience for the first time publicly tied his therapeutic innovations to a whole program of thinking and viewing the world. Likewise the formal psychoanalytic movement arose from other circumstances in Europe. Simultaneously, the lectures in English, along with other

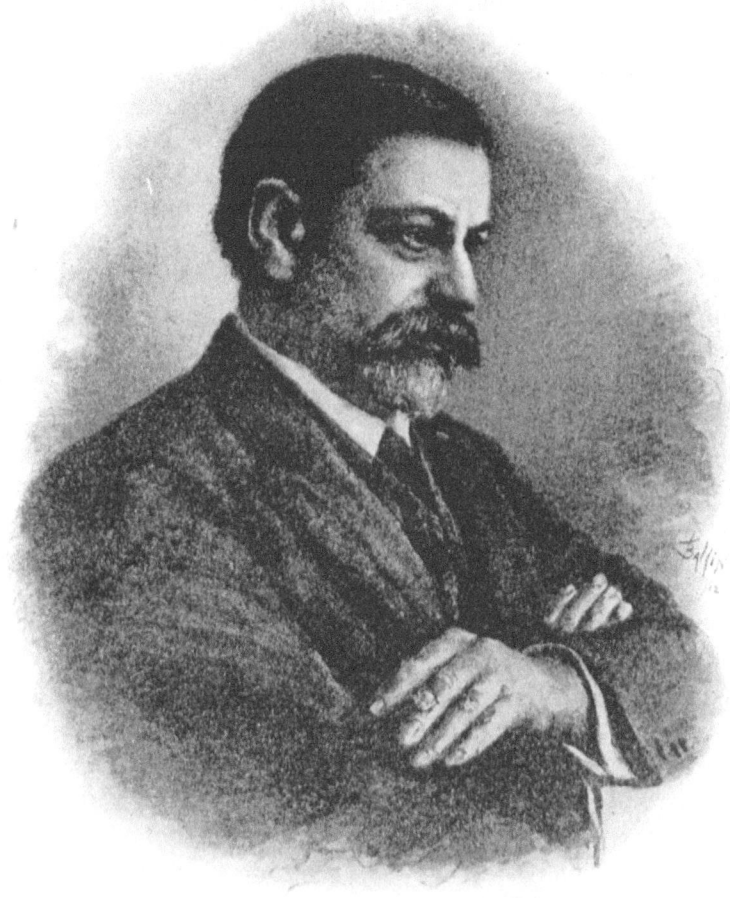

SIGMUND FREUD

I.1. Drawing of Sigmund Freud published as a plate in a medical journal in 1912 as part of the first wave of enthusiastic publicity about psychoanalysis in the years immediately after Freud left. *Medical Review of Reviews* 18 (1912), opposite page 252. Courtesy of Ohio State University Libraries.

translations, began to make Freud and psychoanalysis stand out in the United States among other new types of "modern" thinking.

Freud, however, continued to fix his attention on Europe. Except for an ill-starred attempt to impose a leader on American psychoanalysis at the beginning of the 1920s, Freud tended to ignore American personnel and events. Right up to his death in 1939, he intensified his consciously

Central European contempt for the culture and character of Americans. His American followers, then, knew him mostly only as a symbol or at most a figure understood only through his European adherents. For a generation and more, they were free to find their own ways in psychoanalysis.

Ernst Falzeder documents, dissects, and displays Freud's notorious anti-Americanism. But an underlying theme of Falzeder's paper is how personally irrelevant Freud became to psychoanalysis in the United States. The irony could not be greater: between the wars, Freud, the icon and symbol, was in fact substantially indifferent to the successes that both the formal and the informal versions of psychoanalytic ideas enjoyed in the United States, the home of a culture toward which he was noisily hostile if in fact, as Falzeder shows, ambivalent.[26]

Transnational communication continued, however, as Americans went to European psychoanalytic centers to train or as Europeans traveled to the United States—and sometimes stayed. With the rise of the Nazis in continental Europe, however, a major transfer of the center of psychoanalysis to English-speaking countries began. In some ways the transfer was extremely unusual. There were many individual analysts who took refuge in the United States, it is true, but by 1938–39 substantial parts of entire local European psychoanalytic communities transferred from Central Europe to America. Most notably, Vienna came to New York City and dominated the most central and important center of psychoanalysis. Moreover, Heinz Hartmann and the other new leaders, working with fellow refugees and local analysts already in place, established ego psychology as the defining brand of psychoanalytic practice and, perhaps more importantly, theory, that stood for the most orthodox or pure psychoanalytic practice in North America for four decades.

George Makari uses details of what happened in New York to evoke the individual and institutional events that were so portentous for the general history of psychoanalysis in the United States. He also suggests the personal costs and tragedy involved when established European figures had to adjust—and resisted adjusting—to their new professional and social environment. Makari spells out particularly how analysts were driven by community loyalties that created splits between analysts who were all en-

---

26. The general Central European ambivalence is described in Alf Lüdtke, Inge Marssolek, and Adelheid von Saldern, "Amerikanisierung: Traum und Alptraum in Deutschland des 20. Jahrhunderts," in *Amerikanisierung: Traum und Alptraum im Deutschland des 20. Jahrhunderts*, ed. Alf Lüdtke, Inge Marssolek, and Adelheid von Saldern (Stuttgart: Franz Steiner Verlag, 1999), 7–33.

thusiastically promoting the practice of psychoanalysis and the spread of Freudian ideas.

This major transatlantic relocation had many nuances and many local settings that related to social as well as professional and intellectual circumstances. There were individual achievements and adjustments as well as those within a community. Compared to some cultures, even generally hostile, anti-foreign, anti-Semitic, anti-feminist, and provincial Americans often could be supportive and occasionally welcoming to refugees who embraced various forms of psychoanalysis. Despite high personal costs, many of the refugees became professional leaders for decades into the postwar period, extending varieties of psychoanalytic practice and thinking.

Hale Usak-Sahin describes several cases to suggest the variations from the dominant patterns in which Central Europeans came into the psychoanalytic communities of the United States. She also uses Turkey, the stopping place of two women refugees, to provide a powerful comparison to the relative openness that several women found in the Baltimore area of the United States. Quite independently, once in the United States, those women also formed their own support network to help each other adapt to their new circumstances. She also points out that in Baltimore the psychiatric frame, with a continuing focus on very serious mental illnesses that was not usual among most analysts, could facilitate the transfer of ideas and the ways in which Europeans spread the knowledge and use of psychoanalytic ideas.

The powerful impact that Freud's ideas were having on American intellectuals and leaders became unmistakably obvious in the 1940s. At that point in the story, the narrative implicit in our essays broadens and shifts. Now it becomes necessary to treat psychoanalytic thinking as one of the great forces that helped shape American culture in the war years and for generations afterward. Hence in the second part of the book, the authors approach psychoanalysis from the general perspective of the culture into which proponents of Freud had come. To this partially shifted point of departure, away from the practitioners and institutions of psychoanalysis and to the surrounding culture, the authors writing about the second half of the twentieth century are starting with the high point of the impact of Freud's ideas and moving into events of the later decades of the century. In their essays, then, Dorothy Ross, Louis Menand, Elizabeth Lunbeck, and Jean-Christophe Agnew assess how Freud's ideas interacted with the broader American culture in the mid-twentieth century and after. They do this by calling attention to some different, but connected, cultural contexts:

modernism, Cold War anxiety, the culture of narcissism, and the transition from American triumphalism.

From these essays, it becomes clear that a further decisive shift occurred when psychoanalytic ideas affected and were affected by all of the developments for which we use "the 1960s" as a symbol, the time when "the personal became political." This bursting of boundaries meant that intellectuals took ideas and techniques focused on events interior to a person and endowed them with sociopolitical meanings. Because Freud had had much to say about interior events in people, his work immediately became caught up in the political controversies of the 1960s and 1970s, with reverberations that lasted, along with those controversies, into the twenty-first century.

Modernism was a foundational intellectual movement already in place in the 1930s, but one that grew and then flowered after the war.[27] Only the radical break that led from the 1960s to postmodernism could begin to end the hegemony of modernists among humanistic intellectuals. Psychoanalytic thinking was an essential component of modernism and modernists' concern with subjectivity and the self. Freud's tragic pessimism and resigned courage appealed to many modernists who were affected by the repeated threats of annihilation in the wartime and postwar years. Each variety of modernist could find in Freud refreshing support for personal courage, whether to adapt to an imperfect society or to defy conventional standards. As modernism fell into the hands of political and cultural radicals, both they and their critics could trace that radicalism, especially in the personal and libidinal, to the venerated figure of Sigmund Freud.

Dorothy Ross argues that the rise and fall of Freud's influence among intellectuals can be understood best by following the changes that occurred in their ideas of modernism from 1940 to 1980. She uses her analysis of styles of modernism to show how modernists of every variety reacted to Freudian ideas and appropriated them. Freud was presented as both a rationalistic Apollonian modernist and a romantic Dionysian one. Erik Erikson shaped psychoanalytic ideas into a domesticated modernist quest for authenticity. Not least of those who reacted to psychoanalytic thinking and appropriated it were radicals and feminists who ultimately rejected standard versions of both modernism and psychoanalysis.

World War II, which came into a world already dominated by modern-

---

27. See, for example, Daniel Joseph Singal, "Towards a Definition of American Modernism," in *Modernist Culture in America*, ed. Daniel Joseph Singal (Belmont, CA: Wadsworth Publishing, 1991), 1–27. Zvi Ben-Dor Benite et al., "Historians and the Question of 'Modernity,'" *American Historical Review* 116 (2011): 631–751.

ism, brought with it into the United States another major cultural phenomenon: widespread concern about anxiety. Anxiety in fact became a major American preoccupation in the Cold War period in both highbrow and mass media. Anxiety became a preoccupation among intellectuals in part because of the ingress of existentialism and in part because of attractive but conservative religious themes. French existentialism became trendy as Freudianism did, and many thinkers tried to mix the two in the form of internal conflict and neuroticism. But with the anxiety of the 1950s also came drugs produced commercially to combat anxiety, Miltown (also known as Equanil) and their successors. Thus at the beginning of the era of psychopharmaceuticals, ironically, the promotion of the tranquilizers was framed in Freudian terms—a remarkable demonstration of the ubiquity and power of psychoanalytic thinking. Anxiety, with Freudian content, was also a dominating, often underlying discourse around concern about totalitarianism, until all of the terms of discussion were derailed when the personal became political in the 1970s.

Louis Menand is strikingly original in summarizing the origins of the American preoccupation with anxiety and then following variations of thinking about anxiety as diverse elements of the society, from anguished intellectuals to pill-popping executives, drew directly or often unwittingly on psychoanalytic ideas and assumptions. In showing how ostensibly competing ideas contributed to the high point of psychoanalytic thinking during the Cold War, Menand also shows how psychoanalytic thinking contributed to major shifts in both intellectual and public discourse of the 1940s through 1960s.

The personal took on another label, if not another form, in the 1970s with the age of narcissism. When a rising analyst tried to adapt psychoanalysis to American conditions, it was not to traditional environmentalism per se but to a newly contextualized self. Heinz Kohut, this exemplar of revisionist Freudianism who nevertheless stayed within the institutional boundaries of formal psychoanalysis, undertook to write about a "healthy narcissism." He and others garnered celebrity and publicity for "psychoanalysis" even as the rigid, orthodox practitioners attracted attack and an unfavorable press. Kohut and other "self psychologists" nevertheless also symbolized the fragmenting of institutional psychoanalysis, a fragmenting that took place in the changing intellectual climate in which Freud's ideas had diminishing appeal during and particularly after the 1970s.

Elizabeth Lunbeck, in moving the discussion to the later decades of the century, strikingly sets out her tale of clinical practice and psychoanalytic theory by starting not with technical workers but with that "age of narcissism." Only subsequently does she examine how technical and popularized psychoanalysis played into the new outlook. Indeed, she suggests how traditional reformist, self-improving Americanization enabled Kohut and other self psychologists to extend a version of Freudianism into the new social analysis that still commanded respect as the century came to an end.

Jean-Christophe Agnew concludes the book by tying modernism and Freudianism to the concept of "the American Century." He finds it striking that, as Dorothy Ross argued, in the critical period of the 1960s–1980s, both modernism and psychoanalysis lost authority and explanatory power. What happened, people of the twenty-first century can ask, to the search for "the American character" and the abstinent, disciplined Freudian hero? Both were gone, along with the masculinist old-boy framing of self and society. Nevertheless, Agnew will insist, modernism and Freudianism coexisted with anxiety and faded only with postmodernism and postmodernization late in the century. Even decades later, when the mid-century high point seemed to many commentators to be obscure, distant, and irrelevant, Freudianism and modernism persisted in often unrecognized ways past the end of the twentieth century, perhaps consonant with an inevitable, tragic historical dissolution.

Freud's legacy, then, proceeded from unintentional beginnings in 1909 through the transport of ideas and people and even whole intellectual communities to the United States. The modernization of the "American Century" and the conflicts and anxiety of modernism and other Cold War and 1960s adjustments enveloped a remarkably well-accepted, if variously understood, psychoanalysis. Psychoanalysis had a great run during the century after Freud left, even though many people came to believe that it was, outside of some still substantial academic and clinical sites, irrelevant at the turn of the millennium.[28] Or perhaps much of psychoanalysis had simply become absorbed into American culture to such an extent that it had become untraceable. Freud's ideas, however, had and have an intellectual scaffolding, and as that scaffolding became indistinct, much of the meaning as well as the identity of his work diminished radically.

The essayists in this book therefore establish landmarks by which we can follow this rise-and-fall narrative that had such a fundamental impact on the history of the twentieth century. Where earlier historians often used the coming of psychoanalysis to explore American exceptionalism, more recent scholars can see the process of transnationalization in the interac-

---

28. In 2010, there were more than 3,200 members in the American Psychological Association Division 39, Psychoanalysis.

tion of Freud's thinking with a dynamic local culture. There were specific carriers—individuals and organizations, each with histories. There were intellectual movements and the broader cultural contexts. We underline that these papers are meant to be suggestive so that readers will want themselves to connect the dots and reflect on the different ways in which over a hundred years Freud's thinking came into and interacted with a changing American context.

PART ONE

1909 to the 1940s:
Freud and the Psychoanalytic Movement Cross the Atlantic

INTRODUCTION TO PART I

Transnationalizing

Part I starts with Freud's visit to America in 1909 and then continues to trace how psychoanalytic practices and ideas spread in the four decades that followed. The authors in Part I generally focus on practitioners, those who constituted the front ranks of the formal psychoanalytic movement. Freud dominated the story only briefly, at the very beginning, before other figures carried and spread the ideas and practices in the United States. In the 1930s and 1940s, as leading psychoanalysts fled the Nazis and ended up on American shores, the transnational movement of psychoanalysis from Central Europe to the United States took on a new dimension and scale.

The essayists in Part I write against the background furnished by many historians who have shown that Freud already by 1909 had in his mind the basic components of a distinctive but formidable intellectual worldview based on the education of a cultivated European and centered around his work as a physician and psychotherapist. He had already revealed parts of this schema in German-language publications. The focus of our authors, however, is not so much on Freud personally as on his role and that of many others as carriers of his ideas, and in this case specifically transnational carriers.

This story of the continuing transatlantic transfer of Freud's legacy was not ever a simple one. Our Part I authors distinguish two threads that give continuity to the stories. One is indeed the process of transnationalizing, of which the transfer of psychoanalysis to the United States is a spectacular historical example. The other thread is the importance of local settings and events, as is obvious from the events at Clark University in 1909 to the actual transfer of local groups of practitioners from Europe to new localities in the United States in the face of Nazi persecution. Indeed, general historians of psychoanalysis, too, have very often focused on local events, trying on some level to find universals in very specific happenings, typically in communities such as Vienna, Budapest, or Zürich.

Scholars, not least Nathan G. Hale Jr., have traced in detail how, in the United States, cultural and media leaders before 1950 often mentioned or alluded to psychoanalytic therapy and psychoanalytic ideas. As science and technology appeared with special prominence in intellectual and popular media in the United States in the first half of the twentieth century, so did psychoanalysis. All were particularly part of the interwar fad of "modernity," the popular quest for innovation exemplified in the successive models of new cars that now came regularly out of Detroit each year. American writers urged "modern," educated people to learn about their hidden selves, whether formed from complexes and drives or glandular imbalances or childhood conditioning. By the 1930s, even theatergoers and moviegoers could learn about treatment for neurotic symptoms, treatment most often labeled "psychoanalysis."[1]

The greatest direct impact, however, took place among thinkers—leading intellectuals in all fields, including the arts and literature, but especially the American social sciences.[2] During the 1920s, a number of specific institutions appeared and developed in which the influence of psychoanalytic ideas was explicit. One was the child guidance movement, which originated in Chicago and Boston and spread to the whole world. Another was the Yale Institute of Human Relations. Psychoanalytic ideas were particularly central in the culture and personality studies that dominated much of the social science innovation in the United States from the late 1920s into the 1960s.[3]

---

1. Nathan G. Hale Jr., *The Rise and Crisis of Psychoanalysis: Freud and the Americans, 1917–1985* (New York: Oxford University Press, 1995); John C. Burnham, *How Superstition Won and Science Lost: Popularizing Science and Health in the United States* (New Brunswick, NJ: Rutgers University Press, 1987); Marcel C. La Follette, *Making Science Our Own: Public Images of Science, 1910–1955* (Chicago: University of Chicago Press, 1990); Roland Marchand, *Advertising the American Dream: Making Way for Modernity, 1920–1940* (Berkeley: University of California Press, 1985); John C. Burnham, "The New Psychology: From Narcissism to Social Control," in *Change and Continuity in Twentieth-Century America: The 1920s*, ed. John Braeman, Robert Bremner, and David Brody (Columbus: Ohio State University Press, 1968), 351–98.

2. In another place, Dorothy Ross, "A Historian's View of American Social Science," in *Scientific Authority & Twentieth-Century America*, ed. Ronald G. Walters (Baltimore: Johns Hopkins University Press, 1997), 32–49, especially 38–40, points out that the social sciences in particular were structured around the question of the special circumstances of American society.

3. One contemporary discussion is Clyde Kluckhohn, "Culture and Behavior," in *Handbook of Social Psychology*, ed. Gardner Lindzey, 2 vols. (Cambridge, MA: Addison Wesley Publish-

It was in this intellectual and social milieu that a new generation of American analysts came into prominence in the interwar period. A number trained in Europe and helped carry additional and new psychoanalytic ideas from Berlin or Vienna directly back to the United States. Their patients, like those of the older analysts, included major cultural arbiters, often in literature, the media, and the social sciences. Such powerful leading figures as anthropologist Alfred Kroeber and sociologist William Fielding Ogburn thus gained personal knowledge of psychoanalytic practice and theory without leaving the United States. As our authors show, from the beginning the history of psychoanalytic practice and ideas was cultural as well as technical.

For all of the complexity, the initial event itself—of which these papers mark the centennial—unfolded in a straightforward way in 1909. Versions of the story were recounted by historians over many years, and then in 1992, after decades of research, Saul Rosenzweig published an exhaustive reconstruction of the visit:[4]

February 28. Freud finally accepts the invitation of G. Stanley Hall to speak at the meetings that will celebrate the twentieth anniversary of Clark University.
August 19. Freud travels from his home in Vienna to Bremen.
August 21. Freud, along with his traveling companions, C. G. Jung and Sándor Ferenczi, boards the North German Lloyd liner, the *George Washington*, to travel from Bremen to the New World.
August 29. Freud arrives at a pier in Hoboken, New Jersey, and travels to his hotel in New York City.

---

ing Company, 1954), 2:921–76; or see S. Kirson Weinberg. *Culture and Personality: A Study of Four Approaches* (Washington, DC: Public Affairs Press, 1958). Two recent historical accounts are Dennis Bryson, "Personality and Culture, the Social Science Research Council, and Liberal Social Engineering: The Advisory Committee on Personality and Culture, 1930–1934," *Journal of the History of the Behavioral Sciences* 45 (2009): 355–86; and John S. Gilkeson, *Anthropologists and the Rediscovery of America, 1886–1965* (New York: Cambridge University Press, 2010), especially chap. 3. Edward J. K. Gitre, "Importing Freud: First-Wave Psychoanalysis, Interwar Social Sciences, and the Interdisciplinary Foundations of an American Social Theory," *Journal of the History of the Behavioral Sciences* 46 (2010): 239–62.

4. C. P. Oberndorf, *A History of Psychoanalysis in America* (New York: Grune & Stratton, 1953). John C. Burnham, *Psychoanalysis and American Medicine, 1894–1918: Medicine, Science, and Culture* (New York: International Universities Press, 1967); Nathan G. Hale Jr., *Freud and the Americans: The Beginnings of Psychoanalysis in the United States, 1876–1917* (New York: Oxford University Press, 1971); Saul Rosenzweig, *Freud, Jung, and Hall the King-Maker: The Historic Expedition to America (1909) with G. Stanley Hall as Host and William James as Guest* (St. Louis: Rana House Press, 1992).

September 7–11. Freud delivers five lectures, in German, at Clark University in Worcester, Massachusetts.

September 21. Freud embarks for Bremen on the North German Lloyd liner *Kaiser Wilhelm der Grosse*.

October 2. Freud finally arrives back at Berggasse 19, his home in Vienna.

The authors of the first papers in this section focus on the historical symbol that Freud and his visit became.[5] Any time that one looks closely at such historical memories, one gets into revisionism or myth-busting. As is usually the case, the actual historical details of 1909 are far more informative than any symbolic event. So it turns out in the essays of these authors. The story they uncover provides a fresh account of a familiar narrative, as Richard Skues will note explicitly.

But the authors also raise fundamental questions. Of what did psychoanalysis consist that it could be transmitted and understood—or misunderstood? Sonu Shamdasani provides a point of comparison as he re-creates for us the world of psychotherapy in 1909. Skues spells out not only when the visit became iconic but how Freud's lectures brought a wholly new dimension to what he had to offer to Americans and, indeed, the world, beyond another version of psychotherapy. Ernst Falzeder raises the question of Freud's personal role as a transmitter not only in 1909 but for the next thirty years. Falzeder joins Shamdasani and Skues in implicitly calling attention to the distorting and misleading assumption that the receivers of intellectual transmission in the United States, even those enthusiastic about psychoanalysis, were passive receptacles of doctrine.[6]

Just as Skues's paper follows Shamdasani's inquiries in a natural sequence, so Falzeder next asks about the extent to which Freud was a necessary agent in bringing his ideas to the United States—implicitly, again, the question of Freud's role, or lack of role, as a popularizer of psychoanalysis. To find out, Falzeder looks closely at Freud's antipathy toward America and refines the question why Freud's attitude did so little to slow the transit of his ideas across national cultural boundaries in 1909 and afterward. We already know that Freud's prejudices did influence at least his close asso-

---

5. So iconic had the visit become that in 2006 a novelist used it as the setting for a murder mystery: Jed Rubenfeld, *The Interpretation of Murder: A Novel* (New York: Henry Holt, 2006). Another twenty-first-century follow-up to the visit is George Prochnik, *Putnam Camp: Sigmund Freud, James Jackson Putnam, and the Purpose of American Psychology* (New York: Other Press, 2006). Or see Evaline List, "Sigmund Freud fährt nach Amerika und C. G. Jung kommt mit: Umstände und Folgen einer Reise im Jahr 1909," *Wiener Zeitschrift der Geschichte der Neuzeit* 5 (2005): 67–80.

6. A distortion long since questioned by historians of colonialism.

ciates, many of whom ended up in the New World in the 1930s. Beyond the usual European stereotyping of uncultured Americans, Freud had substantial concerns.[7] Americans' enthusiasm was often just lip service. Many or most Americans were careless of theoretical and technical details. And they were notoriously given to eclecticism, pragmatically taking only parts of psychoanalysis, not the whole, carefully considered edifice. Franz Alexander, who came from Berlin in 1930, blamed the rigid conservatism of later émigré analysts on their knowing "too well" Freud's own "reservations about dilutions in America."[8]

In one dimension, George Makari's tale of the coming of the émigrés to New York involves much personal tragedy. Important historical agents, well established in cultures in which they felt comfortable, respected, and influential, suddenly were thrust into a culture they mostly disdained—but they were without funds and often barred from their accustomed work by technical regulations. To top it off, they were partially disabled by language handicaps and patronized by colleagues of whom they disapproved or whom they considered inferior. Moreover, especially as the dangerous era of the Cold War set in, an important contingent for whom high culture combined with leftist politics fearfully hid their political views, which had been very much a part of their intellectual identity. They thus found themselves falling in with the narrowness they perceived in the medical orientation of organized psychoanalysis in the United States.[9] As Makari shows, the extent to which what could be assumed in Europe could take root in New York was limited and sculpted by circumstance and by the institutions and personnel already present. In the details, Makari presents remarkable vignettes showing exactly how the transfer of intellectual and professional ideas took place and did not take place in the face of cultural and institutional-political constraints.

Hale Usak-Sahin brings in additional specific examples of the variety of routes and agents through which psychoanalysis came into the United States. Both the everyday and comparative aspects demonstrate the com-

---

7. Background is in Andrei S. Markovits, *Uncouth Nation: Why Europe Dislikes America* (Princeton, NJ: Princeton University Press, 2007), especially chap. 2; and Adelheid von Saldern, "Perceptions of European Anti-Americanism in US Magazines of the 1920s," in *Emotions in American History: An International Assessment*, ed. Jessica C. E. Gienow-Hecht (New York: Berghahn, 2010), 139–58.

8. Quoted in Hale, *The Rise and Crisis of Psychoanalysis*, 133.

9. Russell Jacoby, *The Repression of Psychoanalysis: Otto Fenichel and the Political Freudians* (New York: Basic Books, 1983); *Exile, Science, and Bildung: The Contrasted Legacies of German Emigre Intellectuals*, ed. David Kettler and Gerhard Lauer (New York: Palgrave Macmillan, 2005).

plexities in the transfer process. Usak-Sahin's story centers around Baltimore, a reminder that transfer from Europe had multiple entrepots and local settings, and in this case, through Adolf Meyer, a direct connector to Freud's 1909 visit. Some of the agents of cultural transfer from 1909 to the 1940s were absolutely central. Others played much more modest roles. Our authors bring out by example and by historical synthesis the ways in which cultural attributes of professional and general populations within the United States conditioned how, and to what extent, Freud's influence and legacy affected the institutions of mental healing. They also suggest how disagreements about technique could engage not only theory but the changing cultural environment. Many of the carriers and receivers of psychoanalytic ideas were, as our authors make clear, sensitive indicators of trends and changes in the American cultural environment, beginning in 1909.

ONE

Psychotherapy, 1909: Notes on a Vintage

SONU SHAMDASANI

The year is 1909. Henry Ford commences manufacturing the Model T. Marinetti publishes the *Futurist Manifesto*, and Sergei Diaghilev's Ballets Russes took the stage by storm in Paris. In Rome, Joan of Arc was beatified, and the city of Tel Aviv was founded. Henry James's *Italian Hours* appeared, alongside Gertrude Stein's *Three Lives*. The Nobel Prize for literature was awarded to the now long-forgotten Selma Lagerlöf (the first woman to have won it). Notable births include Isaiah Berlin, Benny Goodman, and Lester Young, and in psychotherapy, Rollo May and Jerome Frank.[1]

In the psychotherapeutic world, iconic significance is attached to Freud's 1909 visit to America. But did this have anywhere near the importance subsequently attributed to it? The subsequent rise of psychoanalysis and the psychoanalytic rewriting of history had the effect of obliterating much of the landscape of the world of psychotherapy and dynamic psychiatry that Freud encountered.[2] Before one can assess the effects of Freud's trip, then, one needs to salvage and repopulate this landscape. In the following pages, I plan to give a panning shot of the state of psychotherapy and dynamic psychiatry in 1909, restricting myself to publications and events in 1909 itself, as a synchronic view may highlight features that tend to be obscured by the more usual diachronic perspectives. As the topic of this book is "After Freud Left," my contribution will depict the scene "Before Freud Came."

In the psychological world, the major conference in 1909 was undoubt-

---

1. Of the Bordeaux wines that year, Michael Broadbent notes "Stormy August and hail badly damaged a healthy crop. The vintage was saved by late September sun. Average crop of light wines which are long past their best." *Vintage Wine: Fifty Years of Tasting over Three Centuries of Wine* (London: Websters, 2002), 27.

2. On this issue, see Mikkel Borch-Jacobsen and Sonu Shamdasani, *The Freud Files: An Inquiry into the History of Psychoanalysis* (Cambridge: Cambridge University Press, 2011).

edly the Sixth International Congress of Experimental Psychology in Geneva, held under the presidency of Théodore Flournoy. The list of participants reads like a virtual who's who of psychologists in 1909: James Mark Baldwin, Edouard Claparède, Paul Dubois, Joseph Grasset, Harald Hoffding, Ernest Jones, C. G. Jung, Oswald Külpe, James Leuba, William McDougall, Alphonse Maeder, Morton Prince, Théodule Ribot, Charles Richet, Sante de Sanctis, Albert von Schrenk-Notzing, Charles Spearman, Robert Yerkes, Theodore Ziehen, and so on.[3]

Congress-goers under the presidency of Théodore Flournoy were invited to promenade around Lake Geneva and had an official dinner offered by the state and town of Geneva. For someone deciding their 1909 schedule of which congresses to attend, this would likely to be top of the list. It was also covered in the *New York Times*—the only congress of psychology covered in the paper that year. On 6 August, the *New York Times* ran a piece on the next conference: "The Psychological Congress today accepted by acclamation the American invitation to hold its next congress, which will occur in 1913, at Boston." William James was designated as honorary president. This congress never took place. The *New York Times* also covered the debates at Geneva: "August 14. Scientists returning from the Congress of Psychology at Geneva report a remarkable debate over the question whether animals, including man, move and act of their own volition or from purely mechanico-chemical impulses."

At the congress, themes were chosen for discussion with two reporters designated for each one. These papers were pre-circulated several months before. I focus on one session that has the most direct bearing on psychotherapy, namely, that on the subconscious. This featured papers by Max Dessoir, Pierre Janet, and Morton Prince. Max Dessoir, a neo-Kantian professor of psychology in Berlin, began his paper on the "underconscious," which was basically a restatement of his work in the 1880s and 1890s on the double "I," by indicating how subsequent research had confirmed his earlier investigations.[4]

Pierre Janet has to be considered the most significant figure in psychotherapy in 1909.[5] In 1909, Janet held a prestigious chair of experimental and

---

3. *VIme Congrès internationale de psychologie, tenu à Genève du 2 au 7 Août 1909*, ed. Edouard Claparède (Geneva: Libraire Kündig, 1910), 16–34. These names will be familiar to historians of the psychological sciences even a century or more later.

4. Max Dessoir, "Das Unterbewusstsein," in *VIme Congrès internationale de psychologie*, ed. Claparède, 38.

5. On Janet, see Sonu Shamdasani, "Pierre Janet," in *The Dictionary of Medical Biography*, ed. W. F. and Helen Bynum (Westport, CT: Greenwood Press, 2006), 701–3. On Janet's links with psychotherapy in America, see Henri Ellenberger, "Pierre Janet and His American Friends," in

comparative psychology at the Collège de France. He did not actually attend the conference, as he had to pull out at the last moment, but his paper was pre-circulated and read for him. He began by describing how the old and sterile discussions of the unconscious in the history of philosophy and psychology had been displaced by his own work on the subconscious in the 1880s at Le Havre and then at the Salpêtrière. According to Janet, this meant that the problem of the subconscious was now based on clinical investigations of certain mental troubles, signaling a complete break with the older philosophical notions. He noted that he himself had always used the term "subconscious" in a restricted sense. Others, by contrast, had used the term infinitely more widely, which had simply resulted in a pseudoscience. The main clinical issue that he discussed here was the relation of the subconscious of the hysteric and the depersonalization of the psychasthenic. He concluded by noting that the question of the subconscious was born in the psychiatric clinic, and it was simply not mature enough to leave it.[6]

The other main speaker was Boston psychologist and neurologist Morton Prince. In 1909, he was lecturing in Tufts University and had recently, in 1906, founded the *Journal of Abnormal Psychology*. Like Janet, Prince also had at this point severe qualms about the use of the subconscious. He began by noting:

> It will be agreed that the term *subconscious* is commonly used in the loosest and most reprehensible way to define facts of a different order, interpretation of facts, and philosophical theories. It is often extended in its scope to cover facts of such diverse character that there is no obvious or substantiated ground for including them in the same class and referring them to the same basic principles. The same is true of the term "The Unconscious" (*das Unbewusste*) for which "subconscious" is often used as a synonym.[7]

He could not have put it more clearly than that. Prince then differentiated six different prevalent meanings concerning the subconscious: the portion of our consciousness that is outside the focus of consciousness; the psychological interpretation of certain physiological facts; the same phenomena interpreted physiologically; all past conscious experiences; the subconscious self; and the metaphysical doctrine of the subconscious. He

---

Psychoanalysis, Psychotherapy, and the New England Medical Scene, 1894–1944, ed. George Gifford (New York: Science History Publishers), 63–72.

6. Pierre Janet, "Les problèmes du subconscient," in *VIme Congrès internationale de psychologie*, ed. Claparède, 57–70.

7. Morton Prince, "The Subconscious," in *VIme Congrès internationale de psychologie*, ed. Claparède, 71.

tried to instigate some linguistic reformation in terms of what was actually meant under these terms and their compatibilities and incompatibilities. He concluded: "I would suggest that it would be worthwhile for this Congress to recommend a *terminology* to be adopted by future writers to avoid the confusion which now arises from the various meanings attached to the terms conscious, subconscious, unconscious, etc."[8] His recommendation, of course, never prevailed.

In the *Journal of Abnormal Psychology*, Prince published several chapters of a work in progress on the unconscious, and I shall just refer to those chapters published that year. These concerned experimental and other evidence of conservation of experiences that could not be recalled and the influence of the unconscious on the psychophysical organism. Here, Prince returned to what one could regard as the staple of experimental psychology of the subconscious of the 1880s and 1890s, namely, automatic writing and crystal gazing. He also noted some more recent investigations: "Jung and the Zurich School have, as a result of extensive studies, adduced evidence to show that the delusions, hallucinations, and other symptomatic phenomena of dementia praecox can be traced to past experiences, to complexes formed in the unconscious of which they are the expression."[9]

While signaling his approval of the term "complex" in the general sense, he raised severe misgivings concerning the direction of the new Freudian studies:

> The fundamental basis of Freud's theories is the functioning of unconscious complexes *without* their being awakened in consciousness. . . . The evidence for the relation between the psychical effects and their supposed unconscious causes, as worked out in individual cases by the author of "Psychopathologie des Alltagslebens," is often fantastical and curious rather than scientific, and therefore far from convincing. The use of these theories by the Zurich investigators too often partakes of these characteristics, which mar their otherwise brilliant work.[10]

So while stating a sort of cautious acceptance of general psychological principles of the complex, Prince indicated his misgivings concerning fantasti-

---

8. Ibid., 97.

9. Morton Prince, "The Unconscious: Chapter 3: Experimental and Other Evidence for the Conservation of Experiences that Cannot Be Recalled," *Journal of Abnormal Psychology* 3 (1909): 342.

10. Morton Prince, "The Unconscious: Chapter 4: The Influence of the Unconscious on the Psycho-Physical Organism," *Journal of Abnormal Psychology* 3 (1909): 392.

cal interpretations done by Freud and Jung. He concluded by noting that, properly speaking, there is no subconscious, supplemental, or secondary self. These were merely metaphors.[11]

We return to Janet, whose work extended beyond the Geneva congress. In 1909, he published what, by his standards, was a short book, clocking in at 400 pages. This was a résumé of his earlier work on the neuroses, focusing in particular on hysteria and psychasthenia, bringing them into line with his new conceptions of mental functioning. He considered neuropathic symptoms, fixed ideas and obsessions, amnesias, doubts, troubles of language, choreas, tics, paralyses, phobias, troubles of perception, instincts, visceral functions, hysterical attacks, fugues, crises of agitation, depression, and double personality. In fact, all of us would probably find ourselves in there in some place. This work was nothing less than a general textbook of the neuroses. And he ended with offering, seemingly the first time for Janet, a general definition of the neuroses:

> The neuroses are maladies bearing on diverse functions of the organism, characterized by an alteration of the superior parts of these functions, stopped in their evolution, in their adaptation to the present moment, to the present state of the external world and of the individual and by the absence of the deterioration of the already ancient part of these same functions which could very well exert themselves in an abstract manner, independently of present circumstances. In résumé, the neuroses are troubles of diverse functions of the organism, characterized by the stoppage of development without deterioration of the function itself.[12]

It is evident from this that Janet's nuanced style is something that simply was not going to make much headway in the following decades, which were characterized by the rise of behaviorism. He added that psychological analysis was the point of departure for methods of psychotherapy, which were the only means applicable for the treatment of the neuroses, on which he hoped to concentrate his next volume. The volume in question was nothing less than his master work, *Psychological Medications*, which took a decade to appear.[13] Thus Janet was providing his definition of what the neuroses were and indicating that, in his following work, he intended to show how they should be treated.

11. Prince, "The Unconscious, Chapter 3," 352.
12. Pierre Janet, *Les Névroses* (Paris: Alcan, 1909), 392.
13. Pierre Janet, *Les Médications psychologiques: Études historiques, psychologiques, et cliniques sur les méthodes de la psychothérapie*, 3 vols. (Paris: Alcan, 1909).

The major book on psychotherapy that appeared in 1909 was published by Hugo Münsterberg, then professor of psychology at Harvard. This was another 400-page work—possibly the longest book with the title *Psychotherapy* in the English language up to this point. It met with a rave review in the *New York Times*, entitled "Psychotherapy under analysis: Hugo Munsterberg writes a highly important and illuminating book, dealing with the new psychology."[14] Münsterberg, who was also an M.D., practiced hypnotism for therapeutic purposes for no charge and limited his therapeutic work according to his scientific interests. He began by noting that psychotherapy needed to be sharply distinguished from psychiatry, the treatment of mental diseases, because psychotherapy could also be applied to physical conditions. What was common to all forms of psychotherapy was the method, which he succinctly put as follows: "The psychotherapist must always somehow set levers of the mind in motion."[15] Münsterberg noted that at the current time, there were two predominant schools of psychotherapy: "The one school nowadays lives from the contrast between consciousness and subconsciousness and makes all psychotherapy work with and through and in the subconscious. The other school creates a complete antithesis between mind and body and makes psychotherapy a kind of triumph of the mind over the body."[16] An example of the first would be Pierre Janet, and of the second, Paul Dubois, of whom more anon.

Münsterberg claimed that that both schools were fundamentally wrong. As to the former, he noted: "The fantastic position allowed to a subconscious mind easily gives to the doctrine a religious or even a mystical turn, and the artificial separation between the energies of the mind and those of the body leads easily to a moral sermon."[17] In a lengthy chapter on the subconscious, he began simply by noting: "The story of the subconscious mind can be told in three words: There is none."[18] Slightly less succinctly he continued: "The subconscious mental facts are either not mental but physiological, or mental but not subconscious."[19] He indicated he had already spent several chapters discussing suggestion and hypnotism without any reference to the unconscious. Suggestion and hypnotism played a large role in psychotherapy, as did persuasion, but he argued that there was no strict division between organic and functional diseases. There was much to

---

14. *New York Times*, 1 May 1909.
15. Hugo Münsterberg, *Psychotherapy* (New York: Moffat Yard, 1909), 1.
16. Ibid., 161.
17. Ibid.
18. Ibid., 125.
19. Ibid., 130.

be said for recovering reservoirs of unused energy, a conception stemming from William James in *The Energies of Men*, something we shall take up shortly. He also made passing reference to Freud: "Interest in suggestion does not represent today a last step of psychotherapy. The latest movement, which is entirely in its beginning, the development of which no one can foresee, but which promises wide perspectives, is connected with the name of Freud in Vienna."[20] What was novel about this, he noted, was that for the first time there was in sight a psychotherapy that not only aims to remove symptoms but the disease itself. Given his caustic criticisms of almost any other form of psychotherapy, these endorsements stand out in this book. Münsterberg's general conclusion was that the time had come when every physician should study psychology. Scientific psychology had to furnish the basis for full understanding of psychotherapy. Psychology should be on the medical curriculum, and there should be institutes of psychotherapy.

This project of developing a general science of psychotherapy was the central endeavor in 1909 for August Forel. The main institutional development in psychotherapy that year was Forel's founding, in Salzburg, Austria, of the International Society for Medical Psychology and Psychotherapy. In his memoirs, he recalled:

> That such a society was necessary was shown by the fact that Professors Dubois and Monakow had founded a Neurological Society which was quite a superfluous rival of our Swiss Alienists' Society. Dubois, who knew nothing about hypnotism, spoke of it with disdain, although he himself unconsciously suggested his patients by a so-called "persuasion"! By the confused conceptions of this gentleman a fatal and artificial divorce would have been effected between the actually identical departments of psychiatry and neurology.[21]

In Forel's view, it would be a complete disaster to separate psychiatry and neurology. In August, he sent circulars off to the principal representatives of European psychotherapy, including Freud and Jung, asking them to join. Forel felt that the lack of coordination between different orientations in psychotherapy was a critical problem. He wanted to create order in this "Tower of Babel" by facilitating scientific exchanges and establishing "a clear international terminology, capable of being accepted in a general

---

20. Ibid., 356.
21. August Forel, *Out of My Life and Work*, trans. B. Miall (London: G. Allen and Unwin, 1937), 271.

manner by different people"[22]—in other words, to form one general science of psychotherapy. In his official announcement of its foundation, he stated the following:

> [Psychotherapy] thus comprises, above all, therapeutic suggestion, psychoanalysis and analogous methods, based directly on a well understood psychology.... But scorned and neglected in general by the faculties of medicine, psychology and psychiatry have been studied above all by autodidacts who have formed special or local schools, such as at Paris, Nancy, Vienna, etc., schools which have each developed according to their special ideas, without contact with the others, without in-depth scientific discussions, without agreement on terms.
>
> As a result of this situation, it seems to me that many things are highly necessary.
>
> 1. Obtain an international agreement to help the scientific discussions in the domain which occupies us—agreement on the facts and on the terms.
>
> 2. Unify neurological science and make it known in all its branches by the faculties of medicine.[23]

We see, then, that in 1909, figures such as Prince, Münsterberg, and Forel were militating for a unified, international discipline of psychotherapy.

Freud and Jung had already left to attend the Clark conference meeting in Worcester, and they received Forel's invitation only upon their return. By this time, the society had already been founded. The main event had actually happened in Salzburg and not in Worcester. The formation of this organization placed them in an awkward position. Forel had proposed diverse psychotherapies without according a special status to psychoanalysis. Forel and Ludwig Frank were taking the reins under the banner of a true scientific psychology and were offering Freud and Jung a back seat in the organization. After long hesitation and deliberation, Freud and Jung decided to accept Forel's invitation in November so as not to leave the field to their rivals.[24] However, within a month and a half, Freud had already proposed the idea of a rival association of psychoanalysts, firmly grouping

---

22. August Forel, "La psychologie et la psychothérapie à l'université," *Journal für Psychologie und Neurologie* 17 (1910): 315–16.

23. August Forel, "Fondation de la Société Internationale de Psychologie Médicale et de Psychothérapie," *Informateur des aliénistes et des neurologistes* (supplément mensuel à *L'Encéphale*), 5 (25 February 1910): 44.

24. See the correspondence between Freud and Jung from 1 October 1909 onward in *The Freud/Jung Letters: The Correspondence between Sigmund Freud and C. G. Jung*, ed. William McGuire, trans. Ralph Manheim and R. F. C. Hull (Princeton, NJ: Princeton University Press,

together adherents to his doctrine. This timing was not accidental. But that would take us to 1910.[25]

I return now to the debates within the field of psychotherapy itself. In 1909, a second American edition of Paul Dubois's *Psychic Treatment of the Nervous Disorders, Psychoneuroses and Their Moral Treatment* appeared, with a new foreword. In this book, Dubois, positioned in Berne, had launched a critique of suggestion, claiming that it only increased the state of dependence of patients. Psychoneurotics needed to immunize themselves from suggestion. They should accept nothing but the counsels of reason. Patients needed to regain their self-mastery. In place of suggestion, Dubois spoke of moral persuasion. This debate between suggestion and persuasion was one of the main issues animating the field of psychotherapy in 1909. In his 1909 preface, he noted what he called "suggestive therapeutics, erroneously termed psychotherapeutics."[26] According to Dubois, it was Philippe Pinel who first introduced psychotherapy in the treatment of mental diseases at the time of the French Revolution. Liébault and Bernheim and the whole hypnotic tradition were displaced. The implications were clear. Psychotherapy was simply the new form of "traitement morale."

A parallel critique was launched by Paul-Émile Lévy, a former pupil of Bernheim. In 1909, he published a work, *Neurasthenia and Neuroses: Their Definitive Cure in Free Treatment*. For Lévy, the treatment of neuroses could be summed up by one word: "education"—followed by "dispense with suggestion." Neuroses, Lévy wrote, were the consequences of a lack or error of education, and the goal and the cure was simply education or reeducation. These terms appear like a mantra throughout his work. What was required was to return self-governance to the patient. Like Forel and Münsterberg, Lévy adhered to monism. The sick person in front of me, he noted, is one. It is impossible to distinguish the mental from the physical. Hence there was no need, as with Dubois, to get rid of physical methods. He launched a withering attack on Dubois.

The significance of Lévy's work was such that it was reviewed in the *American Journal of Insanity* by Ernest Jones, who was at that time a demonstrator of psychiatry at the University of Toronto, and soon to become a staunch Freudian. Jones critiqued the book, indicating that as far as he

---

1979 [1974]), 247ff.; and Jung to Forel, 12 October 1909, *August Forel: Briefe Correspondence 1864–1927*, ed. Hans Walser (Bern: Hans Huber, 1968), 403.

25. For a full discussion of this issue, see Borch-Jacobsen and Shamdasani, *The Freud Files*, 77–78.

26. Paul Dubois, *Psychic Treatment of Nervous Disorders [Les Psychonévroses et leur traitement moral]*, trans. S. E. Jeliffe and W. A. White (New York: Funk & Wagnalls, 1909 [1904]), xiii.

was concerned, he saw little difference between Dubois and Lévy. And in quintessentially Jonesean militaristic as well as hyperbolic language, he concluded: "The psychology on which this is based is that of the populace at the time of the French Revolution, that 'Age of Reason,' when the touching belief in the importance of reason as a driving force in the minds of man lasted until its undignified downfall under the wheels of Napoleon's cannon."[27]

Another 1909 work taking up these themes was by a German physician, Wilhelm Hilger, *Hypnosis and Suggestion: Their Nature, Action, Importance, and Position amongst Therapeutic Agents*. This had an interesting preface by Albert van Renterghem, the old hypnotist. Van Renterghem began by launching a critique of the critiques of the critiques of suggestion by Lévy, Déjérine, and Dubois. Of Dubois, he noted, he "was treading in the footsteps of the Nancy school, he has set to found himself a new one and in so doing has industriously made use of the writings of the Nancy master, but without mentioning his name."[28] Hence van Renterghem accused Dubois of plagiarism. In contrast to Dubois, van Renterghem noted that there was something new on the scene: "Freud recognizes the use of all kinds of psychical treatment which can effect a cure. . . . [H]e knows how to value the successes of his colleagues who make use of verbal treatment in a general sense, with or without hypnosis, in the cure of their patients. He proves by this that he possesses a scientific spirit."[29] This was not often said about Freud.

In 1908, W. B. Parker of Boston in the United States started the publication of a multivolume work entitled *Psychotherapy: A Course of Readings in Sound Psychology, Sound Medicine, and Sound Religion*. The title indicated that psychotherapy consisted of sound psychology, medicine, and religion. This three-volume compendium ultimately comprised eighty-five articles. It was a home-study course. Broadly represented were the works of what Morton Prince later called the Boston school of abnormal psychology, or the Boston school of psychotherapy such as has been studied by Eugene Taylor.[30]

This series also marked the controversies surrounding the Emmanuel Movement. In 1906, Elwood Worcester had established a center for free

---

27. Ernest Jones, review of Paul Émile Lévy, *Neurasthénie et névroses: Leur guérison définitive en cure libre*, in *American Journal of Insanity* 65 (1909): 794.

28. Albert van Renterghem, introduction to the Dutch edition in Wilhelm Hilger, *Hypnosis and Suggestion: Their Nature, Action, Importance and Position amongst Therapeutic Agents*, trans. R. Felkin (London: Rebman, 1909), 8.

29. Ibid., 11.

30. Eugene Taylor, *The Mystery of Personality: A History of Psychodynamic Theories* (Dordrecht: Springer, 2009), 36 and passim.

treatments at his church in Boston, the Emmanuel Church. At the end of 1908, his work, *Religion and Medicine*, co-authored by Isador Coriat and Samuel McComb, had been published.[31] In 1909, the Emmanuel Movement was at the height of its controversial existence. It was, as Worcester later recalled, a victim of its own success.[32] The newspapers were full of letters pro and contra the Emmanuel Movement. There were several issues at play. One was what we might call the mediazation of the debate around psychotherapy. Psychotherapy was everywhere. It was in *Good Housekeeping* and other ladies' journals, and it was in the newspapers. "There is perhaps too much talk afloat about psychotherapy, the widest circles cultivate the discussion, the magazines overflow with it," complained Hugo Münsterberg.[33] Another issue was that of medical control, and establishing appropriate relations between psychotherapy and religion, which partly arose as a consequence of the mediazation of psychotherapy.

Within this context, I turn to what was the most significant event in the psychotherapeutic world in 1909 in the U.S., namely, a symposium in New Haven at the meeting of the American Therapeutic Society. Speaking in 1909, Ernest Jones argued that there were two stages in the development of any medical treatment. First, the treatment was seen as an adjunct of the therapeutic armamentarium and applied for the relief of conditions already studied and learned. In the second stage, through applications, conditions came to be studied afresh and new aspects of pathology opened up. Of the present moment, Jones declared:

> Now in psychotherapy, most of the medical world is at present only entering on the first stage. That the medical world of America will definitely enter on this stage as a prelude to further advancement and will, I trust, be one of the results of this afternoon's conference.[34]

Jones was speaking of and at the New Haven congress, and not concerning the Clark conference. Abraham Brill later described this as the first meeting on psychotherapy held in America.[35]

The American Therapeutic Society had been founded in 1901, and by its

31. Isador Coriat, Samuel McComb, and Elwood Worcester, *Religion and Medicine: The Moral Control of Nervous Disorders* (New York: Moffat Yard, 1908).
32. Sanford Gifford, *The Emmanuel Movement: The Origins of Group Treatment and the Assault on Lay Psychotherapy* (Boston: Francis Countway Library of Medicine, 1997), 62.
33. Münsterberg, *Psychotherapy*, vii–viii.
34. Ernest Jones, "Psycho-Analysis in Psychotherapy," in *Psychotherapeutics: A Symposium*, ed. Morton Prince et al. (London: Fisher Unwin, 1910), 108.
35. A. A. Brill, "Psychotherapies I Have Encountered," *Psychiatric Quarterly* 21 (1947): 583.

constitution it was limited to one hundred members at any one time. This symposium took place through its president, Frederick Gerrish, who was professor of anatomy and surgery at Bowdoin College. Gerrish was an enthusiastic advocate of hypnosis. He wrote to members of the society asking them to suggest topics for the three symposia, and several had suggested psychotherapy. He invited eight physicians to speak: "They constitute a galaxy which cannot be duplicated on this continent."[36] He himself then began by giving an opening address pitching the value of hypnotic suggestion. There were three symposia at this annual meeting of the American Therapeutic Society, on diabetes, diet, and psychotherapy. These were not parallel sessions. One did not choose between diabetes, diet, or psychotherapy. One sat through all three.

The symposium on psychotherapy took place at Yale University on Friday, 7 May. In February, Jones had informed Freud that Gerrish had invited whom he considered the most prominent men on the subject in America, and at Jones's suggestion, the papers would be published in the *Journal of Abnormal Psychology*, and then published separately to be sold throughout America "as an official announcement of its best men, (God forgive them!)."[37] In addition, lengthy abstracts were also published in the *Transactions of the American Therapeutic Society*.[38] The other speakers were Morton Prince, Boris Sidis, John Waterman, John Donley, James Jackson Putnam, and E. W. Taylor.

What does this symposium tell us about the state of psychotherapy? First, that hypnosis and suggestion were still prominent and the staple means of practice. Second, that the work of Janet—who had delivered a series of fifteen lectures on hysteria at Harvard in 1906[39]—was considered absolutely fundamental: dissociation was taken as a central principle of psychopathology. Third, that William James's energetics was playing an increasingly prominent role in giving a new conception of how psychotherapy functioned and how it could function to release untapped reservoirs of energy.

36. Frederic Gerrish, "Introduction," in *Psychotherapeutics: A Symposium*, ed. Prince et al., 10. Except for Jones from Toronto, all of the speakers came from Boston or elsewhere in New England.
37. Jones to Freud, 7 February 1909, in *The Complete Correspondence of Sigmund Freud and Ernest Jones 1908–1939*, ed. R. Andrew Paskauskas (Cambridge, MA: Harvard University Press, 1993), 13. For Jones's involvement with psychotherapy in America at this time, see R. Andrew Paskauskas, "Ernest Jones: A Critical Study of His Scientific Development" (Ph.D. diss., University of Toronto, 1985). Jones's own subsequent accounts need to be treated with caution. *Journal of Abnormal Psychology* 4 (1909): 69–199.
38. *Transactions of the American Therapeutic Society*, ed. P. Brynberg Porter (Philadelphia: American Therapeutic Society, 1910).
39. Pierre Janet, *The Major Symptoms of Hysteria* (New York: Macmillan, 1907).

Morton Prince's paper was on "The Psychological Principles and Field of Psychotherapy." He noted that certain general principles governed the field of psychotherapy: complex formation, by which ideas, feelings, and movements became associated together; conservation of what was experienced; dissociation; automatism; and emotional energy. Once again, we find this theme appearing throughout 1909—the search for generic principles to cover the whole field of psychotherapy. Prince highlighted the utilization of emotional energy as one of the principles of psychotherapy, referring to William James's brilliant illumination of this principle. Prince held that this principle accounted for the development both of the neurosis and of states of health, and that it was easy to transform energy levels to hypnosis by bringing certain ideas in the patients' minds to consciousness.[40]

E. W. Taylor gave a paper entitled "Simple Explanation of the Therapeutic Method." He was advocating the use of a psychotherapeutic method involving no special knowledge, a method that was available to all medical practitioners. This simply consisted of analysis of a mental state in searching for causes of the neurosis. Taylor conjectured that many neuroses came about under stress through misinterpretation of other innocuous events. So what was required was simply to trace the neurosis back to its genesis, locate the misinterpretations, and engage in reeducation—a word that comes up here again.

Jones's paper was entitled "Psycho-Analysis in Psychotherapy." The title itself is interesting. It indicates that psychoanalysis could be added on to other methods of psychotherapy. Psychoanalysis was the second stage in the development of psychotherapy, that is, it provided deeper insight into morbid phenomena and hence greater precision in the application of psychotherapy. To carry out psychoanalysis, several procedures could be adopted under special circumstances. Hypnosis had a legitimate place. The "word reaction association method" as developed by Jung was also of high importance. Jones ended with a plea for a greater role for training in psychology in medical education. In his paper, the limit of psychoanalysis was not altogether clear. He was including the practice of hypnosis and also making linkages with Prince's notion of association neurosis and Adolf Meyer's substitution neurosis.[41]

By contrast, Boris Sidis, of Boston, a sometime student of William James, gave a paper that critiqued psychoanalysis. Sidis was focusing on

---

40. Morton Prince, "The Psychological Principles and Field of Psychotherapy," in *Psychotherapeutics: A Symposium*, 11–45.

41. Jones, "Psycho-Analysis in Psychotherapy," 105–18.

his own work with inducing "hypnoid states." Contrary to "the Germans," Sidis argued that tracing the psychogenesis of symptoms did not lead to cure and had no special therapeutic value. The therapeutic effect of psychotherapy rested upon access to hidden reserves of energy provided by the hypnoidal state, which he described as a primordial state of sleep. The theory of reserve energy that he and James had advanced provided an alternative explanation of the therapeutic pretensions of all other schools of psychotherapy. "It is highly probable that Freud's success in the treatment of psychopathic cases is not so much due to 'psycho-analysis,' as to the unconscious use of the hypnoidal state."[42] For Sidis, in psychoanalysis, the couch has more therapeutic efficacy than the analyst, and the talking cure was really a reincarnation of the rest cure.

Like Prince, Sidis was attempting to account for the efficacy of different modes of psychotherapy. If one looks at the citations in this symposium, Freud was cited more than any other figure, 14 times; Dubois, 10 times; Prince, 9 times; with Janet, Jung, and William James, 3 times apiece. So Freud was clearly already present in the psychotherapeutic field in the U.S. before the Clark conference, though in quite a diffuse sense. What does this say about the reception of psychoanalysis? Years ago, John Burnham noted: "Most Americans first heard of Freud's work only as part of the larger psychotherapy movement. Needless to say, this circumstance contributed considerably to the misunderstanding of psychoanalysis; but it also contributed immeasurably to its rapid acceptance"[43]—a statement to which I can subscribe with one qualification, namely, it is not clear what a correct understanding of psychoanalysis could have been, since its limits had not yet been clearly demarcated.

The following are some examples of this. In the *Journal of Abnormal Psychology*, psychologist Walter Dill Scott presented a paper called "An Interpretation of the Psychoanalytic Method in Psychotherapy with a Report of a Case So Treated." This method had become known, as he puts it, "through the writings of Breuer, Freud, Jung, and Riklin," and his conclusion is as follows:

> It seems to be a matter of indifference which means of applying the method is used, whether hypnosis, hypnoidization, or free association. The prin-

---

42. Boris Sidis, "The Psychotherapeutic Value of the Hypnoidal State," in *Psychotherapeutics: A Symposium*, ed. Prince et al., 132.

43. John Burnham, *Psychoanalysis and American Medicine, 1894–1918: Medicine, Science and Culture* (New York: International Universities Press, 1967), 73.

ciple and the result are the same. They all enable the patient to overcome the gaps in memory, to resurrect the disturbing complexes, to unite them with the upper consciousness, and thus allow them to complete themselves normally.... The psycho-analytic method is nothing more than an unusually skillful application of the method of suggestion.... [I]t offers no proof for the existence of subconscious complexes of suppressed emotional ideas.[44]

Scott's critique takes one back to the standard critiques of Freud, such as that made by Gustav Aschaffenburg three years earlier.[45] In his paper, Scott focused on the case of a woman called Mrs. T., who had a phobia of being in a streetcar in a strange place. Scott described how she was subjected to a treatment having the characteristics of the psychoanalytic method: "She was hypnotized and told to call to mind one after another all the instances in which she had been frightened or overcome with dread."[46] He concluded: "The successful application of the psycho-analytic method in psychotherapy does not offer any pragmatic support to the theory of the subconscious assumed in psychotherapy, whether applied in the Emmanuel Church, Boston, or in the clinics of Vienna."[47]

That same year, Ernest Jones himself published a paper, "Report on a Case of Complete Auto-Psychic Amnesia." It dealt with the case of a man who could not remember his name. Jones here used what he called "the 'guessing' device. This consists, as is well known, in getting the patient to recall a given mental experience, under the pretense that he is merely volunteering a guess and is not being expected actually to recall the experience as a personal memory."[48] The following is an example of Jones's procedure: "You say that you can't remember whether you are married or not. Now suppose you had to guess whether you are or not, what would you say?"[49] Also in this paper, Jones was still using hypnoidal states.

Many sources therefore show how it was not altogether clear what psychoanalysis was and where its limits lay. This was because these limits had yet to be demarcated. Could psychoanalysis be incorporated within

44. Walter Dill Scott, "An Interpretation of the Psychoanalytic Method in Psychotherapy with a Report of a Case So Treated," *Journal of Abnormal Psychology* 3 (1909): 372-73.
45. Gustav Aschaffenburg, "Die Beziehungen des sexuellen Lebens zur Entstehung von Nerven- und Geisteskrankheiten," *Münchener medizinische Wochenschrift* 53 (1906): 1793-98.
46. Scott, "An Interpretation," 373.
47. Ibid., 377.
48. Ernest Jones, "Remarks on a Case of Complete Auto-Psychic Amnesia," *Journal of Abnormal Psychology* 4 (1909): 220.
49. Ibid.

a broader framework of psychotherapy, as had been proposed by Forel or Prince? This was a real possibility at the time. In December 1909, James Jackson Putnam wrote a paper, "Personal Impressions of Sigmund Freud and His Work, with Special Reference to His Recent Lectures at Clark University." He began by noting, "I wish to call the attention of the readers of this journal to a recent occurrence at which perhaps few persons save a handful of psychologists, neurologists, and social workers took definite cognizance."[50] Putnam was indicating that in the field of psychotherapy, the Clark conference had been a non-event. He was wanting to draw attention to it, in case it had passed without note. As we have seen, the events that were noted were the Geneva congress of experimental psychology and the New Haven symposium. How the Clark conference subsequently came to be accorded its iconic significance is a theme Richard Skues will take up in his paper, which follows below.

The year 1909 did witness the first translation into English of a book considered to be psychoanalytic—though the work was not one of Freud's, but Jung's *The Psychology of Dementia Praecox*.[51] That Jung was translated into English before Freud was no accident: American physicians had been flocking to Zurich (and not Vienna) to study the new dynamic psychiatry under Bleuler and Jung, and Jung's modification of the word association experiment had spread like wildfire and was widely taken up.[52] In their preface, the translators, psychiatrists Abraham Brill and Frederick Peterson of New York, noted that while the "credit of having introduced new life into psychiatry" went to Kraepelin, it was Bleuler and Jung who had "inaugurated a new epoch in psychiatry by attempting to penetrate into the mysteries of the individual influence of the symptoms."[53] They added that Bleuler and Jung were pioneers, the discoverers having been Breuer and Freud. For psychiatrists, it was clearly the work of Bleuler and Jung that would be of most interest. Thus for psychiatrists and psychologists who

---

50. James Jackson Putnam, "Personal Impressions of Sigmund Freud and His Work, with Special Reference to His Recent Lectures at Clark University," *Journal of Abnormal Psychology* 4 (1909): 293.

51. C. G. Jung, *The Psychology of Dementia Praecox*, trans. A. A. Brill and Frederick Peterson (New York: Journal of Nervous and Mental Disease Publishing, 1909).

52. By 1909, Jung had already published three articles in English: "On the Psychophysical Relations of the Associative Experiment," *Journal of Abnormal Psychology* 1 (1907): 247–55; with Frederick Peterson, "Psycho-Physical Investigations with the Galvanometer and Pneumograph in Normal and Insane Individuals," *Brain* 30 (1908): 153–218; with Charles Ricksher, "Further Investigations on the Galvanic Phenomenon and Respiration in Normal and Insane Individuals," *Journal of Abnormal Psychology* 2 (1908): 189–217.

53. Brill and Peterson, "Translator's preface," in Jung, *The Psychology of Dementia Praecox*, v–vi.

were going to attend the Clark conference, of the European visitors, Jung would have been the draw.[54]

In his landmark history of the emergence of psychotherapy in the United States, Eric Caplan perceptively noted apropos the Clark conference: "When Freud first set foot on American soil, psychotherapy was already integrally woven into the fabric of American culture and American medicine. True enough, psychoanalysis added new textures, new hues. What it did not do, however, was to alter the underlying pattern."[55]

Imagine an onlooker on the American psychotherapeutic scene in 1909 returning today and being told that we are commemorating a congress on psychotherapy and a figure in the field of psychotherapy in the U.S., and being asked to name both. His probable reply: "the New Haven Symposium and Hugo Münsterberg."

---

54. And not just before: on 9 September 1909, Trigant Burrow wrote to Adolf Meyer thanking him for the introduction to Jung and informing Meyer that he had managed to get interviews with both Freud and Jung. He concluded that "it was clear that Dr. Jung was the man for me" and went to study with him in Zurich. Adolf Meyer papers, Alan Mason Chesney Medical Archives, Johns Hopkins University.

55. Eric Caplan, *Mind Games: American Culture and the Birth of Psychotherapy* (Berkeley: University of California Press, 1998), 151.

TWO

Clark Revisited: Reappraising Freud in America

RICHARD SKUES

If coverage in the secondary literature is taken as the primary measure, there can be little doubt that Freud's trip to Clark University in September 1909 was of major importance for the history of psychoanalysis in America. A significant number of specialist explorations of the development of psychoanalysis in the U.S. discuss the Clark visit to a greater or lesser extent,[1] and when to these are added the numerous biographical studies of Freud or histories of psychoanalysis that mention his American trip in passing, it must surely seem that this is one of the more well-trodden aspects of the history of psychoanalysis, about which there can be very little left to say or learn.

Paradoxically, however, it is often the most common features of the historical landscape that also harbor unnoticed tensions or contradictions between the many versions, often between different sources but sometimes even within the same piece. One such tension can be detected as early as Freud's own 1914 account of his visit to Clark. He begins by noting: "The introduction of psycho-analysis into North America was accompanied by very special marks of honour." But later in the same paragraph he records: "To our great surprise, we found the members of that small but highly es-

---

1. C. P. Oberndorf, *A History of Psychoanalysis in America* (New York: Harper and Row, 1953 [1964]); E. Jones, *Sigmund Freud: Life and Work*, vol. 2: *Years of Maturity 1901–1919* (London: Hogarth Press, 1955); D. Shakow and D. Rapaport, *The Influence of Freud on American Psychology* (New York: International Universities Press, 1964); H. M. Ruitenbeek, *Freud and America* (New York: Macmillan, 1966); J. C. Burnham, *Psychoanalysis and American Medicine, 1894–1918: Medicine, Science and Culture* (New York: International Universities Press, 1967); N. G. Hale Jr., *Freud and the Americans: The Beginnings of Psychoanalysis in the United States, 1876–1917* (New York: Oxford University Press, 1971); and S. Rosenzweig, *Freud, Jung, and Hall the King-Maker: The Historic Expedition to America (1909) with G. Stanley Hall as Host and William James as Guest* (St. Louis: Rana House Press, 1992) are just a few of the more substantial works.

teemed University for the study of education and philosophy so unprejudiced that they were acquainted with all the literature of psycho-analysis and had given it a place in their lectures to students."[2]

Even allowing for a small if perhaps understandable exaggeration of the extent to which psychoanalysis was as firmly rooted at Clark in 1909 as Freud implies, there is nevertheless some slight friction here, which commonly finds echoes in later commentaries by others: did his visit to Clark really represent the introduction of psychoanalysis into North America, the germinal beginnings from which its immense success was to grow as a consequence of his presence at the anniversary celebrations? Or did Freud's reception of an honorary degree mark the recognition of a success already achieved, a success denied to him in Europe, perhaps, but constituting a sign that by 1909 Freud and psychoanalysis were sufficiently well established in America to make his invitation there a not altogether surprising event?

A survey of the more serious among the secondary sources reveals a general agreement on this point: while Freud's name was known to a few by 1909, the future of psychoanalysis in America was by no means assured. Freud's psychotherapeutic work had certainly been mentioned in more than a handful of articles in the scholarly medical and psychological journals by 1909, but he had been read and commented on only by those relatively few people who kept up with the latest literature from Europe. Psychotherapy in a medical context was still in its early days, but there were a growing number of people working in the area, and Freud was generally seen as representing just one of a competing number of approaches. Outside the specialist literature his name was not generally known. Freud's presence in America was due to the special interest of one of the few people powerfully enough placed to be able to offer him an invitation, G. Stanley Hall, and it was only after his visit that Freud became famous and psychoanalysis burgeoned into a significant social phenomenon.

If this view is more or less the established one among those who have studied the question, does it follow that Freud's visit was the catalyst for what came afterwards? In the more popular literature on the history of psychoanalysis, it is not uncommon to read claims along the lines that Freud's visit launched psychoanalysis in America, yet, perhaps surprisingly, there appear to be not many serious scholars who would claim this unequivocally. This is not for the reason that they maintain the opposite, but rather because for the most part they do not appear to consider the question very

---

2. S. Freud, *On the History of the Psychoanalytic Movement*, S.E. 14:30–31 (1914).

much at all. The aim of this paper is therefore not so much to contradict what has already been established in the better-quality secondary literature; rather, it is to make explicit some conclusions that might be derived from the evidence adduced there, but which appear not to have been articulated in full in the literature itself.

America before Freud

One obvious method of assessing the nature of Freud's reputation in America and the presence of psychoanalysis as a focus of discussion prior to 1909 is to survey the literature in the specialist medical and psychological journals.[3] So far it has been possible to detect roughly thirty to forty articles or reviews that mention Freud between the turn of the century and 1909, but given the wide variation in the nature of these pieces it is quite difficult to generalize about the overall impression created based on a simple numerical count. John Burnham concludes that "by the end of 1906, the complex, which was understood to develop as a result of an experience or mental association, was the theoretical idea most emphasized by American writers." He notes of course that the concept of the complex played little part in Freud's thought, and then continues: "In 1907 the number of allusions to psychoanalytic ideas or treatment increased perceptibly. In this growing literature the association test took a place alongside the complex as the most conspicuous specific items connected with the term psychoanalysis."[4] This summary, with its reference to the association test (which again played little part in Freud's thought) should draw our attention to the fact it was Jung who was very often the focus of the articles that mention Freud.

Clarence Oberndorf remarked on this as long ago as 1953 when he claimed that "clinical psychoanalysis is an importation from Austria via Switzerland, which began about 1906."[5] When assessing the nature of Freud's reputation prior to 1909, it is important to bear the implications of this in mind. It was of course by means of institutionalized psychiatry at the Burghölzli in Zürich, via the medium of Bleuler and Jung, that psychoanalysis first broke out of its Viennese enclave in Europe, and it is now well established that it was similarly through the psychiatric route that psychoanalytic ideas started to be imported to America by virtue of the strong

---

3. Burnham, *Psychoanalysis and American Medicine*, 13-29; Hale, *Freud and the Americans*, 180-94.
4. Burnham, *Psychoanalysis and American Medicine*, 23.
5. Oberndorf, *A History of Psychoanalysis in America*, 41.

connections between Swiss and American psychiatry.[6] However, the writings of Jung and his colleagues that caught the attention of the Americans were not predominantly psychoanalytic pieces, but works on dementia praecox and the association tests, which, while they leaned to some degree on psychoanalytic notions, nevertheless had their own momentum independently of whatever they drew from Freud. It is certainly the case that many (though not all) of the reviews and discussions of Jung's publications mention Freud somewhere along the way, but there is little sense that this psychiatric and experimental work would have been deprived of its main rationale or credibility if all references to Freud were subtracted from it.

There were three main aspects to Jung's presence in the American literature prior to 1909 that gave his reputation in America a different character from Freud's. First, Jung was working on psychiatric problems in an institutionalized psychiatric context with strong links to a similar network in America, whereas Freud was effectively working as a lone neurologist, and this would inevitably lead to Jung's profile having a greater prominence. Secondly, Jung's work on the association tests gave him a decided advantage in the American context because they were experimental. At a time when experimentalism was beginning to take off as the underpinning ideology of the newly confident and emerging psychological disciplines from around the turn of the century, Jung's work bridged a gap between the scientism of the new psychologies and the more interpretative psychiatric theories that were taking shape around the same time as an alternative to the long-entrenched somaticist tradition. Thirdly, as noted above by Sonu Shamdasani, Jung himself was published in English translation in a way that gave readers direct access to his work. Not only was Jung represented in English as sole author, but his name also appeared in partnership with other, American scholars, and in these works Freud's name is rarely mentioned.[7] Jung indicated in a letter to Freud in January 1909 that the English version of *The Psychology of Dementia Praecox* was due to be published soon, and we know from a review in the July 1909 edition of the *American Journal of Psychology* that it came out before the Clark anniversary event in Septem-

---

6. Burnham, *Psychoanalysis and American Medicine*, 18–19, 128; E. I. Taylor, "Jung before Freud, not Freud before Jung: The Reception of Jung's Work in American Psychoanalytic Circles between 1904 and 1909," *Journal of Analytical Psychology* 43 (1998): 97–114.

7. C. G. Jung, "On Psychophysical Relations of the Associative Experiment," *Journal of Abnormal Psychology* 1 (1907): 247–55. F. Peterson and C. G. Jung, "Psycho-Physical Investigations with the Galvanometer and Pneumograph in Normal and Insane Individuals," *Brain* (July 1907): 153–218. C. Ricksher and C. G. Jung, "Further Investigations on the Galvanic Phenomenon and Respiration in Normal and Insane Individuals," *Journal of Abnormal Psychology* 2 (1907): 189–217. Only the work with Peterson contains a reference to Freud.

ber.⁸ This was the third of a special series of monographs, of which the next was to be the first translation of some of Freud's papers into English. Saul Rosenzweig, however, records that this fourth volume did not appear until 30 September 1909, so that at the time of the Clark celebrations, Freud, unlike Jung, was not published at all in the English language.⁹

The point here is not about the relative statuses of Jung and Freud in American psychology and medicine, although there may be some interesting observations to be made on this topic.¹⁰ The point, rather, is that we must be careful not to read the history of this period in reverse. We know that Jung had scattered numerous favorable references to Freud throughout his published works during this period, had privately pledged his allegiance to Freud, and was to do so again publicly at the Clark event and for a few years afterwards. But that does not mean that allusions to Freud and Jung in the periodical literature at this time can all be seen as references to psychoanalysis. Psychoanalysis formed no coherent body of thought in America before 1909, and Jung's work had an independent existence that cannot be apprehended as a mere reflection of Freud's project.¹¹ If simple mentions of Freud and psychoanalysis in the context of broader discussions are excluded, along with those dedicated to works of Jung, then the articles that were either devoted to reviewing exclusively Freud's work or to discussing it in any depth were exceedingly few, amounting to no more than a handful.¹² If we consider the amount that Freud had published in

---

8. S. Freud and C. G. Jung, *The Freud/Jung Letters*, trans. Ralph Manheim and R. F. C. Hull, ed. W. McGuire (Princeton, NJ: Princeton University Press, 1974), 194. C. G. Jung, *The Psychology of Dementia Praecox*, trans. A. A. Brill and Frederick Peterson (New York: Journal of Nervous and Mental Disease Publishing, 1909). T. Walters, review of Jung, *Psychology of Dementia Praecox*, in *American Journal of Psychology* 20 (1909): 467.

9. S. Freud, *Selected Papers on Hysteria and Other Psychoneuroses* (New York: Journal of Nervous and Mental Disease Publishing, 1909). Rosenzweig, *Freud, Jung, and Hall*, 201.

10. Eugene Taylor's discussion, "Jung before Freud," is a spirited corrective to the idea that Jung's status in America prior to 1909 was as a mere adjunct to Freud.

11. In the January 1909 edition of *The Psychological Bulletin*, E. F. Buchner, a psychologist and professor of education at Johns Hopkins University, published his annual survey of progress in psychology during the previous year: E. F. Buchner, "Psychological Progress in 1908," *Psychological Bulletin* 6 (1909): 1–13. It is notable that he refers to "Jung and his co-workers Peterson, Ricksher and Binswanger" (9) as a preface to a dozen lines recording their work on psycho-galvanic reactions. Freud is nowhere mentioned. Jung receives a second reference later (11) in connection with his work on dementia praecox.

12. In fact, references to "psychoanalysis" are almost nonexistent. Even Putnam's 1906 article mentions it in the title and then only four more times in its adjectival form of "psychoanalytic," but always relating to a method, not a body of thought. J. J. Putnam, "Recent Experiences in the Study and Treatment of Hysteria at the Massachusetts General Hospital; with Remarks on Freud's Method of Treatment by 'Psycho-Analysis,'" *Journal of Abnormal Psychology* 1 (1906): 26–41. At this stage, psychoanalysis in the way we identify it today simply did not

German by 1909 and then ask ourselves how much of this could be reconstructed from accounts published in English by this time, the answer would be very little indeed. Although Freud's work in German was indeed read and reviewed, the number of people doing this was very small. For the vast majority of those who would have read the journals, only a minute part of the totality of what psychoanalysis consisted of by 1909 could have been constructed from what had so far been published in English.

In terms of Freud's standing in America, therefore, it is difficult to see that this could in any way justify the extension of an invitation to speak and to receive an honorary degree if this were to be based on his reputation in English alone. But of course one of the elite group who had been following Freud's work closely in German, who had found it resonant with his own interests, and who was also in a position to extend such an invitation was G. Stanley Hall. Dorothy Ross has discussed in detail the aspects of Freud's work that made it particularly attractive for Hall. Although Hall was always on the fringes of the Boston group, he shared their interest in the latest developments in psychopathology and psychotherapy and was aware of Freud's writings from early on in the century. But what was perhaps more crucial for Hall was the overlap between Freud's studies and his own genetic psychology, underwritten by Haeckel's biology of recapitulation and its relation to child development. When to this is added Hall's strong commitment to the study of sexuality, it is possible to see a convergence of interest that would have made Freud irresistible for him, even though these interests related to aspects of Freud's thought that were by no means the dominant themes featuring in the English-language literature. But in addition to his own personal investment in Freud's work, Hall was no doubt aware of the rising interest in it also shared by those connected with the Boston group, and managing to attract Freud to Clark was a significant competitive statement to Boston and Harvard.[13]

There is no doubt that as far as Hall was concerned, Freud was his most important guest. It was, after all, Freud and Jung out of the four foreign visitors who were Hall's houseguests, and it was Freud who was top of the list

---

exist. Probably the only other substantive discussion of it in English prior to Freud's visit (and even here it is still predominantly a "method") was the paper referred to above by Shamdasani that Ernest Jones presented to the New Haven meeting in May, which was then published in the June/July issue of the *Journal of Abnormal Psychology*. E. Jones, "Psycho-Analysis in Psychotherapy," *Journal of Abnormal Psychology* 4 (1909): 140–50.

13. D. Ross, *G. Stanley Hall: The Psychologist as Prophet* (Chicago: University of Chicago Press, 1972), 368–94, esp. 387. D. Ross, "American Psychology and Psychoanalysis: William James and G. Stanley Hall," in *American Psychoanalysis: Origins and Development*, ed. J. M. Quen and E. T. Carlson (New York: Brunner/Mazel, 1978), esp. 45.

of speakers in the preliminary announcement for the Clark celebration that he published in the *American Journal of Psychology* in the summer of 1909 (p. 469).[14] Rand Evans and William Koelsch have documented the lengths to which Hall went to engineer favorable press coverage for Freud, not only writing a couple of pieces himself, which appeared without his name, and in all likelihood providing summaries of the lectures delivered in German for the local reporters, but also inviting an Austrian journalist, Adalbert Albrecht, to come to his home to interview Freud.[15] Given that history was largely to vindicate his perceptive invitation of his primary guest, along with his most able lieutenant at the time, it is not surprising that there is a marked convergence between Hall's own account of the significance of the event for psychoanalysis and that of some of the briefer versions to be found within standard histories of psychoanalysis.[16]

But what of Freud? What did he make of this unexpected invitation? Did he leap at the chance suddenly offered to him to make his name overseas and to further the interests of the psychoanalytic movement abroad? The primary source of evidence is his correspondence of the time, particularly with Jung, and the trip to America is discussed intermittently throughout the period immediately prior to it.

As is well known, Freud did not feel able to accept Hall's first invitation to him when it came in December 1908 because the projected timing of the event in July of the following year would have meant that he would have had to stop his work with his patients some three weeks earlier than normal, and this he could ill afford to do. But after telling Jung of his decision, he continued: "But I am sorry to have it fall through on this account, because it would have been fun."[17]

In response to Jung's urging him to reconsider, however, Freud shed more light on his reluctance to make any sacrifices for the sake of the trip:

There is a good deal to be said about America. Jones and Brill write often, Jones's observations are shrewd and pessimistic, Brill sees everything through

---

14. Followed by Stern, Jung, and Burgerstein. The remaining four domestic speakers are listed in alphabetical order.

15. R. B. Evans and W. A. Koelsch, "Psychoanalysis Arrives in America: The 1909 Psychology Conference at Clark University," *American Psychologist* 40 (1985): 942–48, esp. 946–47.

16. "The conferences in this department were attended not only by psychologists but by eminent psychiatrists, and the influence of Freudian views in this country, where they had been little known before, from this date developed rapidly, so that in a sense this unique and significant culture movement owed most of its initial momentum in this country to this meeting." G. S. Hall, *Life and Confessions of a Psychologist* (New York: D. Appleton & Co., 1923), 333.

17. Freud and Jung, *The Freud/Jung Letters*, 193.

rose-coloured spectacles. I am inclined to agree with Jones. I also think that once they discover the sexual core of our psychological theories they will drop us. Their prudery and their material dependence on the public are too great. That is why I have no desire to risk the trip there in July. I can't expect anything of consultations.[18]

Once the date of the celebrations had been moved to September, thereby enabling Freud to accept a second invitation, he confessed to Jung:

> I must admit that this has thrilled me more than anything else that has happened in the last few years—except perhaps for the appearance of the *Jahrbuch*—and that I have been thinking of nothing else. Practical considerations have joined forces with imagination and youthful enthusiasm to upset the composure on which you have complimented me.... We shall have a good deal to say about this trip and all its possible consequences for our cause.[19]

Despite this glimmer of ambition for the psychoanalytic cause, nothing seems to have come of it in discussion, and Freud's generally low expectations, which were also shared by Jung, resurface intermittently in the correspondence.

By mid-June, Jung had received his own invitation to Clark University, but as late as July Freud admitted to him:

> I am purposely not thinking very much about America and our trip. I want every pleasant experience to come as a surprise, I am determined not to spoil my enjoyment by hypercathected anticipation and to take all disappointments lightly. Do likewise, don't let the thought of your lectures weigh too heavily on you.

In mid-July Freud was on holiday in Ammerwald and still putting off any serious thought about the trip: "Here I am not planning to do a thing, not even to think of America; I am too tired."[20]

On 13 May Freud had written to Oskar Pfister: "You too must have been impressed by the great news that Jung is coming with me to Worcester. It changes my whole feeling about the trip and makes it important [*be-*

---

18. Ibid., 196.
19. Ibid., 210, translation modified.
20. Ibid., 240, 242.

deutungsvoll]. I am very curious to see what will become of it all."[21] On the boat home immediately after the event, Freud wrote to his daughter Mathilde: "But it was highly interesting and for our cause probably very significant. All in all it has to be considered a great success."[22] But beyond these two minor references, it is very difficult to ascertain why Freud thought the trip might be important, how he planned to make it so, or why after the visit he thought it had been significant for the psychoanalytic cause. There is no doubt that Freud was very much excited by the prospect of his trip and looked forward to it with considerable anticipation, but it appears from his correspondence that this was largely because he was determined not to treat it as something requiring a great deal of labor or where much was at stake. His preparations with Jung for what one might think would be a potentially very important series of lectures seem to have been casual in the extreme, where his main aim seems to have been to make sure that he enjoyed himself. In the end, Freud apparently composed his talks during a walk with Ferenczi just before each lecture.[23] There is little sign here of anything that might remotely approach concerted ambition.

Freud at Clark

Apart from Freud's lectures themselves, the celebrated photograph that has so often accompanied accounts of Freud's entry into America is probably the most significant legacy of the Clark events for historians of psychoanalysis. Properly analyzed, this photograph can yield key pieces of evidence that deepen our understanding of what we see there and perhaps correct some misconceptions about Freud's presence at Clark. But to begin this examination we first need to know something more about how the celebrations were structured.

The phase of the anniversary celebrations in which Freud was involved took place between 6 and 17 September. During these two weeks, each department in the university arranged for a gathering of specialists to give a series of lectures on topics of interest to its own field. Psychology and education held their events throughout the first week, with a ceremony on

---

21. S. Freud and O. Pfister, *Psycho-Analysis and Faith: The Letters of Sigmund Freud and Oskar Pfister* (London: Hogarth Press, 1963), 25.

22. S. Freud, *Unser Herz zeigt nach dem Süden: Reisebriefe 1895–1923*, ed. C. Tögel (Berlin: Aufbau-Verlag, 2002), 312.

23. S. Freud, "Sándor Ferenczi," S.E. 22 (1933).

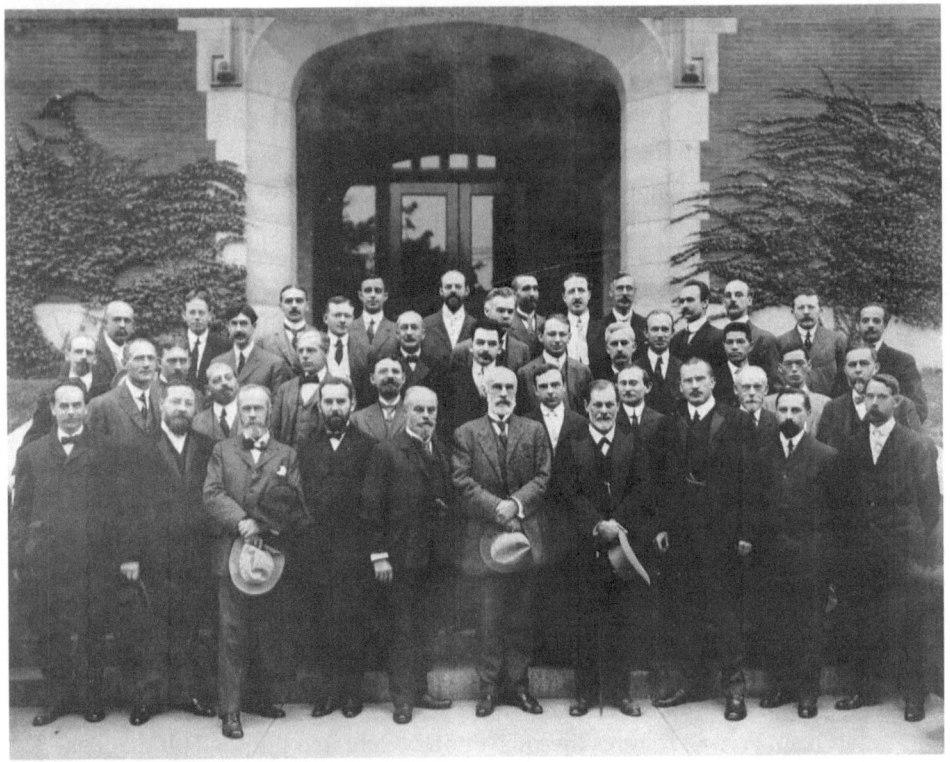

2.1. The often reprinted picture of the lecturers in psychology and pedagogy with some of their colleagues at the 1909 Clark University conference. This version is taken from a print made from the original negative and presented to John Burnham by Dorothy Ross. Courtesy of the Medical Heritage Center, Ohio State University.

the evening of 10 September.[24] Although the two disciplines were formally separated on the program, in practice they were intertwined in their delivery, reflecting the close relationship between psychology and pedagogy at Clark. In addition to the formal lecture sessions, there were subsidiary events organized for some of the afternoons, which mostly took the form of conference-type meetings with papers and discussion organized on a specific theme.[25] The following year the guest lectures in psychology were published in the *American Journal of Psychology* and those in education in the *Pedagogical Seminary* (both journals were edited by Hall), alongside

24. Anon., "The Twentieth Anniversary of Clark University," *Science* 30 (1909): 333–34.
25. Evans and Koelsch, "Psychoanalysis Arrives in America," 945.

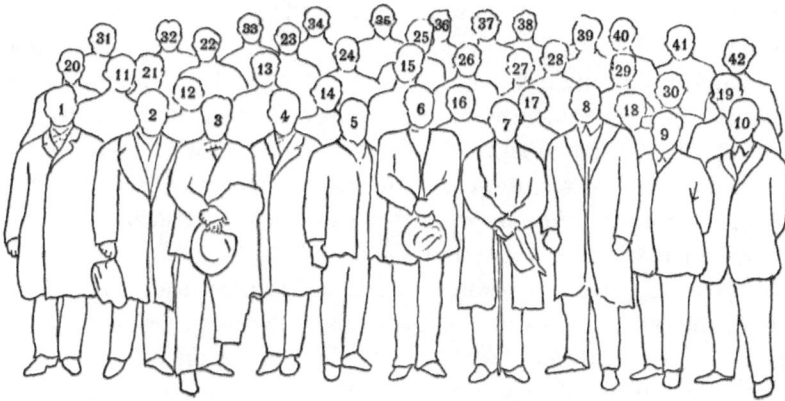

2.2. Identities of figures in the picture of the psychologists and educationalists at the conference at Clark University in 1909, in *Lectures and Addresses Delivered Before the Departments of Psychology and Pedagogy in Celebration of the Twentieth Anniversary of the Opening of Clark University* (Worcester, MA: Clark University Press, 1910), frontispiece. See appendix for key to numbers.

some of the papers that were given at the afternoon conferences. Both sets of papers were then reprinted later in the year in a single volume of *Lectures and Addresses*.[26]

All of those speakers who were invited from outside Clark University to give formal lectures in either psychology or education were awarded honorary degrees. Apart from Freud and Jung, the degree recipients from the psychology and pedagogy groups were the anthropologist Franz Boas from Columbia University; the psychiatrist Adolf Meyer from the Johns Hopkins Medical School; the biologist Herbert S. Jennings from Johns Hopkins University; the psychologist Edward B. Titchener from Cornell University; the school-hygiene specialist Leo Burgerstein from Vienna; and the psychologist William Stern from the University of Breslau.

In light of this, let us return to the photograph. Ignoring for one moment the presence of William James, we can now begin to see that if we set it in the context of these details of the Clark celebration, the front row is quite carefully arranged. There in the center is Stanley Hall, of course, but counterbalancing Freud and Jung on Hall's left are his other two distinguished guests specially invited from abroad, Leo Burgerstein immediately

---

26. Clark University, *Lectures and Addresses Delivered before the Departments of Psychology and Pedagogy in Celebration of the Twentieth Anniversary of the Opening of Clark University, September 1909* (Worcester, MA: Clark University Press, 1910).

to Hall's right and then next to him William Stern. Notwithstanding the fact that he is not exactly a household name today, we must not overlook the significance of the fact that if Freud was Stanley Hall's principal guest for psychology, Leo Burgerstein was his most prestigious invitee in the field of education. While he had originally been trained as a geologist, Burgerstein had turned his attention and his career in the mid-1880s to school hygiene, and by the time he was invited to Clark, he had had for many years an international reputation in the field.[27]

While the speakers from abroad are ranged symmetrically on each side of Hall, the other four degree recipients flank the front row, with two on each side. Herbert S. Jennings is on the far right of the row, and standing next to him is Adolf Meyer. Meyer had close connections with Hall and with Clark University: he had taught at Clark between 1895 and 1902 while he was a pathologist at the nearby Worcester Lunatic Hospital. On the far left of the front row is Franz Boas, who had taught anthropology at Clark between 1889 and 1892, and next to him is Hall's co-editor on the *American Journal of Psychology*, Edward B. Titchener, who had loyally stood by Hall at the time when he had been threatened with losing control over the journal back in 1893.[28]

So what of William James? James was neither a guest speaker nor a degree recipient. In fact we know that he visited the Clark celebrations on 10 September for only one day, having arrived at Hall's home the previous evening in order to meet Freud and Jung.[29] But one would imagine that the standing of James within American psychology and his long (if troubled) relationship with Hall would have been sufficient to ensure that he joined the group photograph on its front row, even at the cost of disrupting its careful symmetry, rather than being relegated to one of the rows behind. In fact, if we look carefully at the photograph, we can see signs of James's late entry after the other principal guests had taken their places: he stands just forward of the others in the front row, his lower body not fully aligned with his upper torso, and Burgerstein has turned to his left to accommodate the additional person, thus ensuring that Stern (with feet closed together) was not too compressed between him and James.

James's presence enables us to date the picture to 10 September, for we know this was the only day he was in attendance. But the fact that, apart from him, the front row comprises all the honorary degree recipients in ad-

---

27. L. Eisenberg, *Das Geistige Wien: Künstler- und Schriftsteller-Lexikon*, vol. 2: *Medicinisch-naturwissenschaftlicher Theil* (Wien: C. Daberkow's Verlag, 1893), 69–71.

28. Ross, *G. Stanley Hall*, 239.

29. Rosenzweig, *Freud, Jung, and Hall*, 80.

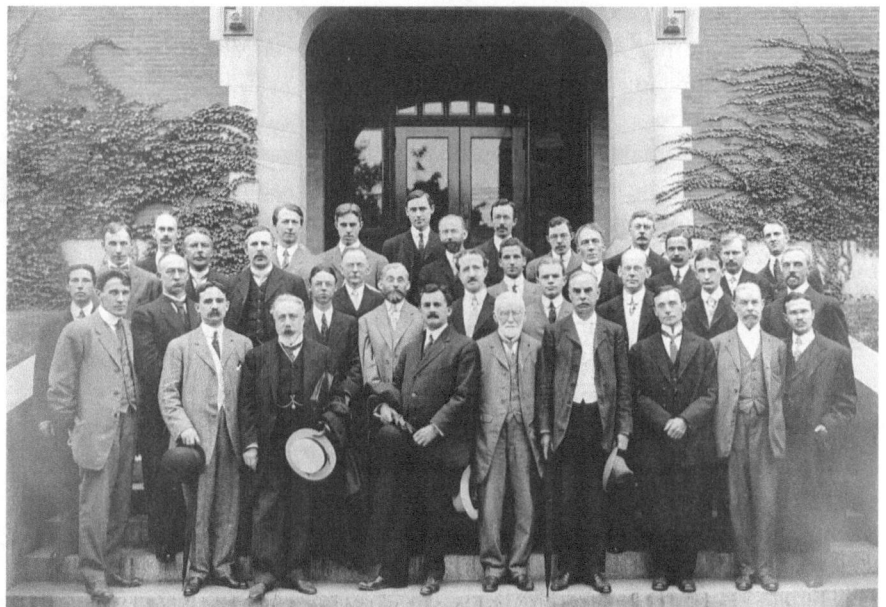

2.3. The lecturers sponsored by the Departments of Mathematics and Physics at the twentieth-anniversary celebration of Clark University in 1909, posed in the same way with members of the audience as were the psychologists and educationalists in figure 2.1. Courtesy and permission of the Clark University Archives.

dition to Hall surely makes it necessary to tie the occasion for the picture to the degree ceremony that was to take place that evening, for given that the ceremony was to be the biggest event of the week, there could have been no better occasion for assembling as many as possible of the distinguished guests and participants.[30]

The presence of eight men standing behind the front row is accounted for by their function at the week's celebrations: six of them (Buchner, Drew, Goddard, Jastrow, Seashore, and Whipple) either presided over, led discussion, or gave papers at the afternoon conferences that were run separately from the main morning addresses, while two others (Porter and Sanford, both at Clark) ran a demonstration session on psychological laboratory equipment on the final day of the event.[31] If we take out these eight and also the eight honorary degree recipients, along with Hall, James, Brill, Fe-

---

30. The Clark University Archives contain another photograph taken of the mathematics and physics group on exactly the same spot. See fig. 2.3.

31. Clark University, *Lectures and Addresses*, part 1, vi; part 2, vii.

renczi, and Jones, this leaves twenty-one individuals in the picture. Twelve of these remaining men had either studied or been employed at Clark University in previous years or were still currently at Clark.[32] The fact that such a large number of people in the picture had connections to Clark University therefore makes it quite probable that it was this fact that either brought them to the celebration event in the first instance or secured their place in the commemorative photograph. But that still leaves nine people unaccounted for.

Like James, five of the remaining nine had connections to Harvard University,[33] and four of those had also conducted work in an area very similar to that covered by Jung. E. B. Holt had completed his Ph.D. at Harvard in 1901 and had been appointed assistant professor in psychology there in 1905, where he was a demonstrator in the laboratory under Hugo Münsterberg. There he had worked alongside the man standing to his left, C. S. Berry, an animal psychologist specializing in imitative tendencies, who had completed his Ph.D. at Harvard in 1907 but who was to make his career in education. Berry, along with Robert Yerkes, another of his Harvard colleagues and also a close colleague of Holt's, published in 1909 an article on association reactions, which was heavily dependent on Jung's association studies.[34] The article discussed experimental support for the effectiveness of the association tests for establishing facts that the subject wished to keep hidden. Jung addressed this very topic in the first of his lectures by recounting how he had used the tests to detect the perpetrator of a crime, a method that was to be replicated and described in an article two years later by E. W. Katzenellenbogen. Katzenellenbogen was an assistant physician at Danvers Insane Hospital, where he was a colleague of Charles Ricksher, one of Jung's collaborators. He also lectured on abnormal psychology at Harvard University, where he worked under Münsterberg alongside Holt.[35]

---

32. Burnham, Chamberlain, Dawson, Hayes, Kakise, Kanda, Karlson, Kirkpatrick, Magni, Schinz, Wilson, Young. L. N. Wilson, *List of Degrees Granted at Clark University and Clark College 1889–1914* (Worcester, MA: Clark University Press, 1914). L. N. Wilson, ed., *Clark University Directory of Alumni, Faculty and Students* (Worcester, MA: Clark University Press, 1915).

33. Baldwin, Berry, Holt, Katzenellenbogen, Wells.

34. R. M. Yerkes and C. S. Berry, "The Association Reaction Method of Mental Diagnosis (*Tatbestandsdiagnostik*)," *American Journal of Psychology* 20 (1909): 22–37.

35. E. W. Katzen-Ellenbogen, "The Detection of a Case of Simulation of Insanity by Means of Association Tests," *Journal of Abnormal Psychology* 6 (1911): 9–32. Katzenellenbogen had what might be regarded only charitably as a checkered career after the period documented here. He left America in 1915 and ended up being tried and sentenced to life imprisonment as a war criminal at Dachau in 1947 for crimes committed at Buchenwald, where he was inmate, camp doctor, and consulting psychiatrist. The sentence was subsequently commuted to fifteen years

F. L. Wells was to follow in Katzenellenbogen's footsteps by also lecturing for a time on abnormal psychology at Harvard, and he too published a number of papers around the time of the Clark event that were closely related to Jung's association and galvanic response studies.[36] B. T. Baldwin had gained his Ph.D. at Harvard in 1905 also on a topic in the area of association studies, which he published a year later.[37]

Of the remaining four, S. C. Fuller was not only a friend of Hall but also reputedly his physician at some time as well as a pathologist at Westborough State Hospital.[38] H. I. Klopp, standing next to Fuller, was one of his colleagues at Westborough and a scientific collaborator. J. M. Cattell had been a student of Hall's when he was at Johns Hopkins.[39] Relations between them had not always been easy, and it is possible that as well as being an invitee, Cattell was there in his capacity as editor of *Science*, the journal of the American Association for the Advancement of Science.[40] This leaves just G. M. Forbes, associated all of his professional life with the University of Rochester, where he was professor of philosophy and pedagogy, and while it has not been possible to find a direct connection between Forbes and Hall, Clark University, or any of the main speakers, there is no real surprise at his attendance given his disciplinary interests.

Once we establish the connections of the individuals in the photograph to Clark or to Hall and also appreciate its purpose,[41] then we can see that it would be a complete misreading to represent it as a picture of Freud and

---

on appeal, and he was released in 1953. Sonu Shamdasani, "A Woman Called Frank," *Spring* 50 (1990): 30, has discovered that in 1955 Katzenellenbogen wrote a letter to Jung, in the course of which he reminded him that Miss Frank Miller, the woman at the heart of Jung's 1912 work, *Transformations and Symbols of the Libido*, had been a patient of his and that through his personal acquaintance with her he could attest to the accuracy of the analysis of her fantasies that Jung had published. He had written to Jung in 1918 to the same effect. Shamdasani also ascertained that the admitting psychiatrist had been none other than Charles Ricksher (32).

36. F. L. Wells, "Some Properties of the Free Association Time." *Psychological Review* 18 (1911): 1-23. F. L. Wells, "A Preliminary Note on the Categories of Association Reactions," *Psychological Review* 18 (1911): 229-33. F. L. Wells, "Practice Effects in Free Association," *American Journal of Psychology* 22 (1911): 1-13. F. L. Wells and A. Forbes, "On Certain Electrical Processes in the Human Body and Their Relation to Emotional Reactions," *Archives of Psychology* 2 (1911): 1-39.

37. B. T. Baldwin, "Associations under the Influence of Different Ideas," in *Harvard Psychological Studies*, ed. H. Münsterberg (Boston: Houghton Mifflin, 1906), 2:431-74.

38. R. H. Sharpley, "Solomon Carter Fuller," in *Psychoanalysis, Psychotherapy, and the New England Medical Scene, 1894-1944*, ed. G. E. Gifford Jr. (New York: Science History Publications, 1978), 194.

39. Ross, *G. Stanley Hall*, 145-47.

40. M. M. Sokal, "*Science* and James McKeen Cattell, 1894-1945," *Science* 209 (1980): 43-52.

41. See Appendix.

his audience. Apart from the small number of obvious exceptions, there is no reason to think that most of the men pictured came to Clark expressly for the purpose of hearing Freud speak. Leaving aside those directly connected with the formalities of the celebrations, most of those in the picture were at some time either students, graduates, or teachers at Clark University, and, judging by their own research publications, even the very small group with connections to Harvard would seem more likely on the face of it to have been more interested in Jung's work than Freud's.

If we are to look for evidence after the event for any possible continuing interest in Freud or psychoanalysis that may have been sparked by hearing him speak, then there seems to be not much to find. It is true that Karlson went on to complete his Ph.D. thesis in 1912 under Chamberlain on the topic of psychoanalysis and mythology and that Holt published a book that was very complimentary towards Freud, though it did not have much to do with psychoanalysis, but this is very little to show for what is often characterized as the launch of psychoanalysis in America.[42] What evidence we do have in firsthand accounts from those who were not already his followers gives little reason to amend this view. Meyer, recording his own memory in 1948, was unimpressed with some aspects of what he encountered: "I remember . . . the apparent self-preoccupation on the part of Freud and Jung, who were sitting before me when I read my paper, without any real response or participation." Meyer nevertheless was prompted by seeing Freud lecture to present a discussion of his work in 1910.[43] F. L. Wells adopted in print a critical, though not dismissive, stance towards psychoanalysis and on more than one occasion recalled that he made himself unpopular with Hall by speaking his mind to him about this at the Clark event.[44] Titchener, for his part, thought that Freud's notion of revolution-

---

42. J. K. Karlson, "Psychoanalysis and Mythology," *Journal of Religious Psychology* 7 (1914): 137–213. E. B. Holt, *The Freudian Wish and Its Place in Ethics* (New York: Henry Holt, 1915). In abstracting Karlson's work in 1922, Ernest Jones ("Applied Psycho-Analysis: K. J. Karlson. Psychoanalysis and Mythology, *Journal of Religious Psychology*, Nov. 1914, Vol. VII, pp. 13–213," *International Journal of Psychoanalysis* 3 [1922]: 365) noted: "The title of this paper is rather a misnomer, for the subject of the paper is not so much the relation of psycho-analysis to mythology as the general psychology of myth-formation, and the mention of psychoanalysis occupies less than a fifth of the whole paper."

43. Meyer, cited in R. Leys, "Meyer's Dealings with Jones: A Chapter in the History of the American Response to Psychoanalysis," *Journal of the History of the Behavioral Sciences* 17 (1981): 460. A. Meyer, "A Discussion of Some Fundamental Issues in Freud's Psychoanalysis," *State Hospitals Bulletin* 2 (1910): 827–48.

44. Ross, *G. Stanley Hall*, 390; J. C. Burnham, "Interviewing as a Tool of the Trade: A Not-Very-Satisfactory Bottom Line," in *Thick Description and Fine Texture: Studies in the History of Psychology*, ed. D. B. Baker (Akron, OH: University of Akron Press, 2003), 33.

izing psychology would set it back about two generations: "And the man wonders that we do not take his psychologising seriously."[45]

On the other hand, we know of course that there were people whom Freud either met or who heard him speak who were neither pictured nor reported as participating in the conference brochure or in the press. Jung wrote in his letters to his wife of the round of socializing that the visit to Clark entailed: "We are gaining ground here, and our following is growing slowly but surely. To-day I had a talk about psychoanalysis with two highly cultivated elderly ladies who proved to be very well informed and free thinking. I was greatly surprised, since I had prepared myself for opposition."[46] But whether this kind of response from the people Freud and Jung met face-to-face implied anything more substantial in the way of new support for psychoanalysis remains at best an open question, given the absence of any specific evidence in its favor.

Who was actually present at Freud's lectures is likely never to become very clear on the basis of the available evidence. Even if one was compiled at the time, there appears to be no surviving record of the audience for any of the lectures, and eyewitness accounts are few and far between.[47] Coriat

---

45. Cited in Evans and Koelsch, "Psychoanalysis Arrives in America," 944–45.

46. C. G. Jung and Aniela Jaffé, *Memories, Dreams, Reflections* (London: Flamingo, 1983 [1963]), 399.

47. Ross, *G. Stanley Hall*, 389. Rosenzweig, *Freud, Jung, and Hall*, 132–34, is one of several commentators who have noted that the celebrated anarchist Emma Goldman was present in Worcester at the same time as Freud and who have speculated not only about the significance of her presence at Freud's lectures but also about the effect of this on what he had to say. Gordon Patterson, "Freud's Rhetoric: Persuasion and History in the 1909 Clark Lectures," *Metaphor and Symbolic Activity* 5 (1990): 227, for example, writes: "It is impossible to know what the audience thought when they saw Emma Goldman enter the lecture hall each morning. . . . It is not far-fetched to imagine that some of the audience may have wondered what Goldman might do in the course of Freud's lecture. Freud was certainly aware of the controversy, and it is my suspicion that he seized on Goldman's unexpected presence in the auditorium for what was indisputably the most extraordinary analogy in the Clark lectures." This of course is the analogy of the process of repression to that of a disruptive person ejected from the lecture room, which Freud employs in his second talk (S. Freud, "Five Lectures on Psycho-Analysis," S.E. 11:25 [1910]).

Goldman did not of course come to Worcester for the purpose of attending the Clark celebration, but was there on tour and just happened to be in the town at the same time. Moreover she had already seen Freud lecture during her stay in Vienna in the mid-1890s and had been impressed by him then (E. Goldman, *Living My Life* [New York: Knopf, 1931], 173) and so had already long been acquainted with the kind of thing he might have to say. However, the contemporary evidence we have from the newspaper reports (see Rosenzweig, *Freud, Jung and Hall*, 132ff.) suggests only that she went to one of the afternoon conferences on pedagogy, and Goldman's own account of the occasion dates from her memoirs published over twenty years later. Here she indeed refers to hearing an address given by Freud at Clark in 1909: "I was deeply impressed by the lucidity of his mind and the simplicity of his delivery. Among the

says that the hall was "well filled," but any further inference about audience size or the level of interest in Freud or psychoanalysis is limited by the format of the presentations.[48] The lectures of all the guests were presented sequentially in the three hours between 9 a.m. and noon. Freud lectured at 11 a.m. every day from Tuesday to Saturday, so he was preceded each day by two other speakers: Burgerstein and Stern on Tuesday; Burgerstein and Titchener on Wednesday; Jung and Titchener on Thursday; Jung and Stern on Friday and Saturday.[49] The extent to which the etiquette of the occasion demanded that people who were present hear the first lecture were constrained to remain in the room for the full three hours is another of those unknowns that makes a clear assessment of the nature of Freud's audience hard to gauge. Although it was recorded that 175 people were present for the opening of the first day, Jung reported in a letter home to his wife that as the first lecture (presumably by Stern) was boring, he and his colleagues soon sneaked out and went for a walk around the outskirts of the town.[50] Freud and Ferenczi too were presumably both absent for most of the morning sessions when they were piecing together what Freud was to say. So if the psychoanalysts felt at liberty to absent themselves from at least some of the proceedings that they felt to be less interesting, others may have felt likewise.

There is one further aspect of the photograph that repays closer questioning. This is the simple fact that Freud and Jung are standing next to one another. We know of course that Freud and Jung traveled to Clark together along with Ferenczi. They were joined by Jones and Brill, and not only do all five feature in the large group photograph, but there was a second picture taken of this psychoanalytic group along with Stanley Hall. There can therefore be little doubt about the fact that, from their respective points of view, both Hall and Freud saw this as at least in some sense a psychoanalytic expedition. Such was his dependence on Jung that Freud had no reason to think that anything other than psychoanalysis was the central

---

array of professors, looking stiff and important in their university caps and gowns, Sigmund Freud, in ordinary attire, unassuming, almost shrinking, stood out like a giant among pygmies" (*Living My Life*, 445–46). However, by the time she wrote this, Freud had become very famous, and even if her reminiscence after such a lapse of time is not slightly tinted by that fact, her reference to university caps and gowns suggests that it was the degree ceremony she was referring to, rather than any lectures. All she mentions in the passage in question is "an address." So although it would be nice to think of Goldman attentively hanging on to every word of Freud's lectures, there is no evidence that she actually attended any of them.

48. I. H. Coriat, "Some Personal Reminiscences of Psychoanalysis in Boston: An Autobiographical Note," *Psychoanalytic Review* 32 (1945): 3.

49. Evans and Koelsch, "Psychoanalysis Arrives in America," 944–46.

50. Ibid., 944. Jung and Jaffé, *Memories, Dreams, Reflections*, 399.

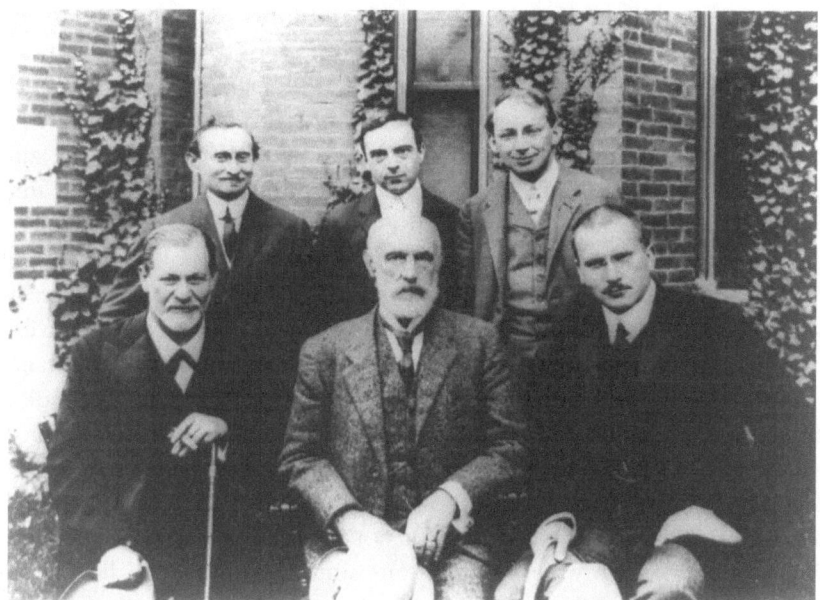

2.4. The psychoanalytic contingent at the Clark meetings posing with G. Stanley Hall. Front row: Freud, Hall, Jung. Back row: Brill, Jones, Ferenczi. Library of Congress.

interest that the Americans would have in them both and in what they had to say in their lectures. The reality is rather more complex.

Rosenzweig discusses at length the apparently anomalous aspects of Jung's invitation. He notes that this was not issued at the same time as Freud's, but only in June 1909, and he also establishes that this happened only after the withdrawal of another of the proposed lecturers, Ernst Meumann, a former student of Wundt and a specialist in experimental pedagogy, who had carried out investigations into learning and memory as applied to childhood education. But Rosenzweig is puzzled why Jung, who had no particular expertise in pedagogy, should be a replacement for Meumann and suggests that the Clark committee on honorary degrees may have had doubts about Jung's suitability for the award, given his relative youth compared with the other candidates and his comparative lack of renown even in the German-speaking world.[51] There is clearly room for doubt about how Jung's invitation came about since no correspondence between Jung and anyone at Clark appears to have survived, and Rosenzweig's puzzlement is understandable: what is Jung doing at an event where

---

51. Rosenzweig, *Freud, Jung, and Hall*, 34–36.

he stands alongside Freud, Ferenczi, Brill, and Jones, but where he is cast as an expert not in psychoanalysis but in education? After all, his lectures were published alongside Freud's in the *American Journal of Psychology*, not in the *Pedagogical Seminary*, where the other educational papers appeared.

What of Jung's own account of how he came to be there? Aniela Jaffé reports that Jung attributed his invitation to the association studies that he had been conducting for some five years or so and which had been reported widely in the American journals, both in papers he himself had written and those written with associates such as Peterson and Ricksher: "It was these association studies which later, in 1909, procured me my invitation to Clark University; I was asked to lecture on my work. Simultaneously, and independently of me, Freud was invited." Later in the book a similar account is given: "I had been invited to lecture on the association experiment at Clark University in Worcester, Massachusetts. Independently, Freud had also received an invitation, and we decided to travel together."[52] Rosenzweig criticizes this account for not being in accord with the facts. First, the invitations were by no means simultaneous, Freud having accepted his invitation some four months before Jung was asked to attend, and secondly Jung inverts the priority of the two invitations: "The impression is conveyed that Freud's invitation was secondary to Jung's when, in fact, the opposite was the case."[53]

However, Rosenzweig's criticism is somewhat misplaced and is perhaps to some extent colored by his own questionable assumption of the centrality of Freud to the whole event. To be sure, "simultaneously" does imply a degree of coincidence that is not quite consistent with a four-month gap, but this is a translation of "gleichzeitig," which could equally well be rendered more loosely as "at the same time," and interpreted idiomatically this would not be at all inconsistent with how things happened. But there is a further sense in which Jung's invitation was perhaps more independent of Freud's own than even he implied, and even when allowance is made for the fact that we cannot be fully confident that Jaffé has represented Jung's account verbatim, we could do worse than to take Jung's statement as it is presented.[54]

In his discussion of the planning of the lecture series, Koelsch establishes that the fact that Jung was invited as a replacement for an education-

---

52. Jung and Jaffé, *Memories, Dreams, Reflections*, 141, 179.
53. Rosenzweig, *Freud, Jung, and Hall*, 38.
54. S. Shamdasani, "Memories, Dreams, Omissions," *Spring* 57 (1995): 115–37.

alist led directly not only to his being cast as an expert in pedagogy but also to his honorary degree being designated as in pedagogy and school hygiene.[55] It seems that each department was allocated up to two slots for foreign visiting speakers, and there was considerable shuffling at the planning stage to make sure that the quotas were both complete and balanced. So, strange as it may appear, Jung's formal status as a specialist in pedagogy runs throughout the formal record of the Clark events. There in the introduction to the *Lectures and Addresses* volume is a list of all the honorary degree recipients and the titles of their awards. Apart from Titchener, who was awarded a Doctorate of Letters, all those in the photograph were made Doctors of Laws, but whereas Boas, Freud, Jennings, Meyer, and Stern were given their degrees in the subcategory of Psychology, both Jung and Burgerstein are listed under the subheading of Education and School Hygiene. Moreover, Hall's introduction to the volume records that overall there were six lectures in Education and fourteen lectures in Psychology. Listing the number of lectures given by each guest, we have Freud, 5; Jung, 3; Stern, 4; Jennings, 1; Meyer, 1; Titchener, 2; Boas, 1; Burgerstein, 3.[56] How do we subdivide these so that they fall into the two categories of fourteen for psychology and six for education? Indeed we can do this sensibly only by dividing them along the lines of the degree classifications and by grouping Jung's three along with Burgerstein's three as part of the education rather than the psychology grouping.

Jung himself alludes to this in the very opening paragraph of his lecture as published: "When I was honored with the invitation from Clark University to lecture before this esteemed assemblage, a wish was at the same time expressed that I should speak about the methods of my work, and especially about the psychology of childhood." Just a few years later, Jung again refers to his Clark lectures near the opening of the lectures that he gave at Fordham University in 1912: "I, too, have already had the great

---

55. W. A. Koelsch, "Freud at Clark: Planning the 1909 Conference," in *Freud in Our Time: A Seventy-Fifth Anniversary Symposium*, ed. W. A. Koelsch and S. Wapner (Worcester, MA: Clark University Press, 1988), 61.

56. Clark University, *Lectures and* Addresses, vi–vii. In fact only one of Titchener's two lectures is published in the Clark series. The second was a talk on "The Experimental Psychology of the Thought Processes," given a day after the first (Evans and Koelsch, "Psychoanalysis Arrives in America," 945). The reason for the non-publication of this lecture is most probably the fact that Titchener had given a series of five lectures on precisely this topic at the University of Illinois the previous March and these all appeared in a published volume that very year. E. B. Titchener, *Lectures on the Experimental Psychology of the Thought-Processes* (New York: Macmillan, 1909).

honour of lecturing in America, on the experimental foundation of the theory of complexes and the application of psychoanalysis to education [*Erziehung*]."[57]

E. C. Sanford and W. H. Burnham published a report on the Clark gathering in the first issue of the *Journal of Educational Psychology*, launched in 1910. After noting that most of the lectures and discussions were concerned with subjects represented by the journal, they proceeded to summarize some of the psychology contributions, commenting that recent progress in this field was marked by a trend towards useful applications and analysis of the more complex mental phenomena. But mention of these characteristics led not to a summary of Freud's lectures but rather to those of first Stern and then Titchener. When they moved on to the lectures in the department of education—which "treated especially school hygiene and mental hygiene"—it was Leo Burgerstein's work that was mentioned first, followed by a short paragraph on Jung:

> Lectures on the Psychology of Association and Mental Hygiene were given by Dr. C. G. Jung of the University of Zürich. In this course Dr. Jung presented and illustrated his *diagnostische Assoziationsmethode*. Interesting as these lectures were for the direct results presented, they were still more significant, perhaps, because they suggested the possibility of establishing a truly mental hygiene based upon scientific principles.

Finally, right at the end of the piece, Freud's lectures are mentioned: "Even the lectures in psychiatry given by Prof. Sigmund Freud of the University of Vienna were not without educational and hygienic as well as psychological significance. Special interest attached to these lectures in large part on account of the interesting personality of the lecturer."[58] The authors then quote from a report from the "correspondent of the New York Nation," giving a flattering overview of Freud's intellectual history and psychological system, which was in fact written by Stanley Hall himself and which may even have been inserted here at Hall's instigation.[59]

So while it is clear that from the point of view of the educational psychologists, Jung's presence at the celebrations was more apposite than Freud's, there remains a curious ambiguity, nevertheless, about what he was doing

---

57. Clark University, *Lectures and Addresses*, 39. C. G. Jung, *Symbols of Transformation*, in *Collected Works of C. G. Jung*, vol. 5 (Princeton, NJ: Princeton University Press, 1956 [1913]), 88.

58. E. C. Sanford and W. H. Burnham, "Twentieth Anniversary of Clark University," *Journal of Educational Psychology* 1 (1910): 34–35.

59. Evans and Koelsch, "Psychoanalysis Arrives in America," 946.

there at all. Putting all this together, it suggests that Jung's attendance and the content of his lectures covered a patchwork of interests and functions.

Jung is surely correct that it was his work with the association studies that qualified him to be invited in the first place, and he spoke of these in his first lecture, giving a general overview of his word-association methods. Yet Hall had needed a replacement for an educationalist, and this would have prompted him specifically to request that Jung speak not just about his general association method but also about the psychology of childhood. Jung fulfilled this part of his obligation in the final lecture, where he looked at the psychic life of the young child through an anonymized account of his experiences with his own daughter. The second lecture concerned how similarities between generations in reaction patterns could be detected by the association tests and how they demonstrated that family constellations could effectively transmit complexes from one generation to the next, and this lecture constituted a thematic bridge between the topics of the other two. His status as a psychiatrist no doubt enhanced his standing as one well qualified in the eyes of Sanford and Burnham to link discussions of upbringing and education in the broadest sense with practical issues relating to mental hygiene, at that time a very topical issue and one with which both William James and Adolf Meyer were actively concerned.[60] Yet neither Jung's formal position within the program of lectures, nor his reputation among most of those present, nor even his honorary degree had any direct connection with psychoanalysis.[61]

After hearing him speak, of course, no one present would have had any doubts as to where his allegiances lay. Not only did Jung make his theoretical dependence on Freud's psychoanalysis quite explicit in his third lecture; he also made his personal commitment plain in his speech of thanks for the honorary degree: "My work is identical with the scientific movement inaugurated by Professor Freud, whose servant I have the honour to be."[62] So while the formal proceedings of the Clark celebrations presented Jung to his audience as a specialist in education and mental hygiene, with a strong experimental bent to his general approach, this is not what has been left to us in conventional histories of the event.

60. G. Grob, *Mental Illness and American Society, 1875–1940* (Princeton, NJ: Princeton University Press, 1983), 144–78.
61. Koelsch, "Freud at Clark," 65, surmises that as Hall probably delegated the invitations in the education area to Burnham, this explains why there is no evidence of correspondence between Jung and Hall. Burnham's files have not survived.
62. "Dankesrede," cited in S. Shamdasani, *Jung and the Making of Modern Psychology: The Dream of a Science* (Cambridge: Cambridge University Press, 2003), 137.

If Freud and Jung each had his own reasons and motives for allowing their joint presence to be seen as a tightly bonded double act, Stanley Hall certainly had a significant part to play in this. Given that Freud was booked as his own star turn, he would doubtless have been quite happy to collude with the idea of Jung's lectures being construed as a supporting performance, and having heard the two sets of lectures, there is no reason to suppose that he would have had any great difficulty in publishing them together in the *American Journal of Psychology* rather than placing Jung's in the *Pedagogical Seminary* along with the other educational papers. The key image that sets this in the historical record is the photograph of Hall in the middle of the psychoanalytic group of five, which then so easily becomes superimposed on our reading of the other, larger photograph of the forty-two participants and shapes it quite misleadingly as a record of a chiefly psychoanalytic event.

From Freud's point of view, Jung was unquestionably there as a confirmed representative of psychoanalysis and also to act as his principal lieutenant. Jung's third lecture on the psychic life of the child was quite clearly designed as a substantiating exemplar for Freud's discussion of infantile sexuality delivered later that same morning, though rather than Jung's engineering the content of his lecture so as to support Freud's general theses, as Rosenzweig supposes, it is perhaps more likely that Freud arranged his own discussion of infantile sexuality to coincide with Jung's talk and to draw support from it.[63] The point, however, is that whereas Freud's audience would all be expecting him to devote his lectures to the topic of psychoanalysis, if Jung had happened never to mention it, probably very few people present would have thought it strange or expected anything different. From the point of view of most people there, psychoanalysis would by no means have been the principal reason for Jung's presence.

Having dwelt at length on the photographic record of Freud's and Jung's visit to Clark, there is one more piece of evidence that repays attention if we are to evaluate Freud's standing at the event. During the preparations for the week's events, a ten-page brochure was published, advertising details of the speakers and the conferences. The Department of Psychology has the first section, where the general purpose of the gathering is heralded, followed by a separate subsection detailing the guest lecturers. At the top of the list is William Stern, who is given ten and a half lines of biographical detail and an indication of his lectures. This is followed by a simple listing

---

63. Rosenzweig, *Freud, Jung, and Hall*, esp. 135–63.

of the American guests: Titchener, Boas, Jennings, and Meyer. Freud's name appears nowhere. A further subsection of six paragraphs follows, where an outline is given of the planned conferences and demonstrations, an indication of how to obtain lodgings for the event, and information about dining facilities. The final paragraph consists of two lines: "In Psychiatry a series of lectures will be given by Dr. Sigmund Freud. Subjects to be announced later." There then follows a section for the Department of Pedagogy and School Hygiene, where Burgerstein and then Jung each receive half a dozen lines of introduction. Jung's reads:

> Dr. C. G. Jung, Privatdozent in Psychiatry in the University of Zürich, Switzerland, will give three lectures on Mental Hygiene or related topics. Dr. Jung is the well-known specialist in the study of Association Processes and in the method of *Assoziation-Diagnostik*. He is also editor of the *Jahrbuch für Psychoanalytische und Psychopathologische Forschungen*.

In explaining the brevity and placing of Freud's billing, Koelsch has managed to piece together that at one time it appears that Hall considered placing him as a neuropathologist at the head of a series of lectures in biology. The basic outline of the proofs of the brochure, which had been constructed at that early stage, were simply rolled forward into the final version, so Freud's billing seems to have fallen victim to the complications that arose in planning the celebration.[64] This was not helped by the fact that owing to Hall's request for the information not reaching him, Freud gave no indication to Hall of the topic of his lectures or how many there would be until five days before the start of the event.[65] But whatever the reason for it, the brochure would have given no one the impression that Freud was in any sense the leading guest at the proceedings, and it is something of a historical irony that while the association tests are clearly Jung's principal drawing point, it is against his name and not Freud's that the only reference to psychoanalysis is made.

We should not neglect to take into account that there were two individuals who were subsequently to maintain a lifelong involvement with psychoanalysis who heard Freud speak at Clark but who were not represented in the photograph: Isador Coriat and James Jackson Putnam. Coriat later said that although Freud's lectures "crystallized a latent interest in psycho-

---

64. Koelsch, "Freud at Clark," 60–61.
65. Rosenzweig, *Freud, Jung, and Hall*, 355.

analysis," it was only "several years later that I was able to accept its fundamental concepts."[66] By contrast, meeting Freud was immediately of great importance to Putnam. Not only did he invite Freud, Jung, and Ferenczi to spend a few days at the Putnam Camp in Keene Valley in the Adirondacks during the following week, but thereafter there was a correspondence with Freud that lasted until Putnam's death in 1918. But before meeting him at Clark, Putnam had already publicly committed himself to "the genius of Freud" when he presented a paper at the New Haven symposium on psychotherapeutics in May 1909. Furthermore it is evident from the paper he gave to the American Neurological Association in May 1910, discussing his own personal experience with Freud's psychoanalytic method, that Putnam had begun working with patients in this manner about a year previously, and therefore several months before he met Freud.[67] It was Ernest Jones, not Freud himself, who was mainly responsible for convincing Putnam of the merits of psychoanalysis and for leading him to go beyond his previously receptive, but nonetheless skeptical, attitude. Putnam's meeting with Freud at Clark added a personal dimension to an intellectual commitment that was already well established.

If we are to understand fully the significance of Freud's visit to Clark, we must therefore recognize a number of its aspects that have generally remained unremarked in discussion of the event, although the evidence for these conclusions has long been available. First, while Hall's role in issuing the invitation is almost universally acknowledged, the fact that it was due to the power, influence, and efforts of this one man also means that his high evaluation of Freud or familiarity with his work was not necessarily matched elsewhere in the broader medical or psychological fields, or indeed within his own university. Freud was certainly not unknown, but given the nature of his own work, Jung was probably at least as familiar a figure as Freud, and quite probably more so, to most of those who attended the lecture sessions. Second, the celebrated photograph is of little significance as documentary evidence about the psychoanalytic movement in America. Most of those represented were there to attend the twentieth-anniversary celebrations, not to hear Freud, and very few of them would have found their own intellectual interests overlapping with what he had to say. Third, there is no specific evidence of any great clamor or rush to join the ranks of psychoanalysts that followed as a result of his visit. The reports in the

---

66. Coriat, "Some Personal Reminiscences," 2.
67. J. J. Putnam, "The Relation of Character Formation to Psychotherapy," in *Psychotherapeutics: A Symposium*, ed. M. Prince et al. (Boston: Richard G. Badger, 1910), 189. J. J. Putnam, *Addresses on Psycho-Analysis* (London: Hogarth Press, 1951), 31, 39.

local newspapers were largely planted by Hall and would in any case have had only local effects. But even in the local area, there is no evidence of an upsurge in interest in psychoanalysis. It was not until 1914 that Putnam founded the Boston Psychoanalytical Society with Coriat as secretary, and even then, in its first incarnation, it did not survive Putnam's death in 1918.

After Clark

Yet looking at the historical record, it does nevertheless appear that the months immediately following the Clark conference constituted a period marked by a sudden rise in interest in Freud and psychoanalysis, a trend that can be seen in journal publications, meetings of professional bodies, and so on. If Freud's visit to America did not bring this about, what did?

First of all, and probably most importantly, there is the appearance of Freud translated into English. Before the Clark conference, no one who did not have access to German could have read Freud in his own words. As already noted, Freud's first works in English (*Selected Papers on Hysteria and Other Psychoneuroses*) were published at the end of September 1909, and then in 1910 there appeared not only the *Three Essays on the Theory of Sexuality* but also Freud's Clark lectures themselves. Up to then, Freud had had a curiously muted attitude towards publishing in his own name in America. Jones reports that as early as August 1905 Morton Prince had written to Freud and invited him to submit a paper for the first issue of his new *Journal of Abnormal Psychology*, but nothing came of this.[68] Then in November 1908, Jones wrote to Freud that he and Brill had been invited by Prince to write a series of articles on Freud's work for his journal, and he asked for Freud's opinion on this, adding that "there is a great call for your work in America, especially in New York and Boston." Freud replied, giving his assent, but also suggesting: "It might be the best way to introduce my work to your countrymen, perhaps much more efficacious than a translation of my papers."[69] So Freud seemed to have been in no hurry to rush into print in the English-speaking

---

68. Jones, *Sigmund Freud: Life and Work*, 2:31. Paskauskas, in S. Freud and E. Jones, *The Complete Correspondence of Sigmund Freud and Ernest Jones*, ed. R. A. Paskauskas (Cambridge, MA: Harvard University Press, 1993), 8 n. 10, records that Freud had refused to contribute but cites no evidence for this nor gives any indication as to why Freud might have done so. In his paper "Who Founded the American Psychopathological Association?" *Comprehensive Psychiatry* 27 (1986): 439–45, Taylor claims that Freud's refusal was due to the fact that Prince's journal was not to be purely psychoanalytic (441), though this on the face of it seems unlikely, for at that time there were no psychoanalytic journals anywhere. Freud's relationship with Prince stands in need of further research.

69. Freud and Jones, *The Complete Correspondence*, 7, 9.

world, either through the translation of works already published or by writing pieces especially composed for the American market.

The publication of his five Clark lectures was undoubtedly a particularly important factor in spreading Freud's name.[70] In fact, these lectures have a significance in the development of psychoanalysis that has perhaps up to now not been sufficiently appreciated. It is notable that when Freud is mentioned in the American journals in connection with psychoanalysis prior to 1909, it is usually along the lines of his being a psychotherapist who has adopted a new method, which he calls "psychoanalysis," and which has led to some interesting findings. But with the publication of the lectures, this changed, because for the first time in either German or English, "psychoanalysis" started to include not just a method but also a set of results and conclusions. In short, this was the point at which psychoanalysis began to become not merely a method, but also a body of thought.[71]

For here, as well as relating the historical origins of psychoanalysis as a method of psychotherapy, Freud set out in a single work his findings on neurosis, dreams, jokes, slips, sexuality, and so on in such a way that even today it remains arguably the best introduction to all things Freudian for any novice in the field. This exposition gave psychoanalysis a form of coherence that it had previously lacked, and within which particular findings became associated with Freud's name beyond the "trauma and catharsis" work that he had done with Breuer fifteen years earlier and which had still been the dominant theme in many reviews of his studies. At the same time, of course, this provided a sound base for controversy, as psychoanalysis shifted from being seen as a new method of psychotherapy with potentially open-ended outcomes to a set of distinctly "Freudian" conclusions deriving from that method.

But although the publication of his five lectures was important in furthering Freud's reputation in America and was also a significant landmark for psychoanalysis in general, the fact that this followed as an immediate consequence of his visit to the Clark celebrations is somewhat incidental.

---

70. In one of the earlier retrospective accounts of psychoanalysis in America, Junius F. Brown, "Freud's Influence on American Psychology," *Psychoanalytic Quarterly* 9 (1940): 283, states his view that "except for a handful of people Freud was unknown and without influence in American psychology until his addresses of 1909 had been published in the *American Journal of Psychology* the ensuing year."

71. Apart from a minor piece originally given as a lecture three years earlier, Freud's *Five Lectures on Psycho-Analysis* (originally published in English as *The Origin and Development of Psychoanalysis*) constitute the first freestanding work by Freud to contain "psychoanalysis" in its title; cf. S. Freud, "Psycho-Analysis and the Establishment of the Facts in Legal Proceedings," S.E. 9 (1906).

For if he had been so minded, Freud could quite easily have written and published a similar exposition in America or elsewhere without actually going there, and this would most likely have had a comparable effect. The lectures were important not because they constituted a written record of Freud's prestigious visit to Clark but as a publication in their own right. In fact, the visit to Clark has perhaps through an act of displacement been attributed a significance in retrospect that it would never have had if it had not been for the publication of the lectures that he gave there.

A second key factor in the sudden growth in psychoanalysis in America at this juncture is the success of others, apart from Freud, who were working to further its reputation. Here it appears that their effects were quite disproportionate to their numbers, since prior to Freud's Clark visit, it is only possible to include Ernest Jones and Abraham Brill in this category. In the period before Freud's visit, Brill was largely engaged in translating Jung's work, and later, of course, Freud's writings, and he himself published little in his own name. On the other hand, Jones, once he was based at Toronto, worked forcefully and tirelessly in support of Freud's work, initially through the Boston group, where he made systematic inroads in raising the profile of psychoanalysis through personal contacts, discussion and meetings, and so on, including persuading Putnam to commit himself to the cause.

But Jones also made significant interventions in the public domain in print. A glance at his bibliography reveals just one psychoanalytic publication in 1908, two in 1909, and then a veritable explosion of about a dozen in 1910.[72] Jones was vociferous and combative, and his success in raising the profile of psychoanalysis should not be underestimated. Much has been written over the years about the proselytizing and abrasive style of some of those committed to the psychoanalytic cause in the early years of its history in America, but it is sometimes difficult to avoid the conclusion that this image is largely based mainly on Jones, who seems to have become almost an archetypal figure in the mythology of the psychoanalytic movement, as the way he carried out his role as the leading spokesman for the cause in America appears to have produced reflections affecting the perception of the whole movement.

But if the sudden growth of psychoanalysis after 1909 can be accounted for by factors other than Freud's own visit, does this therefore mean that Freud's trip to America must be deemed a failure? The answer to this question largely depends on what aims Freud had in going there in the first

---

72. E. Jones, "Bibliography of the Scientific Publications of Ernest Jones, M.D.," *International Journal of Psychoanalysis* 10 (1929): 363–82.

place. Had he seen it as a primary opportunity to build support for psychoanalysis and to further the spread of the movement in the New World, then there is little direct evidence of success. But then we have already seen in examining his correspondence of the time that this did not appear to be his aim at all. This seems to have been Jones's main purpose in life. Freud's own hopes seem to have been twofold. First to enjoy himself and the experience of traveling to a distant place to which he had not been before. Secondly, to bask in the recognition that the invitation afforded him. It is notable that this is the aspect that comes to the fore when he recalls his trip in later years:

> In Europe I felt as though I were despised; but over there I found myself received by the foremost men as an equal. As I stepped on to the platform at Worcester to deliver my *Five Lectures on Psychoanalysis* it seemed like the realization of some incredible day-dream: psychoanalysis was no longer a product of delusion, it had become a valuable part of reality.[73]

Ferenczi's astute observation is very much to the point here. Referring to the weakness displayed by Freud when he attempted to repress his "American vanity," Ferenczi speculates on the psychodynamic involved:

> "How could I take so much pleasure in the honors the Americans have bestowed on me, when I feel such contempt for the Americans?" Not unimportant is the emotion that impressed even me, a reverent spectator, as somewhat ridiculous, when almost with tears in his eyes he thanked the president of the university for the honorary doctorate.[74]

Freud's dominant reaction to his visit to America was about ambition fulfilled, not ambition for what was to come.[75] One aspect of Freud's disaffection with America (discussed below by Falzeder) and his lack of optimism about its future prospects for psychoanalysis meant that in the preparations for his visit to Clark and also in the immediate aftermath, he did not devote a great deal of energy or ambition to furthering the cause there,

---

73. S. Freud, "An Autobiographical Study," S.E. 20:52 (1925).
74. S. Ferenczi, *The Clinical Diary of Sándor Ferenczi*, ed. J. Dupont (Cambridge, MA: Harvard University Press, 1985), 184.
75. The awarding of the degree seems to have had a strangely significant effect on Freud. Just two years later, he began a letter to Ludwig Binswanger: "I know of no better way of celebrating the second anniversary of the doctorate I received at Worcester than by answering your letter." S. Freud and L. Binswanger, *Freud-Binswanger Correspondence 1908–1938*, ed. G. Fichtner (London: Open Gate Press, 2003), 73.

preferring to leave this to his acolytes such as Brill and Jones. It is notable, for example, that in his correspondence with Putnam, whom Freud regarded as a particularly prestigious and valuable representative in America, there is very little discussion at all of the politics of the movement or of any sustained effort to further its interests through him.[76]

So what final observations on the early history of psychoanalysis in America might we be drawn to by these considerations? From one point of view, Freud's visit to Clark might be seen as an exemplary case of the psychoanalytic movement in operation: the ambitious Freud, accompanied by a small band of devoted followers and opportunistically making the most of a fortuitous invitation, takes the stage in America before a prestigious audience and lays his wares before them, resulting in a great upsurge in commitment to psychoanalysis and thus building the launchpad from which it was to become such a dominant cultural force. This is of course pure fantasy. As we have noted, Freud seems to have been occupied with very little in the way of ambitious planning before his trip and still less in the way of expectation about what might be achieved. But the idea that Freud's visit to Clark might still nevertheless mark a decisive event in the history of psychoanalysis in America can seem intuitively persuasive, and this is perhaps dependent on a common notion of how psychoanalysis is propagated that needs to be reconsidered.

It is exceedingly common in both the primary and secondary literature to see references to people being "converted" to psychoanalysis. Jones himself used the term regularly but also saw some of the difficulties of it: "I use the word 'convert' advisedly, for approach to psychoanalysis cannot be effected by reason alone, however much it may speak the final word; it is necessarily an emotional process involving important inner mental changes of a more than coldly rational order." One of the difficulties he notes is that it becomes easy to dismiss this as a kind of religion, "since religion is the final example we have of an emotional process which transcends reason."[77] A consequential problem is that if one sees the spread of psychoanalysis primarily in terms of conversion experiences, then this is simply the mirror image of those critics of the psychoanalytic movement who regard it as a "cult." Typically of course such "conversions" primarily operate through personal, face-to-face contacts of the kind that it is easy in the abstract to imagine taking place when Freud and his followers descended on Clark University in 1909.

---

76. N. G. Hale Jr., *James Jackson Putnam and Psychoanalysis* (Cambridge, MA: Harvard University Press, 1971).

77. E. Jones, *Free Associations: Memories of a Psycho-Analyst* (London: Hogarth Press, 1959), 212.

But while the idea of "conversion" may aptly be used metaphorically as a description of how some people on some occasions become convinced to subscribe to a particular body of thought, it is much less useful as a general explanation of why people adopt certain ideas rather than others. Such a notion usually presupposes either (positively) that there is something special about the ideas in question that goes beyond mere "rational persuasion" (along the lines of the standard religious model, or Jones's conception) or (negatively) that there is something erroneous or quasi-pathological about the beliefs adopted such that anyone who subscribes to them must do so as a result of some exceptional process or mental condition. The main problem with this is that such judgments about beliefs are essentially contestable and cannot be regarded as in any way settled outside the terms of the judgments themselves; there is no neutral way to use the term "conversion," whether applied to religion or psychoanalysis. To employ it on the assumption that this is somehow to adopt a "value-free" psychological explanation of the spread of an idea is to be drawn unwittingly onto the disputed terrain on which the debates and disagreements about those very ideas take place. For example, one might look for particular reasons why Putnam "converted" to psychoanalysis at the point that he did,[78] but if one is to be even-handed, it might also be asked why at an earlier point he had "converted" from a somatic to a functional neurology, or after that why he "converted" to the Emmanuel Movement.

There are two further reasons why seeing the spread of psychoanalysis immediately after 1909 in terms of conversions is unhelpful. First, if there is one thing that is clear from the serious literature on the development of psychoanalysis in America, it is that assimilation occurred though a process of eclecticism, dilution, distortion, and redefinition.[79] This is because psychoanalysis did not enter America as a brand-new element in an uncontaminated environment; American culture was already heavily populated with comparable and potentially competitive therapeutic and psychological enterprises as well as its own distinctive cultural conditions.[80]

---

78. E. I. Taylor, "James Jackson Putnam's Fateful Meeting with Freud: The 1909 Clark University Conference," *Voices* 21 (1985): 78–89, explores this line of reasoning: "It is my contention that if the agenda is not to document or justify psychoanalysis, then the claim of scientific validity alone as the reason may not be wholly justified. Instead, personal, subjective considerations were the dominant factor" (79). In shifting the grounds of what might be an acceptable explanation, Taylor is simply moving from one non-neutral position to a different one.

79. E.g., Burnham, *Psychoanalysis and American Medicine*, esp. chap. 5; Hale, *Freud and the Americans*, esp. chap. 13.

80. This much is quite clear just from the outlines of "precursors and anticipations" from the early histories (Oberndorf, *A History of Psychoanalysis in America*, 6–39) through the stan-

By far the majority of those who became enthusiastic about psychoanalysis did so because they saw some, but by no means all, aspects of it that they thought useful or that could serve their purpose. Such individuals for the most part do not fit well the standard image of the "convert" in Jones's sense. In fact, psychoanalysis was able to advance as far as it did in such a short period of time in part because key individuals were prepared to give it house room in their publications and their own institutions despite the fact that they were not prepared to embrace it as a totality—Prince and Meyer are obvious examples. Nor was it the case that any notion of doctrinal purity or test of degree of commitment was a prerequisite for membership of the early psychoanalytic associations founded from 1911 onwards.[81] Freud's view of the prospects and fate of psychoanalysis in America was always fairly pessimistic in terms of the preservation of his key ideas, but it is by no means clear that his expectations were unrealistic or unjustified given the form that the spread of his theories took once they had crossed the Atlantic.

Secondly, this means that the growth of the psychoanalytic movement can in no sense be measured by the number of "conversions" that were effected. While the beliefs of individuals are one factor that might enter any estimate of expansion, there are all kinds of other considerations that are not reducible to subjectivities, whether "converted" or not: organizational membership, educational and training practices and curricula, publications on psychoanalysis by opposed or neutral parties, journal circulation, variety of article-placement locations, non-psychoanalytic use of psychoanalytic concepts, and so on. In practice of course all these kinds of things feature in descriptive histories of psychoanalysis, yet there is very often a tendency to overemphasize "conversions" as the key variable in assessing the success of the movement.

This may in part account for the often unspoken assumptions about the effects of the Clark celebrations on the progress of the psychoanalytic movement. If interpersonal encounters are presumed to be the basic cur-

---

dard studies and collections (Burnham, *Psychoanalysis and American Medicine;* Hale, *Freud and the Americans;* Gifford, *Psychoanalysis, Psychotherapy, and the New England Scene*) to more recent explorations of the pre-psychoanalytic environment such as E. Caplan, *Mind Games: American Culture and the Birth of Psychotherapy* (Berkeley: University of California Press, 1998) and E. I. Taylor, *Shadow Culture: Psychology and Spirituality in America* (Washington, DC: Counterpoint, 1999).

81. Hale, *Freud and the Americans*, 436–37, stresses the importance of not adopting anachronistic notions of "orthodoxy" when looking at this period. Oberndorf, *A History of Psychoanalysis in America*, 114, notes that in looking at the earliest membership lists of the New York Psychoanalytical Society "it is apparent that a goodly number of the members had little acquaintance with or sustained interest in psychoanalysis."

rency of the whole endeavor, then how could a face-to-face meeting with the man who stands as the origin of this movement not have a significant effect on those who were present during those fateful few days? Given how easy it is to idealize such a figure, it is hard to resist reading history backwards and projecting onto the photograph the sense that those who were in the presence of the "great man" in that photograph must have been equally overawed by him. It can be somewhat sobering to research the details of the event as pictured and to realize how little this is likely to have been the case. So while it is quite appropriate that we record Freud's presence at Clark University in the history of psychoanalysis in America, not least for the somewhat fortuitous occasion it provided for the production of one of Freud's best summary works of psychoanalysis, let us be prepared nevertheless to recognize the symbolic, iconic standing of his visit without necessarily being led thereby into assuming there were consequences stemming from it that it quite possibly never had.

Appendix

This is not intended as a full biographical sketch of each of the individuals in the photograph but as a record (as it stood in 1909) of aspects of their professional and academic background relevant to their presence at the Clark anniversary event. Professional or academic connections to Clark University or Hall are particularly noted. In view of the fact that some of the participants lectured in German, evidence of proficiency in the German language is indicated where known. Numbers refer to fig. 2.2.

1   Franz Boas b. 9 Jul. 1858 d. 21 Dec. 1942
    Honorary degree recipient. Docent at Clark University, 1889–92. Professor of Anthropology at Columbia University. German extraction.
2   Edward Bradford Titchener b. 11 Jan. 1867 d. 3 Aug. 1927
    Honorary degree recipient. Ph.D. under Wundt in Leipzig 1892. Sage Professor of Psychology, Cornell University. Co-editor with Hall of the *American Journal of Psychology*.
3   William James b. 11 Jan. 1842 d. 26 Aug. 1910
    Psychologist and philosopher. Supervised Hall's Ph.D., Harvard, 1878.
4   William Stern b. 29 Apr. 1871 d. 27 Mar. 1938
    Honorary degree recipient. Psychologist. Extraordinary Professor of Philosophy, University of Breslau.
5   Leo Burgerstein b. 13 Jun. 1853 d. 12 May 1928
    Honorary degree recipient. Specialist in School Hygiene. Royal Professor in the Oberrealschule Vienna.
6   Granville Stanley Hall b. 1 Feb. 1844 d. 24 Apr. 1924
    President of Clark University.
7   Sigmund Freud b. 6 May 1856 d. 23 Sep.1939
    Honorary degree recipient.

8   **Carl Gustav Jung b. 26 Jul. 1875 d. 6 Jun. 1961**
    Honorary degree recipient.
9   **Adolf Meyer b. 13 Sep. 1866 d. 17 Mar. 1950**
    Honorary degree recipient. Docent at Clark University, 1895–1902. Director of the Pathological Institute of the New York State Hospital. Professor of Psychiatry, Johns Hopkins Medical School. Swiss extraction.
10 **Herbert Spencer Jennings b. 8 Apr. 1868 d. 14 Apr. 1947**
    Honorary degree recipient. Studied in Jena with Verworn, 1896. Professor of Experimental Zoology at Johns Hopkins University.
11 **Carl Emil Seashore b. 28 Jan. 1866 d. 16 Oct. 1949**
    Presided over afternoon psychology conference on "Elementary Psychology in the College." Psychologist. Studied in Germany, summer 1895. Director Psychological Laboratory, University of Iowa.
12 **Joseph Jastrow b. 30 Jan. 1863 d. 8 Jan. 1944**
    Gave afternoon lecture at psychology conference. Ph.D. under Hall at Johns Hopkins University, 1886. Professor of Psychology, University of Wisconsin. German extraction.
13 **James McKeen Cattell b. 25 May 1860 d. 20 Jan. 1944**
    Fellow at Johns Hopkins with Hall, 1882–83. Ph.D. under Wundt in Leipzig, 1886. Professor of Psychology, Columbia University.
14 **Edward Franklin Buchner b. Sep. 1868 d. 22 Aug. 1929**
    Presented paper and led discussion in afternoon pedagogy conference on "Education as a College Subject." Docent in Philosophy at Clark University, 1901–3. Professor of Education at Johns Hopkins University.
15 **Edwin Wladyslaw Katzenellenbogen b. 22 May 1882 d. 1955**
    Assistant physician at Danvers Insane Asylum. Docent in abnormal psychology at Harvard University, 1909–10. Austrian/Polish extraction.
16 **Ernest Jones b. 1 Jan. 1879 d. 11 Feb. 1958**
    Accompanied Freud and Jung to Clark University.
17 **Abraham Arden Brill b. 12 Jul. 1884 d. 2 Mar. 1948**
    Accompanied Freud and Jung to Clark University.
18 **William Henry Burnham b. 3 Dec. 1855 d. 25 Jun. 1941**
    Ph.D. under Hall at Johns Hopkins University. Professor of Pedagogy and School Hygiene at Clark University.
19 **Alexander Francis Chamberlain b. 12 Jan. 1865 d. 8 Apr. 1914**
    Anthropologist. Ph.D. at Clark under Boas, 1892. Assistant Professor of Anthropology at Clark. Fluent in German.
20 **Albert Schinz b. 9 Mar. 1870 d. 19 Dec. 1943**
    Honorary Fellow in Psychology and Instructor in French at Clark University, 1897–98. Associate Professor of French literature from 1899 at Bryn Mawr College.
21 **John A. Magni b. ca 1868**
    Psychologist of religion and specialist in child linguistics. Ph.D. Clark University, 1909.
22 **Bird Thomas Baldwin b. 31 May 1875 d. 12 May 1928**
    Educational and child psychologist. Ph.D. in psychology, Harvard University, 1905. Studied with Wundt in Leipzig 1906. Lecturer in Psychology and Education, Swarthmore College and University of Chicago.
23 **Frederic Lyman Wells b. 22 Apr. 1884 d. 2 Jun. 1964**
    Ph.D. under Cattell at Columbia University, 1906. Assistant in pathological psychology, McLean Hospital, Waverley, Mass. Fluent in German.
24 **George Mather Forbes b. 1853 d. 30 Oct. 1934**
    Professor of Philosophy and Pedagogy at Rochester University. Studied for a time in Germany.
25 **Edwin Asbury Kirkpatrick b. 29 Sep. 1862 d. 4 Jan. 1937**
    Scholar in psychology, 1889–90, and Fellow, 1890–91, at Clark University. Director, Psychology and Child Study Department, Fitchburg Normal School, Mass.

26 Sándor Ferenczi b. 7 Jul. 1873 d. 22 May 1933
   Accompanied Freud and Jung to Clark University.
27 Edmund Clark Sanford b. 10 Nov. 1859 d. 22 Nov. 1924
   Conducted demonstration of psychology equipment at afternoon event. Ph.D. under Hall at Johns Hopkins University, 1888. Professor of Experimental and Comparative Psychology at Clark University, 1900–1909.
28 James Pertice Porter b. 23 Sep. 1873 d. 5 Sep. 1956
   Conducted demonstration of psychology equipment at afternoon event. Comparative psychologist. Ph.D., Clark University, 1906. Lecturer in psychology at Clark University.
29 Sakyo Kanda b. 1874 d. 1939
   M.A. in psychology, Clark University, 1909. Comparative psychologist and physiologist. Eventually specialist in bioluminescence.
30 Hikozo Kakise b. 13 Sep. 1874 d. 23 Apr. 1944
   Ph.D., Clark University, 1909. Japanese psychologist from Tokyo University. Student of Jujiro Motora, who had studied under Hall at Johns Hopkins University.
31 George E. Dawson
   Ph.D., Clark University, 1897. Professor of Psychology, Hartford School of Religious Pedagogy, Conn.
32 Samuel Perkins Hayes b. 17 Dec. 1874 d. 7 May 1958
   Studied psychology at Clark University, 1902–3. Studied in Berlin, 1903–4. Professor of Psychology, Mount Holyoke College, South Hadley, Mass.
33 Edwin Bissell Holt b. 21 Aug. 1873 d. 25 Jan. 1946
   Psychology Ph.D., Harvard University, 1901. Assistant Professor of Psychology at Harvard.
34 Charles Scott Berry b. 1875 d. 13 Sep. 1960
   Ph.D. in psychology, Harvard University, 1907. Assistant Professor of Education, University of Michigan. Studied in Berlin, 1906.
35 Guy Montrose Whipple b. 12 Jun. 1876 d. 1 Aug. 1941
   Presided over afternoon psychology conference on "The Teaching of Psychology in Normal Schools." Delivered paper on the instruction of teachers in school hygiene. Scholar and assistant in psychology at Clark University, 1898. Professor of Education, Cornell University.
36 Frank Drew
   Delivered paper on teaching psychology in normal schools at afternoon conference. Ph.D., Clark University, 1895. Superintendent of Schools, Granville, Mass. Professor of Psychology at State Normal School, Worcester, Mass.
37 Jacob William Albert Young b. 1865 d. 1948
   Mathematician. Studied in Germany, 1888–89. Ph.D., Clark University, 1892. Associate Professor of Pedagogy of Mathematics, University of Chicago.
38 Louis Napoleon Wilson b. 5 Sep. 1857 d. 15 Jul. 1937
   Librarian of Clark University. Studied in Germany.
39 Karl Johan Karlson b. 1877 d. 1948
   B.A., Clark College, 1909; M.A., Clark University, 1910. Student of Chamberlain. Ph.D. in psychology, 1912, on psychoanalysis and mythology.
40 Henry Herbert Goddard b. 14 Aug. 1866 d. 18 Jun. 1957
   Delivered paper on research into school hygiene at afternoon conference. Ph.D., Clark University, 1899. Director of Psychological Research at Vineland Training School, N.J.
41 Henry Irwin Klopp b. 1 Jan. 1870 d. 7 Mar. 1945
   Psychiatrist. Assistant superintendent, Westborough State Hospital for the Insane. Worked with Fuller on research into Alzheimer's disease.
42 Solomon Carter Fuller b. 11 Aug. 1872 d. 16 Jan. 1953
   Friend of Hall. Homeopathic pathologist at Westborough State Hospital for the Insane. Studied in Germany with Kraepelin and Alzheimer in 1904.

THREE

"A Fat Wad of Dirty Pieces of Paper": Freud on America, Freud in America, Freud and America

ERNST FALZEDER

Introduction: Freud's Antipathies

It has been said that Sigmund Freud was a great hater. His follower Isidor Sadger, for instance, wrote in his memoirs that he "had always been a ferocious hater. He could always hate much more powerfully than he could love."[1] Another follower, Alfred Winterstein, even let Freud know in the daily newspaper to which he, Freud, subscribed, that Freud was, "as the English use to say, a good hater."[2] According to the late Paul Roazen, he "was among the world's great haters," someone "who never forgave [his] opponents."[3]

And indeed, there are a great many persons, things, fashions, attitudes, and beliefs that Sigmund Freud seems to have hated. Among the persons he hated most were those who had once been his followers, or likely candidates to be persuaded to join his Cause, but who then defected. Even if the troop he commanded was a "wild horde," for him authority and loyalty were as important as in a regular army.[4] Freud could bear such an unforgiving grudge against those who had left him and psychoanalysis that he wouldn't hear their names uttered in his house. For example, Minna Bernays told psychoanalyst Else Pappenheim, a friend of hers, that the name

---

1. ". . . daß Sigmund Freud allzeit ein grimmer Hasser war. Stets hat er weitaus mächtiger hassen als lieben können." Isidor Sadger, *Recollecting Freud*, ed. Alan Dundes (Madison: University of Wisconsin Press, 2005). Sigmund Freud, *Persönliche Erinnerungen*, ed. Andrea Huppke and Michael Schröter, Quellen und Abhandlungen zur Geschichte der Psychoanalyse 4 (Tübingen: edition diskord, 2006), 78.

2. Alfred Winterstein, "Sigmund Freud," *Neue Freie Presse*, 8 February 1924.

3. Paul Roazen, *Freud: Political and Social Thought* (New York: Alfred A. Knopf, 1968), 313.

4. Sigmund Freud and Georg Groddeck, *Briefwechsel*, ed. Michael Giefer (Frankfurt am Main: Stroemfeld / Roter Stern, 2008 [1974]), 59.

of Adler was not to be mentioned in Freud's presence after the break.⁵ In 1931 he drew up a "hate list"—"Not many, seven or eight names in all"— but we do not know whose names were on that list.⁶

He was also opposed to many modern trends or innovations of his time, from modern art and music to fashion fads such as the so-called *Bubikopf*, a kind of pageboy haircut popular in the 1920s.⁷ He "hated the telephone and avoided its use whenever possible."⁸ He "hated bicycles," that is, until motorcycles appeared, which then won his detestation. There is also a widespread belief that Freud hated philosophy, music, and Vienna. Not to mention Christianity.⁹ And finally, there seems to be a consensus that Freud hated America.

Some of these popular beliefs have been put into perspective. We know that as a student Freud was eminently preoccupied with philosophical problems,¹⁰ but neither did he completely lose this interest in his later

---

5. Pappenheim later told Bernhard Handlbauer this in an interview and also confirmed it in writing. Else Pappenheim, *Hölderlin, Feuchtersleben, Freud: Beiträge zur Geschichte der Psychoanalyse, der Psychiatrie und der Neurologie*, ed. Bernhard Handlbauer (Graz: Nausner & Nausner, 2004), 39.

6. Sigmund Freud and Max Eitingon, *Briefwechsel 1906–1939*, ed. Michael Schröter, 2 vols. (Tübingen: edition diskord, 2004), 747.

7. "Filmmaking can be avoided as little as—so it seems—bobbed hair, but I myself won't get mine cut, and don't intend to be brought into personal connection with any film." Sigmund Freud and Sándor Ferenczi, *The Correspondence of Sigmund Freud and Sándor Ferenczi*, vol. 3: *1920–1933*, ed. Ernst Falzeder and Eva Brabant (Cambridge, MA: Belknap Press of Harvard University Press, 2000), 222.

8. According to his son, for Freud "conversation had to be a very personal thing. He looked one straight in the eye, and he could read one's thoughts. . . . Father, aware of his power when looking at a person, felt he had lost it when looking at a dead telephone mouthpiece." Martin Freud, *Sigmund Freud—Man and Father* (London: Angus and Robertson, 1957), 38, 106; cf. Detlef Berthelsen, *Alltag bei Familie Freud: Die Erinnerungen der Paula Fichtl*, 2d ed. (München: Deutscher Taschenbuch Verlag, 1989 [1987]), 28.

9. "Freud hated Christianity, he hated all that it stood for." J. N. Isbister, *Freud: An Introduction to His Life and Work* (Cambridge: Polity Press, 1985), 179.

10. For example, in his encounter with the ideas of Schopenhauer and Nietzsche in the *Leseverein der deutschen Studenten Wiens*, a Germanophile literary and philosophical circle, of which he was a member between 1872 and 1878. Horst-Peter Brauns and Alfred Schöpf, "Freud und Brentano: Der Medizinstudent und der Philosoph," in *Freud und die akademische Psychologie: Beiträge zu einer Kontroverse*, ed. Bernd Nitzschke (München: Psychologie Verlags Union, 1989), 55; and also through his encounter with Franz Brentano (1838–1917), then professor of philosophy in Vienna. For four semesters, he had enrolled in the courses of "this splendid man, scholar and philosopher" and even attended other courses given by him without enrolling in them. Brentano also recommended that Freud and his friend Paneth study Kant, and Freud's library indeed contains a copy of *The Critique of Pure Reason* with many notes in his hand. Sigmund Freud, *The Letters to Eduard Silberstein 1871–1881*, trans. Arnold J. Pomerans, ed. Walter Boehlich (Cambridge, MA: Harvard University Press, 1990), 5 November 1874; cf. J. Keith Davies and Gerhard Fichtner, eds., *Freud's Library: A Comprehensive Catalogue* /

years, as he so often alleged. Why else would he have had Rank send him Schopenhauer's works to Badgastein during his vacation?[11] Why else, to name but one other example, had he quit reading Nietzsche because of "an *excess* of interest"?[12]

While the legend of Freud's philosophical ignorance has since been variously treated, and at least partly refuted, in the scholarly literature,[13] the beliefs in his alleged disdain for music and Vienna respectively still seem mostly to hold their ground. This is not the place to go into detail, but let me just mention that in the letters he sent home to his family from his various travels, he reported no fewer than five visits to the opera house.[14] John M. Dorsey recalled that during a session Freud was "leaning over the couch to sing [!] one or two strains to me from Mozart's *Don Giovanni*."[15] Toward one female patient, who recited a long list of men from various countries (Luxembourg, Norway, Sweden, Holland . . .) whom she had found attractive, he dryly remarked: "This is exactly like Leporello's aria

---

Freuds Bibliothek: Vollständiger Katalog (London: The Freud Museum; Tübingen: edition diskord, 2006). To Fliess he wrote that he "most secretly nourish[ed] the hope of arriving . . . at my original goal of philosophy. For that is what I wanted originally"; and: "As a young man I knew no longing other than for philosophical knowledge, and now I am about to fulfill it as I move from medicine to psychology." Sigmund Freud, *The Complete Letters of Sigmund Freud to Wilhelm Fliess, 1887–1904*, ed. Jeffrey M. Masson (Cambridge, MA: Belknap Press of Harvard University Press, 1985), 159, 180.

11. Sigmund Freud and Anna Freud, *Briefwechsel, 1904–1938*, ed. Ingeborg Meyer-Palmedo (Frankfurt am Main: S. Fischer, 2006), 232. This was in preparation for *Beyond the Pleasure Principle* (1920). Incidentally, Freud quoted Schopenhauer twenty-six times in his works, constantly underlining that he considered him a great thinker. Cf. Samuel A. Guttman et al., eds., *Concordance to the Standard Edition of the Complete Psychological Works of Sigmund Freud*, 6 vols. (New York: International Universities Press, 1983). Samuel A. Guttman et al., eds., *Konkordanz zu den Gesammelten Werken von Sigmund Freud*, 6 vols. (Waterloo, ON: North Waterloo Academic Press, 1995).

12. Herman Nunberg and Ernst Federn, eds., *Minutes of the Vienna Psychoanalytic Society*, vol. 1: *1906–1908* (New York: International Universities Press, 1967), 359, italics added. The fact that Otto Rank gave him, as a birthday present for his seventieth birthday and as a parting gift, the recently published complete works of Nietzsche, twenty-three volumes bound in white leather, is of course not in itself a proof of Freud's interest; Paul Roazen, *Freud and His Followers* (New York: New American Library, 1976), 412. However, it "is significant that Freud, who could bring only part of his library out of Vienna, chose to include Rank's gift"—and probably not just out of affection for Rank. E. James Lieberman, *Acts of Will: The Life and Work of Otto Rank* (New York: Free Press, 1985), 436–37.

13. André Haynal, "Freud's Relation to Philosophy and Biology as Reflected in His Letters," in *100 Years of Psychoanalysis: Contributions to the History of Psychoanalysis*, ed. André Haynal and Ernst Falzeder (Geneva: Cahiers Psychiatriques Genevois, 1994).

14. Sigmund Freud, *Unser Herz zeigt nach dem Süden: Reisebriefe 1895–1923*, ed. Christfried Tögel, with the collaboration of Michael Molnar (Berlin: Aufbau-Verlag, 2002).

15. John M. Dorsey, *An American Psychiatrist in Vienna, 1935–1937, and His Sigmund Freud* (Detroit: Center for Health Education, 1976), 51.

in *Don Giovanni,*" not without adding the name under which this aria is known among music connoisseurs—"the catalogue aria, it's called."[16] There's even an apocryphal anecdote that, when once challenged because of the obvious discrepancy between his proclaimed dislike of music and his love of Mozart, particularly his operas, he is said to have said: "Ah, but Mozart is something else." The often-quoted anecdote that Freud had insisted that the piano, which had been rented for his sister Anna, be removed because her practicing broke his concentration during his studies, might rather be due to the quite understandable irritation by endless and far from faultless repetitions of the same pieces—something everybody can identify with whose neighbor's child practiced "Für Elise" for the umpteenth time—than the action of a serious music hater.[17] After all, during those studies schoolboy Sigi was used to humming Viennese folk songs himself in his own room: "There's one thing, dear Lord, I'm asking for, though, send me a fiver, I'm needing some dough."[18]

I am not claiming that Freud was a music *lover*, however. He much preferred dramas or texts set to music, such as in operas or songs (he adored Yvette Guilbert, for instance),[19] over music without words, such as symphonies, etc., and his taste was quite conventional (*Don Giovanni, Carmen*). His claim of not liking music should also, in my opinion, be seen against the background of the average bourgeois academic in contemporary Vienna, for whom the *Staatsoper* was often like a second living room, who played an instrument himself, and whose children all had to learn to play an instrument. Before the rise of the gramophone and the radio, piano arrange-

---

16. "Das ist die reinste Leporelloarie aus *Don Juan*. Registerarie heißt sie."—In this aria ("Madamina, il catalogo è questo"—My little lady, this is the catalogue), Leporello unfolds a ("Leporello"-folded) list of Don Giovanni's lovers and sings of their numbers and countries of origin: 640 in Italy, 231 in Germany, 100 in France, 91 in Turkey, and 1,003 in Spain . . . Anna Koellreuter, "Wie benimmt sich der Prof. Freud eigentlich?" *Ein neu entdecktes Tagebuch von 1921 historisch und analytisch Kommentiert* (Gießen: Psychosozial-Verlag, 2009), 64.

17. E.g., Anna Freud-Bernays, *Eine Wienerin in New York: Die Erinnerungen der Schwester Sigmund Freuds* (Berlin: Aufbau Verlag, 2004), 214. In fact, in his own later household there seems to have been a piano: in a letter to his daughter Mathilde of 19 March 1908, he writes of "the piano in our apartment." Sigmund Freud, *"Unterdeß halten wir zusammen": Briefe an die Kinder*, ed. Michael Schröter, with the collaboration of Ingeborg Meyer-Palmedo and Ernst Falzeder (Berlin: Aufbau Verlag, 2010), 47.

18. "'Um was ich dich bitt,' lieber Herrgott, schick mir a[n] Fufziger, ich brauch a klan's Geld." Freud-Bernays, *Eine Wienerin in New York*, 221.

19. In 1927, Freud attended all three of Guilbert's performances in Vienna, on a seat in the first row reserved for him by the singer herself, and "utterly enjoyed it" (Freud and Eitingon, *Briefwechsel*, 566). He also went to performances in 1929, 1930, and 1931, and recorded this in his diary. Freud, *The Diary of Sigmund Freud, 1929–1939: A Chronicle of Events in the Last Decade*, ed. Michael Molnar (London: Hogarth Press, 1992), 47, 62, 87, 114.

ments for two and four hands played the major role in distributing classical and popular music, and the households of the Vienna middle classes resounded with the music played on their upright pianos. Freud certainly did not comply with this standard, but this does not make him a music hater.

As to his attitude toward Vienna, his son Martin has put this into commonsense, and I find quite cogent, perspective: "I am not convinced that Sigmund Freud's often-expressed dislike of Vienna was either deep-seated or real. It is not difficult for a London man, or a New York man, both devoted to their respective home cities, to say, 'How I hate London; how I loathe New York.'"[20] Viennese in particular are famous for railing against their home city, in a grumpily devoted and almost tender way. But you should see them race to Vienna's defense if someone from out of town should dare and do the same. From his exile in London, Freud wrote to Eitingon: "The triumphant feeling of liberation is too much mixed with the work of mourning since, after all, one still loved the prison very much from which one was released."[21]

Freud's hatred of America and the Americans was so often expressed, and is so well documented, however, that there seems to be no doubt about his feelings. On the other hand, however, we also find occasional statements of Freud's, in which he had positive things to say about America, or even expressed his admiration. Various historians and scholars have tried to explain Freud's alleged hatred of America without taking into account the other side of his ambivalence. What we lack until now, in my opinion, is a satisfactory explanation of Freud's obviously more complex relationship to the United States and its citizens.

In what follows I will first give some choice examples of negative things Freud had to say and write about America, then give a few examples of positive remarks, discuss some of the peculiarities of Freud's attitude, and finally have a look at his possible motives, including one that was first mentioned by Ferenczi but is rarely mentioned in the literature in this con-

---

20. Martin Freud, *Sigmund Freud*, 48.
21. "Das Triumphgefühl der Befreiung vermengt sich zu stark mit der Trauerarbeit, denn man hat das Gefängnis, aus dem man entlassen wurde, immer noch sehr geliebt" (Freud and Eitingon, *Briefwechsel*, 903). Also quoted by Ernest Jones, *The Life and Work of Sigmund Freud*, 3 vols. (New York: Basic Books, 1953–57), 3:230, who writes about Freud's "deep love" of that city, which "was kept so hidden," however. Bruno Bettelheim suggests that "Freud's supposed 'hatred' of Vienna was probably the expression of a deep early love that became frustrated by anti-Semitism in the early twentieth century, a frustration the more keenly felt as the earlier love was never given up." Bruno Bettelheim, *Freud's Vienna and Other Essays* (New York: Alfred A. Knopf, 1990), 46.

text.²² In assessing the impact of Freud on America, it might help to try and understand Freud's own changing attitudes toward the culture into which he tried to introduce his ideas.

Freud's Negative Attitude toward America

To begin with, let me quote three eminent Freud scholars. Ernest Jones called Freud's attitude toward America a "prejudice," and "so obviously unfair on the subject" that it "actually had nothing to do with America itself." Peter Gay, who gave a long (though not exhaustive) compilation of Freud's invectives against America and the Americans in his Freud biography, wrote: "Whatever guise the American assumed, saint or moneygrubber, Freud was ready to write him off as a most unattractive specimen in the human zoo." He slashed "away at Americans wholesale, quite indiscriminately, with imaginative ferocity."²³ Patrick Mahony: "Whereas Freud changed his mind on many topics, he never altered his vehement anti-Americanism which came from the depths of his being. No matter what genre Freud wrote in—scientific treatise, dialogue, history, biography, autobiography, letters, case-history narratives, you name it—America came to his mind as a ready example of what was bad. And no matter what subject Freud discussed—dreams, clinical theory, psychoanalytic treatment, history, or social issues—America emerged as an immediate association of what was bad."²⁴

It is true that Freud hardly missed an occasion to express his derision, ridicule, or scorn concerning the Americans. Here are a few examples.

In 1915, with regard to his love of and addiction to tobacco: "I actually know of no other apology for Columbus's atrocity" [ich für die Untat des

---

22. Sándor Ferenczi, *Ohne Sympathie keine Heilung: Das klinische Tagebuch von 1932*, ed. Judith Dupont (Frankfurt am Main: S. Fischer, 1988 [1985]); *The Clinical Diary of Sándor Ferenczi*, ed. Judith Dupont (Cambridge, MA: Harvard University Press, 1988).

23. Jones, *Life and Work of Sigmund Freud*, 3:59. Peter Gay, *Freud: A Life for Our Time* (New York: W.W. Norton, 1988), 562–70, quotations from 562, 567. Gay's use of the words "human zoo" is quite in line with Freud's general misanthropy for mankind in general, and, occasionally, patients in particular. To Eitingon, Freud wrote, for example: "My zoo now comprises two Americans and an Englishman, a second specimen of the latter kind is announced for the beginning of April. The supplier is Jones" [Mein Tiergarten umfaßt jetzt einen Amerikaner und einen Engländer, ein zweites Exemplar letzterer Art ist für Anfang April vorgemerkt. Lieferant ist Jones] (Freud and Eitingon, *Briefwechsel*, 191).

24. Patrick J. Mahony, "A l'écoute de l'autre Freud," in *Penser Freud avec Patrick Mahony*, ed. Louise Grenier and Isabelle Lasvergnas (Montréal: Edition Liber), 23–45. (Quoted from the author's own, unpublished English version of this paper, as delivered at the Austen Riggs Center, November 13, 2003.)

Kolumbus eigentlich keine andere Entschuldigung weiß]—namely, to have discovered America.[25]

In 1923, he chided Brill for having "submitted far too much to the two big vices of America, the greed for money and the respect of public opinion."[26]

In 1924: The only reasonable way to bear a "sojourn among such savages," he wrote to Rank, would be "to sell one's life as dearly as possible" [die einzig vernünftige Art des Benehmens . . . , die dem Aufenthalt unter diesen Wilden entspricht: sein Leben möglichst theuer zu verkaufen].[27]

In 1925: "The Americans transfer the democratic principle from politics into science. Everybody must become president once, no one must remain president; none may excel before the others, and thus all of them neither learn nor achieve anything" [Die Amerikaner übertragen das demokratische Prinzip aus der Politik in die Wissenschaft. Jeder muß einmal Präsident werden, keiner darf es bleiben, keiner sich vor dem andern auszeichnen und somit lernen und leisten sie alle mit einander nichts].[28]

In 1925: "I recently offended an American with the suggestion that the Statue of Liberty in New York harbor should be replaced by a monkey holding up a Bible. I.e., I tried [to offend him]; he didn't seem to understand me at all" [Unlängst kränkte ich einen Amerikaner durch den Vorschlag, die Freiheitsstatue im Hafen von New York durch die eines Affen zu ersetzen, der eine Bibel hochhält. D.h. ich versuchte, er schien mich gar nicht zu verstehen].[29]

In 1927, he gave the following reasons for the Americans' opposition to so-called lay analysis: "The analysts' lack of authority, the inability of the American public to make sound judgments, and the low standard of public morals in God's own country, looking the other way, particularly where matters of earning money are concerned—the counterpart to American sanctimoniousness and moral hypocrisy. (I do not invent these things *ad*

---

25. Freud and Ferenczi, *The Correspondence*, 2:58.
26. In English in the original. Library of Congress.
27. Lieberman, *Acts of Will*, 228; original in Library of Congress. And again, in 1928: "These savages have little interest in scholarship that cannot be immediately put into practice" [Diese Wilden haben für Wissenschaft, die sich nicht unmittelbar in Praxis umsetzt, wenig übrig] (to Wittels; Library of Congress).
28. Letter to Radó; in Gay, *Freud: A Life for Our Time*, 566; original in Library of Congress.
29. Freud and Ferenczi, *Correspondence*, 3:227. This was probably an allusion to the notorious Scopes or "Monkey" trial in Tennessee earlier in the same year (1925), testing whether the state could forbid the teaching of Darwinism. The trial was widely publicized, and Freud could well have learned of it from the press or his Anglo-Saxon followers. With thanks to the gentleman (whose name I unfortunately do not remember) who drew my attention to this possibility.

hoc; they are admitted and fought by quite a number of courageous American intellectuals.)" [Ihr (d. h. der Analytiker) Mangel an Autorität, die Urteilslosigkeit des amerikanischen Publikums, und der niedrige Stand der öffentlichen Moral in God's own country, die besonders, wenn es sich um Gelderwerb handelt, beide Augen zudrückt, Gegenstück zur amerikanischen Frömmigkeit und Moralheuchelei. (Das sind Dinge, die ich nicht ad hoc erfinde, die von einer ganzen Reihe tapferer amerik. Intellektueller eingestanden und bekämpft werden)].[30]

In 1929 (with regard to a planned source book of Freud's psychoanalytic writings for American audiences): "Basically, the whole matter is quite distasteful to me as being so very American. You may rest assured that once such a 'source-book' is available, no American will ever consult an original text" [Im Grunde genommen ist mir die ganze Sache als echt amerikanisch recht zuwider. Man kann sich darauf verlassen, daß wenn ein solches "source book" vorliegt, kein Amerikaner je ein Original zur Hand nehmen wird].[31]

In 1929: ". . . the American pattern of replacing quality with quantity."[32]

In 1930: America is "Dollaria."[33]

In 1930 (in print): Americans "make a hotch-potch out of psychoanalysis and other elements and quote this procedure as evidence of their *broad-mindedness*, whereas it only proves their *lack of judgment*" [(Die Amerikaner) schaffen sich einen Mischmasch aus Psychoanalyse und anderen Elementen und geben dieses Vorgehen als Beweis ihrer broadmindedness aus, während es nur ihr lack of judgment beweist].[34]

---

30. Letter to Brill, Library of Congress.

31. Sigmund Freud and Ernest Jones, *The Complete Correspondence of Sigmund Freud and Ernest Jones, 1908–1939*, ed. R. Andrew Paskauskas (Cambridge, MA: Belknap Press of Harvard University Press, 1993), 657; trans. modified.

32. To Frankwood Williams; in Gay, *Freud: A Life for Our Time*, 566–67.

33. Sigmund Freud and Oskar Pfister, *Briefe 1909–1939*, ed. Ernst L. Freud and Heinrich Meng (Frankfurt am Main: S. Fischer, 1963), 135. *Psychoanalysis and Faith: The Letters of Sigmund Freud and Oskar Pfister* (New York: Basic Books, 1963). This contemptuous term for the United States was evidently common among Central European intellectuals. As early as 1921, Albert Einstein, writing about an upcoming trip to America, expected a correspondent, Fritz Haber, to be familiar with a reference to "Dollaria." Albert Einstein to Fritz Haber, 9 March 1921, in *The Collected Papers of Albert Einstein*, ed. Diana Kormos Buchwald et al., trans. Ann M. Hentschel (Princeton, NJ: Princeton University Press, 2009), 12:127. Reference through the great courtesy of Professor Diana Kormos Buchwald.

34. Sigmund Freud, "Introduction to the Special Psychopathology Number of *The Medical Review of Reviews*," S.E. 21:254–55. To Wittels he wrote in 1928: "The worst thing about the American bustle is their so-called broadmindedness, with which they feel superior to us

In 1937: "There is going through my head an advertisement which I think is the most daring and felicitous piece of American publicity: 'Why live, if you can be buried for ten dollars?'" [Mir geht ein ‚advertisement' im Kopf herum, das ich für das kühnste und gelungenste Stück amerikanischer Reklame halte: 'Why live, if you can be buried for ten dollars?'].³⁵

In short, America is "Dollaria," "ruled" not by authority but "by the dollar";³⁶ it is an "Anti-Paradise," that "damned country!"³⁷ "Yes, America is gigantic, but a gigantic mistake."³⁸

American men are savages; they are stupid, ignorant, shallow, uncultivated, egoistic,³⁹ sanctimonious, hypocritical, prudish, money-grubbing, anal,⁴⁰ dishonest,⁴¹ arrogant, inferior, falsely democratic,⁴² stiff, spiritless,

---

narrow-minded Europeans, while in reality this is merely a cover-up of their complete lack of judgment" [Das Ärgste am amerikanischen Betrieb ist ihre sog. broadmindedness, bei der sie sich noch großartig und uns engherzigen Europäern überlegen vorkommen, in Wirklichkeit nur eine bequeme Verschleierung ihrer vollkommenen Urteilslosigkeit]. Library of Congress.

35. Letter to Marie Bonaparte; in Jones, *Life and Work*, 3:465; trans. modified.

36. Freud, *The Complete Letters of Sigmund Freud to Wilhelm Fliess*, 457.

37. Sigmund Freud and Arnold Zweig, *The Letters of Sigmund Freud and Arnold Zweig*, ed. Ernst L. Freud (New York: Harcourt, Brace and World, 1970), 170. Freud and Ferenczi, *The Correspondence*, 3:320.

38. Ernest Jones, *Free Associations: Memories of a Psycho-Analyst* (London: Hogarth Press, 1959), 191.

39. "Unfortunately I trust the Americans least to have a sense of solidarity, an ability to organize, and an inclination to mitigate competition out of consideration for the common cause" [Leider traue ich den Amerikanern am wenigsten Gemeinsinn, Eignung zur Organisation und Neigung zu, die Härte der Konkurrenz durch Rücksicht auf die gemeinsame Sache zu mildern]. To Irmarita Putnam, probably 1932; Library of Congress.

40. "Nowhere is one so overwhelmed by the senselessness of human doings as there, where even the pleasurable gratification of natural animal needs is no longer recognized as a life's goal. It is a crazy anal *Adlerei*" [Nirgends wird man von der Sinnlosigkeit des menschlichen Treibens so überwältigt wie dort, wo auch die lustvolle Befriedigung der natürlichen animalischen Bedürfnisse nicht mehr als Lebensziel anerkannt wird. Es ist eine verrückte anale Adlerei]. To Rank; in Sigmund Freud and Otto Rank, *Inside Psychoanalysis: The Letters of Sigmund Freud and Otto Rank*, ed. E. James Lieberman and Robert Kramer (Baltimore: Johns Hopkins University Press, forthcoming). The Americans have "no time for the libido." Sigmund Freud and Carl Gustav Jung, *The Freud/Jung Letters: The Correspondence Between Sigmund Freud and C. G. Jung*, ed. William McGuire; corr. ed. (Cambridge, MA: Harvard University Press, 1988), 256.

41. Jelliffe was "one of the worst American businessmen, translate: crooks, Columbus has discovered." Sigmund Freud and Karl Abraham, *The Complete Correspondence of Sigmund Freud and Karl Abraham, 1907–1925: Completed Edition*, ed. Ernst Falzeder (London: Karnac, 2002), 162. *Briefwechsel 1907–1925: Vollständige Ausgabe*, ed. Ernst Falzeder and Ludger M. Hermanns, 2 vols. (Vienna: Turia + Kant, 2009).

42. In answer to an American Jew's criticism of analysis, Freud wrote: "I had overlooked what the effect must be of a conjuncture of American-democratic outlook and Jewish-Chutzpah" (Jones, *Life and Work*, 3:451).

loud, anti-Semitic,[43] and dominated by their women, whom they do not know how to put in their right place.

In America there is a "rule by women" [Frauenherrschaft].[44] American women "make fools" of their men; they "are an anti-cultural phenomenon [*eine kulturwidrige Erscheinung*]. . . . In Europe, things are different: men take the lead and that is as it should be."[45] "In America the father ideal appears to be downgraded, so that the American girl cannot muster the illusion that is necessary for marriage."[46] To Blumgart he wrote: "None of you [Americans] has ever found the right attitude toward your women."[47]

Does all this reflect pure, unambivalent, and unadulterated hatred? Was Freud really such a simple man? Is a prejudice sometimes simply a prejudice? Or is "the fellow . . . actually somewhat more complicated"?[48] Could this be a case of the Professor doth protest too much, methinks?

Peculiarities of Freud's Attitude toward America

On a closer look, three things about Freud's America-bashing are somewhat peculiar and stand out. First, that he greatly stepped up his attacks after his trip to the United States. Before, his anti-American utterances were not significantly different from those of the average Central European bourgeois academic of his time.[49] Michael Molnar writes that "Freud's persistent and ungracious denigration of America" had "many of the hallmarks of a commonplace European prejudice of the times. . . . The United States was projected as a monstrous twin and parody of Europe. A conquistador approach towards them was justified, they, the apparent exploiters, are them-

---

43. He wrote of the "redskins": "American anti-Semitism, gigantic in its latency" (Freud and Eitingon, *Briefwechsel*, 801). To Wortis he said: "Every country has the Jews it deserves," and "America certainly hasn't encouraged the best kind of social conduct." Joseph Wortis, *Fragments of an Analysis with Freud* (New York: Simon and Schuster, 1954; reprint, Northvale, NJ: Jason Aronson, 1994), 145.

44. Freud, *Future of an Illusion*, S.E. 21:49, trans. modified. In the S.E. translated as "petticoat government."

45. Wortis, *Fragments of an Analysis*, 98.

46. Herman Nunberg and Ernst Federn, eds., *Minutes of the Vienna Psychoanalytic Society*, vol. 3: *1910–1911* (New York: International Universities Press, 1974), 14.

47. A. A. Brill Library, New York Psychoanalytic Institute.

48. Sigmund Freud, *The Letters of Sigmund Freud*, ed. Ernst L. Freud (New York: Basic Books, 1960; reprint, 1975), 402.

49. However, it should be noted that we have significantly less documentation in general on the years before he began to correspond regularly with his major followers (that is, up until about 1907 or 1908).

selves only fit to be exploited."⁵⁰ After his visit, however, Freud's scorn was spiked with even more vitriol than was usual in Central European circles.

Second, even if one is thus forced to conclude that it was precisely his experiences during that trip that made him form such an unforgiving opinion (and he himself *later* stated numerous times that this was so), the letters he sent to his family *from* America sound much more positive. They sound like what one would expect from someone traveling for the first time to a foreign country and culture: there were things that impressed him, positively or negatively, things he liked and didn't like, conveniences he enjoyed or missed. Quite understandably, he also had difficulties in adjusting to the unfamiliar food and in understanding the American accent.⁵¹

There are actually a number of quite positive remarks:⁵² "One quickly gets accustomed to the city [New York]," for instance; or even: "One also understands the moneymaking [!], seeing what one can get for money, and what can be done with it." When he wrote that he "marvel[ed] at the famous sky-scrapers," and added "I will not let myself be impressed, and I insist on having seen so much more beautiful things, albeit nothing greater and wilder," this sounds like a conscious effort to distance himself from the great impression these things did make upon him, to sober up, so to speak, from the intoxicating impact of New York City. He even wrote: "Within two weeks one would feel at home, and wouldn't want to leave [*und wollte nicht wieder weg*]." One wouldn't want to leave! Why write this about a country that he allegedly hated so much? Why don't we take this statement as seriously as the one he wrote on board the ship on his way back: "America was a crazy machine [*eine tolle Maschine*]; I am very glad that I am out of it, and even more so that I don't have to live there . . . East, West—Home best. I won't object to be again sitting in our little quarters in the 9th district

---

50. Michael Molnar, unpublished manuscript, undated.

51. He was not the only one; immigrants from the German-speaking countries often struggled with the language. Even though they read English, they often understood and spoke the language poorly. Martin Grotjahn tells the amusing story of Otto Fenichel's visit to the Menninger Clinic in Topeka. Having been asked to give a lecture, he "wanted to talk about something he called 'penis envoy.' That did not sound right to us and I tentatively suggested to use the words 'penis ivy.'" Another émigré did suggest "penis envy," but this was "rejected as too unlikely" by Fenichel and Grotjahn. So Fenichel "rushed with great enthusiasm into the matter, respected by all and understood by none. 'Penis envoy' finally brought the house down." Martin Grotjahn, *My Favorite Patient: The Memoirs of a Psychoanalyst* (Frankfurt am Main: Peter Lang, 1987), 148–49.

52. The following quotes are from his travel diary and letters sent to his family (all in Freud, *Unser Herz zeigt nach dem Süden*, 273–318). Some passages from these documents were already quoted by Rosenzweig in his book (1992), occasionally in a questionable or wrong translation.

[of Vienna]"? In fact, this sounds like a textbook example of ambivalence: "One wouldn't want to leave" versus "I'm glad to be out of it." And finally, his lectures at Clark University, as Skues notes in his essay, were all as successful as he could reasonably have hoped for. All in all, judging from these letters, one cannot but get the impression that he seems to have thoroughly enjoyed himself. Perhaps too much so, for his own taste. He nearly seems to have been swept away by all those powerful impressions, only sobering up once he was out of the crazy machine again, and then blaming the whole country for his own loss of self-control.

Sure, there are some remarks in which he made fun of America and the Americans. He complained about the scarcity of public toilets, for instance: "They escort you along miles of corridors and ultimately you are taken to the very basement where a marble palace awaits you, only just in time." As to his difficulties in understanding the American accent, there was that episode when "one American asked another to repeat a remark he had not quite caught," upon which "Freud turned to Jung with the acid comment: 'These people cannot even understand each other.'" [53] When he visited the Canadian side of the Niagara Falls, he commented: "There the people at once speak a clearer English."[54] To Max Schur he once remarked: "This race is destined to extinction. They can no longer open their mouths to speak; soon they won't be able to do so to eat."[55]

The tone of these remarks, however, rather strikes me as nearly playful, a bit tongue-in-cheek, as if writing with a wink to his wife and children from a highly cultured gentleman's expedition to a savage and primitive, yet strangely successful tribe—so if there is an admixture of condescension in these remarks, there is nothing to foreshadow his later unrelenting malice. So what did really happen that, in his later memory, made America such a horrible place?

Freud himself always blamed his firsthand and first-bowel experience of America for his disdain of it, and also for the whole "medley of . . . [his] transatlantic complaints—destroyed health in general, chronic indigestion, intestinal disorders, prostatitis, appendicitis, writer's cramp, and bad handwriting[!]"[56] And this, Mahony continues, although the medical records left by his personal physician do not confirm such a prostate condi-

---

53. Jones, *Life and Work*, 2:60.
54. Freud, *Unser Herz zeigt nach dem Süden*, 307.
55. Undated, in Gay, *Freud: A Life for Our Times*, 567.
56. Mahony, "A l'écoute de l'autre Freud." After the trip, Freud wrote to Ernest Jones (in English): "My handwriting has deteriorated so very much since the American trip" (Freud and Jones, *The Complete Correspondence*, 42).

tion, and he had had attacks of writer's cramp as far back as in the 1880s.[57] We know that he had digestive troubles all his adult life; in fact, in a letter to his daughter Mathilde written shortly *before* the departure to America, he already complained about his "rebellious stomach." Other countries, too, caused such troubles in him. After returning from the International Psychoanalytic Congress in the Hague in 1920, he wrote to his son Ernst that he had "brought back a ruined stomach" with him—but this certainly did not make him hate Holland.[58] As to his handwriting, if this was not actually meant as a joke entirely, which I doubt, there are certainly no signs that it "deteriorated" after the journey.

The third peculiarity about Freud's attitude toward America is the intriguing fact that the things he hated and criticized most (the materialistic worldview, the greed for money, the rule of the dollar) struck a not unambivalent chord in himself. After all, money was "laughing gas" to him. "I know from my youth that once the wild horses of the pampas have been lassoed, they retain a certain anxiousness for life. Thus I came to know the helplessness of poverty and continually fear it."[59] Before this background, it is interesting to see what Freud had to say about money in his notes during the trip: "From time to time I take out the portefeuille and look at the three big banknotes and the small pile of dirty-green 5-dollar notes that I changed, poor images of the mightiest god—to bring me back again to reality." "In my billfold there reigns polytheism: [Austrian] Crowns, [German] Marks, and now the mightiest god, the Dollar." The quote in the title of my paper is taken from the following: "F[erenczi] has a fat wad of dirty pieces of paper with him, black on one side, green on the other, bearing a picture in the middle of something like a buffalo or of other animals. These are dollar notes with a denomination of 10 or 50."[60] It is interesting that Freud also counted the other currencies among the "gods," although in his opinion none was as powerful as the new god, the dollar.

Freud *was* ambitious, he *wanted* to become independent, rich, and famous, despite his loud protestations to the contrary. At the beginning of his medical career, he had even had "the intention of going to America, when the three months for which [he] had made sufficient provision failed to begin very auspiciously."[61] But why to America, if he really hated it so

57. Jones, *Life and Work*, 3:236; cf. 1:169.
58. 7 October 1920, in Freud, *Unterdeß halten wir zusammen*, 308.
59. Freud, *The Complete Letters of Sigmund Freud to Wilhelm Fliess*, 374.
60. These are in Freud, *Unser Herz zeigt nach dem Süden*.
61. Freud and Ferenczi, *The Correspondence*, 2:348. Already as a boy, Freud "knew much about America and American authors," his favorite being Mark Twain (Freud-Bernays, *Eine*

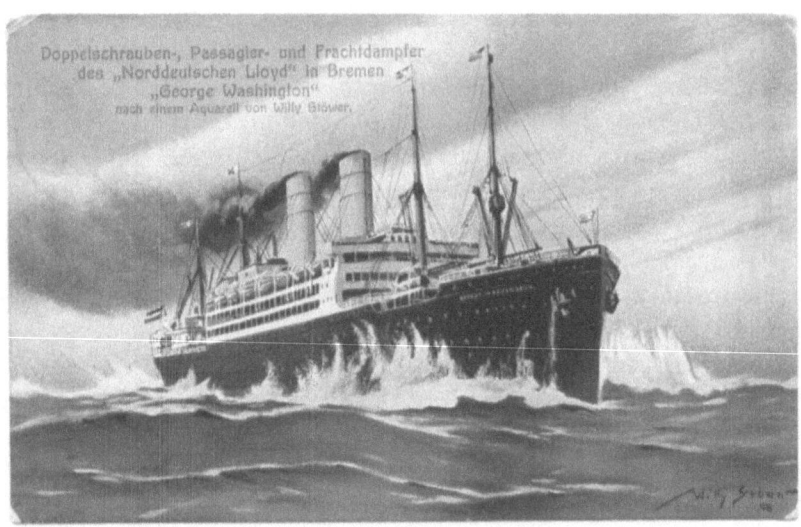

3.1. When Freud was in Bremen departing for North America in 1909, he sent this postcard to his daughter, showing the North German Lloyd ship, the *George Washington*, that carried him to the pier in Hoboken, New Jersey, where he began to form his firsthand impressions of the United States. Courtesy of the Library of Congress Duplication Services, from the Freud Archives in the Manuscript Division of the Library of Congress.

much? Why not to his beloved England, for example, where he also had relatives who could have helped him? Or to Germany? He implies it himself: because he believed he could make money in the New World, more or easier money, that is, than if he stayed on in the Old World. So why despise a whole nation for allegedly being after something he himself wanted to achieve?

As to his claim not to be ambitious at all, Jung's friend and pupil Edward A. Bennet recounts what Jung had told him: "When their boat was approaching New York with its famous sky-line, Jung saw Freud gazing—as he thought—at the view and spoke to him. He was surprised when Freud said, 'Won't they get a surprise when they hear what we have to say to them'—referring to the coming lectures.[62] 'How ambitious you are!' ex-

---

Wienerin in New York, 220). When Mark Twain gave a public lecture in Vienna, Freud "greatly enjoyed" listening to it. Jones, *Life and Work*, 3:329.

62. In another version Freud is said to have said: "Don't they know that we're bringing them the plague?" For example, Richard Noll, *The Jung Cult: Origins of a Charismatic Movement*, 2d ed. (New York: Free Press, 1997 [1994]), 47. According to Elisabeth Roudinesco, *Jacques Lacan: Esquisse d'une vie, histoire d'un système de pensée* (Paris: Librairie Arthème Fayard, 1993); *Jacques Lacan: Bericht über ein Leben, Geschichte eines Denksystems*, trans. Hans-Dieter Gondek (Köln: Kiepenheuer & Witsch, 1996), 398, this anecdote goes back to what Jacques Lacan claimed

claimed Jung. 'Me?' said Freud. 'I'm the most humble of men, and the only man who isn't ambitious.'[63] Jung replied: 'That's a big thing—to be the only one.'"[64]

Freud's critique boils down to his allegation that the Americans do not appreciate the *real* values (ethical norms, classical education, honest work, appreciation of the intellectual elite, etc.), but would do nearly anything for the *false* ones in the interest of their god, the dollar, while maintaining a hypocritical, sanctimonious façade—monkeys holding up the Bible, indeed. Even if there might be a kernel of truth in his criticisms,[65] his attitude bears all the hallmarks of a prejudice. In fact, interestingly enough, his main criticism—greed for money—is one of the most common *anti-Semitic* prejudices.[66] Freud's view was generalized, it did not change in the light of new experiences, and it was singularly aimed at one nation and its inhabitants (or one "race").

As if Freud could not have found such an attitude (and all the other things he accused the Americans of in his sweeping wholesale attack) also much closer to home! It is true, he often enough criticized culture or civi-

---

Jung had told him. Lacan had visited Jung in 1954 to ask him about his relationship with Freud. In a seminar given in Vienna the following year, on 7 November 1955, in German (!), Lacan then declared publicly that Jung had allegedly told him about that statement of Freud's. Roudinesco notes that Lacan's word is the only evidence we have that this might actually have happened. Other sources (Jones, Schur, Ellenberger, Brome, Oberndorf, Roazen, Hale, Gay, or the above-quoted Bennet) only report that Freud said something like: "They will be quite surprised at what we will have to say to them!" In his interview with Eissler, Jung has the following to say: "When we entered the harbor of New York, we were standing on the bridge, and Freud said to me: 'If they only knew what we are bringing them!' [*Wenn die wüßten, was wir ihnen bringen!*] I thought: Well, we will soon see what the Americans will do, won't we?! (laughs)."

63. Probably meaning: among the three of them, Freud, Jung, and Ferenczi.

64. Edward Armstrong Bennet, *C. G. Jung* (London: Barrie and Rockliff, 1961; reprint, with a foreword by Sonu Shamdasani, Wilmette, IL: Chiron Publications, 2006), 43.

65. Not even paranoiacs, when "they project outwards on to others what they do not wish to recognize in themselves, . . . project it into the blue, so to speak, where there is nothing of the sort already," as Freud once stated. "Some neurotic mechanisms in jealousy, paranoia and homosexuality" (S.E. 18:226).

66. I am indebted to David Lotto, who, after having heard this paper, sent me an unpublished paper of his, in which he makes the following point: "Freud's accusations about Americans' alleged preoccupation with making money and using dishonest methods to acquire wealth are uncomfortably close to the traditional anti-Semitic accusations so frequently made about Jews. Thus Freud's passionate prejudice against Americans can be seen as an attempt at overcompensation by adopting values and ways of behaving that serve to refute the stereotypical canard." In his accompanying e-mail message of 7 October 2009, Lotto added: "I do think that combating anti-Semitism was one of the strongest sources that fueled Freud's vitriol toward America. His anger was displaced (although one could argue about how much distortion this involved) from anti-Semites to Americans."

lization in general, and occasionally made a deprecatory aside about other nations, such as Italy, Hungary, Germany, etc., and above all Austria (and its capital, Vienna), but he certainly did not purely hate these countries as such, and no other nation ever gave rise to so much derision in him as America. So were the Americans Freud's scapegoats for something he could not admit in himself?

Freud's Attitude toward Particular Groups of Americans

Freud reserved some special scorn for particular groups of Americans, for instance, businessmen, journalists, publishers—and psychoanalysts. To one Edward Petrikovitch he wrote: "I may assume that you are a compatriot. If you have been living in America for a long time I am surprised that you still believe anything at all written in an American newspaper. . . . With one single exception I have . . . not seen an interviewer in the last years. Most of all I am wary of Americans or correspondents for American papers."[67] Or: "American publishers are a dangerous sort of human beings" [Amerikanische Verleger sind . . . eine gefährliche Menschensorte].[68] His own publishers Boni and Liveright he called "two crooks" [die beiden Gauner].[69]

A chapter in itself would be Freud's unrelenting criticisms of American psychoanalysts. A long list of these complaints can be found in a postscript to his article on the question of lay analysis. This postscript was originally intended for print, but he eventually withdrew it from publication, obviously out of political and diplomatic considerations. There he writes, for instance, of "the Americans' dread of authority, their tendency to exert their personal independence in the few areas that are not yet occupied by the relentless pressure of public opinion"; he states that "the level of general education and of the intellectual capacity to absorb is by far lower than in Europe, even in persons who went to an American college"; or "that the American has no time. True, time is—money, but one does not really understand why time has to be converted into money in such haste. It would retain its monetary value anyway, even at a slower pace, and one should also suppose that the more time one invested to begin with, the more money would come out of it in the end." "The American super-ego seems to lower its severity against the ego very much in matters of financial interest." And Freud ends his tirade with the following words: "But perhaps my

---

67. 17 January 1928, Library of Congress.
68. Letter to Helen Downey; Library of Congress.
69. Freud and Rank, *Inside Psychoanalysis*.

readers will find that I have said enough bad things about this country, to which we have learned to bow in the last decade."[70]

The most devastating example of Freud's unsuccessful efforts to deal with the psychoanalytic movement and institutions in America is arguably his effort to make Horace Westlake Frink the leader of American psychoanalysis. Frink, a native American and co-founder of the New York Psychoanalytic Society, suffered from a manic-depressive psychosis, homosexual conflicts, and confusional states, and became Freud's patient in 1921. A married father of two children, Frink fell in love with his rich patient Angelika (Angie) Bijur, also married. Bijur went to Vienna in the summer of 1921 and saw Freud several times about a possible marriage with Frink. She reported Freud's position this way: "He advised my getting a divorce because of my own incomplete existence—and because if I threw Dr. F. over now, he would never again try to come back to normality and probably develop into a homosexual, though in a highly disguised way." To Frink Freud wrote: "[I requested Mrs. Bijur] not to repeat to foreign people I had advised her to marry you on the threat of a nervous breakdown. It gives them a false idea of the kind of advice that is compatible with analysis and is very likely to be used against analysis. May I still suggest to you that your idea Mrs. B had lost part of her beauty be turned into having part of her money. . . . Your complaint that you cannot grasp your homosexuality implies that you are not aware of your phantasy of making me a rich man. If matters turn out all right, let us change this imaginary gift into a real contribution to psychoanalytic funds." Shortly after both had divorced their partners, Frink underwent a second analysis with Freud, during which he decompensated and suffered from psychotic hallucinatory episodes. He recovered, however; Freud said he felt the analysis to be completed, and Horace and Angie went to Paris and married. Back in America, after some time Frink's condition worsened again. He was hospitalized, recovered, released, made two suicidal attempts, was again hospitalized, and Bijur undertook divorce proceedings.[71]

---

70. Ilse Grubrich-Simitis, *Zurück zu Freuds Texten: Stumme Dokumente sprechen machen* (Frankfurt am Main: S. Fischer, 1993), 226–29; *Back to Freud's Texts: Making Silent Documents Speak*, trans. P. Slotkin (New Haven, CT: Yale University Press, 1996).

71. There were further ramifications of this episode, e.g., the scandal that threatened to break out when Bijur's first husband wanted to make this public in the *New York Times*. Dr. Thaddeus Ames, who was the president of the New York Psychoanalytic Society and also the analyst of Angie's husband, sent that projected public letter to Freud, and added: "Mr. Bijur has placed his affairs in the hands of his lawyers who on sufficient provocation are to air in the newspapers all the details and attack Dr. Frink and psychoanalysis. . . . I am sorry to trouble you with all these details, but I feel that this episode is more far-reaching than just the Frink-Bijurs.

Freud's efforts to make Frink the leader in American psychoanalysis, despite the latter's personal difficulties and the opposition against him in his home country, together with Freud's boundary violations in the analysis, certainly did not help to improve the already strained transatlantic relations. The Frink episode shows, apart from Freud's misjudgment of people, how his anti-Americanism also clouded his judgment of the institutional and political situation in America. So now we may finally ask, what were actually the reasons for Freud's negative attitude toward America?

Possible Reasons for Freud's Attitude toward America

There is no doubt that Freud had a complex attitude toward money. He was extremely touchy when it came to borrowing or accepting money from others (for example, from Josef Breuer), in other words, to depend on others and lose his independence. This was particularly so when the money came from people Freud did not like or even considered enemies. In 1938, he was approached by Franz Riklin Jr., a relative of Jung's, who had been "chosen by some exceedingly rich Swiss Jews to go into Austria *at once*, with a very large sum of money, to do all that he could to persuade leading Jews to leave the country." When he called on Freud, all the latter told him was: "I refuse to be beholden to my enemies."[72] Significantly, in his later years Americans were among those of his analysands and supporters on whose payments he depended most for his personal income, and he found it "sad" that he was "materially dependent upon these savages, who are not better-class human beings" [Ist es nicht traurig, daß wir von diesen Wilden, die keine besseren Menschen sind, materiell abhängen?].[73]

If this becomes public, the members of the New York Psychoanalytic Society are likely to be opposed to Frink if they think that his notoriety will mean fewer patients and less money for them." On the Freud/Frink disaster, see especially Lavinia Edmunds, "Freud's American Tragedy," *Johns Hopkins Magazine* 30 (1988): 40–49; Silas Warner, "Freud's Analysis of Horace Frink, M.D.: A Previously Unexplained Therapeutic Disaster," *Journal of the American Academy of Psychoanalysis* 22 (1994): 137–52; and Arthur Zitrin, "Freud-Frink-Brill: A Puzzling Episode in the History of Psychoanalysis," *Bulletin of the Association for Psychoanalytic Medicine of the Columbia University Psychoanalytic Center*, 1998, 1–19. Mahony, "A l'écoute de l'autre Freud," has given an overview on the basis of these three sources. The quoted letters and other materials (here quoted after Mahony) are held by the Alan M. Chesney Archives at Johns Hopkins University.

72. Barbara Hannah, *Jung: His Life and Work: A Biographical Memoir* (Boston: Shambhala, 1976), 254–55. Jung was repeatedly reproached "for not doing more to help Freud leave Austria." He "always replied: '[Freud] would not take help from me under any circumstances.' It is rather ironic that when Freud did go to England . . . , he had to owe his satisfactory house in London to a Jungian: Dr. E. A. Bennet."

73. To A. Zweig, in Gay, *Freud: A Life for Our Time*, 563–64. "Unfortunately, I am forced . . . to sell the rest of my sparse working time dearly. I would have to charge a German 250 Marks

Americans were good only for being milked for their money. "What is the use of Americans, if they bring no money? They are not good for anything else."[74] He always begrudged Jung the success the latter had in securing huge sums from American benefactors (the McCormicks, the Mellons, for example) for the promotion of Analytical Psychology: "Rockefeller's daughter presented Jung with a gift of 360,000 francs for the construction of a casino, analytic institute, etc. So, Swiss ethics have finally made their sought-after contact with American money. I think not without bitterness about the pitiful situation of the members of our Association, our difficulties with the *Verlag* [the psychoanalytic press], etc."[75] "All the popularity in America has not produced for analysis the goodwill of *one* of the dollar uncles there."[76] Let us also not forget that it was only after Stanley Hall raised the honorarium that he accepted the invitation to Clark University at all: "America should bring in money, not cost money."[77]

This brought Freud into a dilemma. One the one hand, as he wrote, "money is a means of unchaining slaves; . . . one obtains freedom in exchange for money," but, on the other hand, as he continued, one also "sacrifices freedom for money."[78] Thus one both obtains and sacrifices freedom for money. Freud seems to have dealt with this dilemma by freely accepting, and actively encouraging, donations from followers (e.g., Anton von Freund or Max Eitingon), but only for "the Cause," and never for himself—with one exception: He 'allowed' a woman, Marie Bonaparte (but by no means Franz Riklin Jr., let alone C. G. Jung), to fund his emigration by advancing the so-called *Reichsfluchtsteuer*[79]—but took pains to repay this to her in the following summer after arriving in England.[80]

---

per hour, and therefore I prefer Englishmen and Americans who pay the hourly rates usual in their own countries. That is, I do not prefer them, I just have to take them on, rather than others" [Ich bin . . . leider genötigt, den Rest meiner kargen Arbeitszeit teuer zu verkaufen. Ich müsste einem Deutschen mk 250 für die Stunde anrechnen u ziehe darum Engländer u Amerikaner, die nach ihren heimischen Sätzen zalen, vor. D.h. ich ziehe sie nicht vor, ich muß sie bloß eher annehmen]. Freud to Meng, 21 April 1921; Library of Congress.

74. Freud and Jones, *The Complete Correspondence*, 552.
75. Freud and Ferenczi, *The Correspondence*, 2:126.
76. Ibid., 3:78.
77. Ibid., 1:33.
78. Freud, *The Complete Letters of Sigmund Freud to Wilhelm Fliess*, 321.
79. The *Reichsfluchtsteuer*, the Reich Flight Tax or Fugitive Tax, was "a measure taken in 1931 to prevent wealthy persons from leaving the country and taking their capital with them but was transformed in 1934 into an instrument for despoiling emigrating Jews. It was to prove a very lucrative tax. In 1935/36, 45 million RM were collected. 342 million RM were collected in 1938/39 and 300 million RM in 1939/40" (http://goliath.ecnext.com/coms2/gi_0199-6455152/The-Economics-of-the-Final.html; 23 September 2009).
80. Jones, *Life and Work*, 3:223.

In all probability, Freud's anti-Americanism was not caused by one single factor. In addition to the already mentioned factors, various further possible motives can be found. His complicated relationships with relatives who had emigrated to the States (Eli Bernays, for example) probably played a role.[81] He had also pinned high hopes on President Wilson and his so-called Fourteen Points and was very disappointed when the Treaty of Versailles did not fulfill the promises held out therein.[82] Undoubtedly, his later experiences with the development of psychoanalysis in America, and particularly the Americans' opposition against so-called lay analysis, as well as, as he saw it, the unsatisfactory standard of psychoanalytic training and understanding there were important factors. He also linked the stay—and success—in America of some of his followers with their defection or alleged shortcomings. He found that they had "succumb[ed] to the American 'dollar compulsion' [*Dollarzwang*]."[83]

Peter Gay writes that "Freud and his adherents were copying, often in so many words, the condescending pronouncements that cultivated Europeans had been uttering for years," and then asks "why Freud should so uncritically swallow this potent, but by his time musty, mixture of tendentious observation and unmitigated cultural arrogance. What happened was that his conformity and his radicalism oddly worked together to keep his

---

81. Saul Rosenzweig, *Freud, Jung, and Hall the King-Maker: The Historic Expedition to America (1909), with G. Stanley Hall as Host and William James as Guest* (Seattle: Hogrefe and Huber, 1992), argues that Freud's animosity was the product of a displaced sibling rivalry with Eli Bernays. About Eli's son, Edward, the famous "father" of public relations, Freud wrote: He was "an honest boy when I knew him. I know not how far he has become Americanized." Gay, *Freud: A Life for Our Time*, 568.

82. Reverberations of this disappointment may have influenced his judgment in the book he drafted with William C. Bullitt: Sigmund Freud and William C. Bullitt, *Thomas Woodrow Wilson, Twenty-Eighth President of the United States: A Psychological Study* (Boston: Houghton Mifflin, 1967).

83. To Rank, 4 August 1922, in Freud and Rank, *Inside Psychoanalysis*. Jung first spoke in detail of his differences with Freud's theories in his lectures at Fordham University in New York (Jung, 1913), boasting to Freud—much to the latter's displeasure—"that his modifications of psycho-analysis had overcome the resistances of many people who had hitherto refused to have anything to do with it." Carl Gustav Jung, *The Theory of Psychoanalysis*, CW 4. Sigmund Freud, "On the History of the Psycho-Analytic Movement," S.E. 14:7–66. Freud took badly Rank's success in America and linked it with the latter's defection. He also had reservations against Ferenczi's prolonged stay in New York and wrote him after his return: "I find *you* more reserved than you were before America. Damned country!" (Freud and Ferenczi, *The Correspondence*, 3:320). When Franz Alexander left Berlin in 1930 to take a position as Visiting Professor of Psychoanalysis at the University of Chicago, Freud's parting words were: "I hope America will leave something intact of the real Alexander." Franz Alexander, *The Western Mind in Transition* (New York: Random House, 1960), 101; cf. Erika S. Schmidt, "Franz Alexander und die Berliner Tradition in Chicago," *Jahrbuch der Psychoanalyse* 57 (2008): 95–116.

anti-Americanism alive. As a . . . European bourgeois, he thought about Americans as others thought. . . . [A]s a radical antibourgeois in his ideal of free sexual relations, he found Americans the very model of sexual hypocrisy."[84]

Patrick Mahony has put forward the hypothesis that Freud displaced the feelings he had for the pre-oedipal mother onto America: "Freud's biographers err in writing he rarely spoke of the pre-oedipal mother. The overdetermined fact is that he felt always compelled to speak about her, disguised as America. Her demonic power made him regress into an infantile, paranoid state of aggrievement and petulancy that lasted all his life. He tried to control the oedipal but especially pre-oedipal mother by spatially constricting her in his symbolic geography."[85]

Howard L. Kaye argues that what was at the bottom of Freud's hatred of America was "the problem of authority. Freud saw in America something that he had not anticipated, a disturbing disregard for scientific, political, and familial authority that he . . . attributed to American egalitarianism. . . . [T]he American principles of equality and competition . . . seemed to Freud to stifle the independence of thought he had hoped to find."[86]

The Incident on Riverside Drive

Here I would like to suggest another possible motive, based upon the observation that Freud's criticisms became so much sharper after the trip. There was one experience he had in America that must have been utterly humiliating to him, and that undoubtedly left a strong impression. As far as I know, there is one short reference to this event in Ferenczi's *Clinical Diary* and two more detailed accounts of it, both going back to C. G. Jung. One is an interview he gave to Saul Rosenzweig in 1951, who then wrote about it in his book on the psychoanalysts' expedition to America. The other is the account Jung gave Kurt Eissler, when the latter interviewed him for the Freud Archives in 1953.[87]

Ferenczi—obviously an eyewitness—simply mentions Freud's "hys-

---

84. Gay, *Freud: A Life for Our Time*, 569–70.
85. Mahony, "A l'écoute de l'autre Freud."
86. Howard L. Kaye, "Why Freud Hated America," *Wilson Quarterly* 17 (1993): 121–22.
87. Ferenczi, *Ohne Sympathie keine Heilung*; Rosenzweig, *Freud, Jung, and Hall the King-Maker*. A transcript of the Eissler interview is available at the Library of Congress, but it may not be photocopied until 2013 (see the "Register of his papers in the Sigmund Freud Collection in the Library of Congress"). Jung also alluded to this incident in a talk with E. A. Bennet: "In New York Freud spoke to Jung of personal difficulties—Jung did not talk of these—and asked his help in clearing them up." Bennet, *C. G. Jung*, 42.

terical symptom" of "incontinence on Riverside Drive," a "weakness that he could not hide from us and himself."[88] Rosenzweig tells the story as follows:

> [In the interview, Jung] described one aspect of the American journey in detail.... [T]here was a visit ... to the Columbia University Psychiatric Clinic.... While looking at the Palisades Freud suffered a personal mishap.[89] He accidentally urinated in his trousers and Jung helped him out of this embarrassment.... Freud entertained a fear of similar accidents during the time of the lectures at Clark University. So Jung offered to help Freud overcome this fear if Freud would consent to some analytic intervention. Freud agreed and Jung began the "treatment."[90]

It was then that the following famous incident occurred: Jung asked Freud to give him some intimate personal details, and Freud refused on the grounds that he could not "risk his authority." It was precisely at that moment, as Jung later said and wrote various times, that Freud lost his authority altogether.[91]

In his interview with Eissler, Jung also mentions the Palisades.[92] There was no public toilet in the vicinity, and Freud—always according to Jung—was suddenly afraid he wouldn't be able to hold his water, upon which he promptly wet his pants, and they had to get a cab to go back to the hotel. Freud was extremely embarrassed but also feared that this was a sign of approaching senility, a symptom of a paralysis, to which Jung replied, nonsense, that would simply be a neurotic symptom. But, Freud asked, of what? Everybody can see that you are extremely ambitious, Jung retorted,

---

88. Ferenczi, *Ohne Sympathie keine Heilung*, entry of 4 August 1932.

89. Rosenzweig comments that this reference to the Palisades was at first puzzling to him, but he then concluded that the mishap must have happened "on the occasion of the group's visit to Columbia University.... The group were on Riverside Drive ... while visiting the Clinic and could see the distant Palisades on the other side of the Hudson river" (Rosenzweig, *Freud, Jung, and Hall the King-Maker*, 292). Rosenzweig's conclusion that this happened on Riverside Drive is proven by Ferenczi's remark quoted above (first published seven years before Rosenzweig's book, but obviously overlooked by the latter).

90. Rosenzweig, *Freud, Jung, and Hall the King-Maker*, 64–65.

91. E.g., C. G. Jung, *Memories, Dreams, Reflections*, recorded and edited by Aniela Jaffé (London: Fontana Press, 1995 [1962]), 182.

92. Jung's repeated mentioning of the Palisades seems to lend credibility also to other details in his two nearly identical accounts. Why else mention such a detail, unimportant in itself, on two different occasions? We may question some of the slant Jung gives the event, however. I find it hard to imagine, for instance, that Freud actually agreed to submit to a "treatment" conducted by Jung.

which Freud vehemently denied.⁹³ Still, he told Jung that he would be immensely relieved if this were "only" a neurotic symptom. So Jung offered to analyze him and asked him to tell him some dreams. He analyzed them up to the point, at which—and here Jung again tells the story quoted above—Freud refused to give him further details of a very intimate nature. When pressed by Eissler, Jung then hinted at family affairs, with a thinly veiled reference to Martha Freud and Minna Bernays. Still, Jung maintained, the little analytic work they had done was enough to make this symptom disappear for the duration of their trip.

One wonders, by the way, if Ferenczi and possibly also Brill and/or Jones were also witnesses to the conversation and "analysis" between Jung and Freud. At least for Ferenczi, the question of Freud's "authority" certainly played an important role in their relationship. Neither he, nor Brill, nor Jones ever mentioned Jung's attempt to analyze Freud, however.

In any case, Ferenczi was the first to raise the possibility that this incident might have something to do with Freud's attitude toward the Americans: "It is possible that his [Freud's] disdain for the Americans is a reaction to the weakness that he could not hide from us and from himself. 'How could I take so much pleasure in the American distinctions, when I actually despise the Americans so much?' Not unimportant is his emotionality when he, nearly with tears in his eyes, thanked the president of the university for the diploma of his honorary degree—which made a somewhat ridiculous impression even on me, the reverential spectator."⁹⁴

The idea that Freud's enuretic symptom had something to do with his ambitiousness, with his fervent wish to come to something, inevitably brings to mind the scene he tells in *The Interpretation of Dreams*:

> When I was seven or eight years old . . . [o]ne evening before going to sleep I disregarded the rules which modesty lays down and obeyed the calls of nature in my parents' bedroom while they were present. In the course of his reprimand, my father let fall the words: "The boy will come to nothing." This must have been a frightful blow to my ambition, for references to this scene are still constantly recurring in my dreams and are always linked with an

---

93. Psychoanalytic theory linked enuresis to excessive (repressed) ambitiousness. On Freud's denial of being ambitious, see also above.

94. Ferenczi, *Ohne Sympathie keine Heilung*, 184 (entry of 4 August 1932; trans. modified). Skues in his previous essay quotes this passage in another context. Kaye, "Why Freud Hated America," 121, finds "Ferenczi's suggestion that Freud's anti-American animus was a defensive reaction against his 'American vanity,' inspired by the honors he received during his visit" "unpersuasive," but does not take into account the possible link with the incident on Riverside Drive.

enumeration of my achievements and successes, as though I wanted to say: "You see, I *have* come to something."[95]

This weakness, which Freud could not hide from his fellow travelers, certainly had also reverberations in his later relations with them. How could Freud ever forgive Jung for having been witness to this humiliating incidence? Especially when, shortly before their final break, Jung used this episode to rub Freud's nose in it, asking: *"Who's got the neurosis?"* "I am not in the least neurotic," Jung added, giving further fuel to the flames: "You know, of course, how far a patient gets with self-analysis: *not* out of his neurosis—just like you."[96]

Conclusion

Freud's anti-Americanism seems to revolve around two powerful pairs of opposites: ambition and humiliation, and envy and gratitude. He seems to have been tempted to give in, as it were, to the American way of life. Then he ridiculed and despised what had threatened to seduce him. He strove for money, wealth, fame, and independence, but he did not want to be beholden to those who could make this possible.

America is the country in which Freud's ideas enjoyed their greatest success, an observation common to several of the essays in this book. One could say that the Americans loved Freud. But he always maintained that they only loved him because they did not, indeed could not, understand him. Therefore, they were only good for bringing in money, and even this they did not do to the extent he hoped, while lavishing money on Jung, whose "Swiss ethics" thus "made their sought-after contact with American money."[97]

But who were most successful in making money in America? Note the irony in Freud's words when he writes of a visit to the Hammerstein roof gardens in Manhattan and the "vaudeville show on the roof of a skyscraper, *naturally* owned by an Austrian Jew, Hammerstein."[98] Freudian slip or wrong information—it is quite fitting that Freud called Hammerstein an *Austrian* Jew, even if he was in fact a German one. The implicit conclusion is this: in Freud's view, Austrian Jews—like himself—can outdo the Ameri-

---

95. Sigmund Freud, *The Interpretation of Dreams*, S.E. 4 and 5:216. Cf. Leonard Shengold, *"The Boy Will Come to Nothing": Freud's Ego Ideal and Freud as Ego Ideal* (New Haven, CT: Yale University Press, 1993).
96. Freud and Jung, *The Freud/Jung Correspondence*, 535.
97. Freud and Ferenczi, *The Correspondence*, 2:126.
98. Freud, *Unser Herz zeigt nach dem Süden*, 305; italics added.

cans anytime—*if they want*. For this, however, they would have to sacrifice their old values on the altar of the "mightiest god," the dollar.[99]

Freud's negative attitude was not only his private quirk, for it also had an undeniable influence on the reception and development of psychoanalysis in America. Americans who had to deal with the original source of psychoanalytic ideas had also to deal with a combination of Freud's personal attitudes and the Central European stereotypes and prejudices that so often complicated transatlantic relationships (not only) in the first half of the twentieth century.

So why did Freud hate America? Psychobiographical speculations are always tricky; Freud himself can no longer be asked, and we are always in danger of projecting our own fantasies onto him. Perhaps it is safe to say that Freud's attitude toward America is more complex than simply hateful, that he had a deep-seated *ambivalence*, of which one side—his love of America, his temptation to give in to the seduction of making money the easy way, by bending the rules a little—was repressed, while the other side, the hatred, metastasized into a gigantic prejudice by way of an anticathexis.

But let us stay humble and cautious. Even if Freud's sweeping wholesale attacks were unjustified in their generalization, and we therefore may take some gleeful delight in looking for unconscious motives in the father of psychoanalysis, let us not forget that such an attitude in someone else would almost certainly have never elicited such attention and scrutiny. We may perhaps also understand how the same man, who, on the one hand, was impressed by the reality of the America he encountered, was, on the other hand, sharing the European prejudices against a different culture and civilization, which many Europeans perceived and resented as an alien one. It is ironic that nevertheless, and notwithstanding his negative attitude, by coming to America, Freud in fact helped to close a cultural gap and contributed to a new view and understanding of human beings—in Europe *and* in the United States.

Acknowledgments

I would like to thank John Burnham, André Haynal, Howard Kaye, James Lieberman, David Lotto, Patrick Mahony, and Richard Skues for their helpful comments and suggestions.

---

99. Thus also Freud's occasional disdain for Brill, a poor fellow Jewish boy, who, after the first years of studying and working when he could barely make ends meet, was very successful in New York.

FOUR

Mitteleuropa on the Hudson: On the Struggle for American Psychoanalysis after the *Anschluß*

GEORGE MAKARI

Sigmund Freud's visit to Clark University can be seen as a pivotal moment that defined a still protean psychoanalytic scene in America. However, to understand more fully the shape of things to come after 1909 in the United States, we must move beyond a focus on Freud, Putnam, James, and Jung and track different psychoanalytic communities as they grew and changed during the first decades of the twentieth century. Specifically, we must closely attend to the shifting dynamics of the field in Europe, for, I shall argue, those conflicts would traverse the Atlantic and utterly transform Freud's American followers.[1]

What follows, then, is an account of cultural crossings, interchanges between intellectual communities from, on the one hand, a select group of influential European urban centers and, on the other, New York, the key port of entry for these immigrants. In Europe, analysts had developed specific discursive communities with borders and domains that were the result of some three decades of growth, schism, and controversy. When these uprooted analysts took refuge in New York, they sought to remake their lost world, and intense conflict ensued. In this way, American psychoanalysis after World War II, I shall argue, was forged from this critical encounter between analysts who shared the same name but differed intensely over their identities.

An oscillating dynamic of hybridization, crisis, and purification was not new to psychoanalysis. Rather, it was constitutive of the field. Freud's psycho-

---

1. G. Makari, *Revolution in Mind: The Creation of Psychoanalysis* (New York: HarperCollins, 2008). Much of the later part of this paper is taken by permission from the epilogue of the book, 473–85.

sexual synthesis emerged from his immersion in three disparate French and German intellectual communities, each of which supplied the Viennese doctor with new allies and enemies. The first Freudians grew from these roots. In Vienna and Zurich, they were a loose band of enthusiasts; if one accepted any part of Freud's work, whether it derived from French psychopathology, German biophysics and psychophysics, or sexology, s/he was offered entry. There were no other hard-and-fast litmus tests; eclectic debate was the order of the day. However, at the Nuremburg meetings of 1910, foreshadowed in Shamdasani's and Skues's papers above, the International Psychoanalytical Association (IPA) was formed to rein in wild analysts and explicitly consolidate a strictly Freudian community. After that momentous meeting in 1910, for those who wanted to be Freudians, the rules had altered. Now one had to accept psychosexual theory in its fullest elaboration. Instead of consolidating the Freudian community, however, this demand led to great strife and fragmentation. And so, the great schisms began.[2]

If the IPA's 1910 strictures led Bleuler, Stekel, Adler, and Jung to depart, however, that group's hegemony never seemed to fully cross the Atlantic, where even the Professor's most illustrious followers were known to mix ideas from the heretical and the orthodox. And in part for that reason, the Americans earned the contempt of their European colleagues. Like Freud, the elite power-brokers of the field commonly derided the Americans as money-hungry hucksters and theoretical dunces, people who couldn't tell their Adler from their Freud, but surely could tell a ten-dollar bill from a twenty. As Ernst Falzeder makes clear, years after Freud's visit to Clark University, the Americans still had done little to controvert Freud's and his inner circle's prejudice that the New World was a hopeless place for scientific work. In 1925, reviewing his own nation's contributions to psychoanalysis, Clarence Oberndorf glumly admitted that there had been little original work, that is, work that would gain respect in European psychoanalytic circles.[3]

Meanwhile, during that same period, the psychoanalytic field in Europe had changed drastically. After the ravages of World War I, Freud's authority diminished, and in its place four great urban centers for analytic thought and practice emerged in London, Berlin, Vienna, and Budapest. Each of these communities had distinct theoretical proclivities. Yet they all remained held together by a number of shared commitments, including a

---

2. For a full historical delineation of this argument, please see ibid., 1–292.

3. C. P. Oberndorf, *A History of Psychoanalysis in America* (New York: Grune and Stratton, 1953), 179.

new, bureaucratized training process and an increased focus on matters of technique. In Europe, the interwar period was one of massive growth and intellectual richness, thanks in part to this dissemination of authority from one individual to these more diverse communities.[4]

Because this generation of analysts believed that psychoanalysis had grown out of the cultural heritage of European civilization, they viewed themselves as not just physicians but as the vanguard of their culture. The rise of National Socialism in Germany, however, began to change the circumstances in which psychoanalysis and its institutions were flourishing. After 1930, Berlin—arguably the most powerful analytic community in the world, one that frequently took issue with Freud and the Viennese, and prided itself on its scientific character and independent thought—faced annihilation. In 1933, the rise of Hitler led rapidly to the Aryanization and destruction of the mostly Jewish Berlin Psychoanalytic Society, with the few remaining analysts swallowed up into the Nazi Mattias H. Göring's German Medical Association for Psychotherapy.[5]

Due to this political catastrophe, America, a land of refuge far away, began to receive some of the most influential psychoanalysts of Europe. The first wave included the Berlin elite—Franz Alexander, Sándor Radó, Karen Horney, and Hanns Sachs. Led by these newcomers, the once easily dismissed Americans became emboldened. After a few years, they even began to go so far as to imagine the future of the field was theirs. In 1937, Sándor Radó argued that a break from the International Psychoanalytical Association would pose no danger, since the strength of psychoanalysis had been "concentrated in America for many years."[6] In 1938, Franz Alexander delivered as his presidential address "Psychoanalysis Comes of Age" to the members of the American Psychoanalytic Association. The Chicago-based analyst announced that a new American direction would make psychoanalysis a discipline with one foot in medicine and another in the social sciences. In the New World, psychoanalysis would rid itself of obscure theoretical superstructures and be given a new foundation in observation. It would no longer be a Weltanschauung, but would assume a "more scientific character."[7]

4. Makari, *Revolution in Mind*, 322–404.

5. On the analysts who remained in Germany after the Nazis, see G. Cocks, *Psychotherapy in the Third Reich: The Göring Institute* (New Brunswick, NJ: Transaction Publishers, 1997).

6. Sándor Radó to David Levy, 27 May 1937, David Levy Papers, Oskar Diethelm Library, Weill Medical College of Cornell University. Hereafter: David Levy Papers.

7. F. Alexander, "Psychoanalysis Comes of Age," *Psychoanalytic Quarterly* 7 (1938): 299–306.

As their confidence grew, the Americans became less willing to bend to the will of the Europeans and the IPA. The two groups had been stuck in a long-standing dispute over lay analysis. In the wake of the 1910 Flexner report, the Americans wanted to insist that all analysts be physicians, a position famously rejected by Freud and many others, especially in Vienna. In January 1938, the president of the New York society, Lawrence Kubie, and its educational director, Sándor Radó, met with four other analysts appointed by the American Psychoanalytic Association. Kubie's committee had been asked to deal with the problems between the Americans and the IPA. They decided to resolve these conflicts once and for all: they would break from the IPA over the issue of training requirements. And so they did that summer in Paris.

However, if that was the committee's main problem when it met in January, it was not two months later when the annexation of Austria unfolded before their eyes. Kubie hurriedly reconvened the group so they could take up the dire issue of saving their European colleagues from the Nazis. On March 19 the committee formed an Emergency Committee on Relief and Immigration to face this urgent task.

And so, the very same American renegades who had decided to declare their independence and defy the IPA, thereby undermining and perhaps even destroying that bureaucratic embodiment of European predominance, suddenly were thrust into the role of saviors. The problems the committee faced were daunting. In the decade leading up to 1938, a total of some 1,400 German, Austrian, and Italian doctors had immigrated to the United States, but after the annexation of Austria, the number of refugees who landed in America surged to over 1,400 in 1938 alone. While America was a vast space, forty-two of its states prohibited foreign medical doctors from practicing until they became citizens, a five- or six-year process that effectively limited immigrants to a small number of places, most often their port of entry, New York. Kubie recognized that the concentration of specialists in one place could be economically disastrous and started to plan for seeding analysts throughout the country.[8]

Further complicating matters, the United States State Department demanded affidavits and security deposits of $5,000 for an immigrant family of three or four. Kubie pleaded with American analysts: money had to pumped in if they were to save the European analysts. Many analysts contributed five, ten, or twenty dollars a month, but the need outstripped

---

8. American Psychoanalytic Association Archives, Oskar Diethelm Library, Weill Medical College of Cornell University, File Box 9–10.

these resources. As the Nazis moved into other parts of Europe, desperate requests came from Holland and the vestiges of free France. In the end, the Emergency Commission secured over $47,000. Working with Ernest Jones in the UK, Kubie and the Americans gave financial support to some 68 individuals, provided affidavits for 82, and were in contact with another 136. By 1943, 149 exiled psychoanalysts and psychiatrists had been relocated somewhere in the United States.[9]

The exodus brought, among others, some of the most successful Viennese psychoanalysts to America. They had few possessions and little money, but they carried with them a proud identity. They were ambassadors of a great civilization. Now a dark age had engulfed their homes and threatened the culture that made their work possible. Many like Otto Fenichel believed that it was their task to make sure psychoanalysis did not die in America, this money-crazed foreign place. For the Americans, who believed they were the future of the field, the newly arrived Europeans seemed to have arrogated to themselves the rights of a dispossessed royalty. There was bound to be trouble.

The main center of psychoanalysis in America was at the New York Psychoanalytic Society, and events there symbolized what took place in other parts of the country, not least because analysts in New York exerted a leadership role in the United States. The New York Society had opened its training institute in 1931. Two years later, Sándor Radó, who had been brought from Berlin to be Education Director, took over the teaching of theory. Radó's lectures were supplemented by the work of Americans like Abram Kardiner, David Levy, George Daniels, and Bertram Lewin. While these men had varied interests, they—along with Kubie, Alexander, and Paul Schilder—shared a desire to make psychoanalysis more scientific. Kubie was interested in merging Pavlov's reflexology with analysis; Kardiner hoped to use anthropology to enhance psychoanalytic theories; David Levy had conducted extensive research on young children; and Radó himself had become interested in Walter B. Cannon's physiology of emotion, the so-called fight-or-flight reactions, and had used it to model how the ego defended itself against anxiety.

Like others on the American scene, Radó spoke with great enthusiasm about the future of psychoanalysis as a natural science and worked to advance this perspective in the classroom. He was determined to reform psychoanalysis and avoid the fractures that had ripped it apart in the past. Why, Radó demanded, did schisms take place in psychoanalysis and not in physics and chemistry? When theory outweighed facts, then science be-

9. Ibid.

came a matter of opinion, and differences were transformed into a battle of wills. "Competing authorities do not like to dwell under the same roof," he continued. "One of them has to get out. And when he does he founds a school of his own in which he can be just as authoritarian as is his opponent in the school which he left."[10]

In America, Radó hoped to alleviate the situation by underplaying theory and stressing the critical, empirical, and scientific. Only a few years after he arrived, his European colleagues raised their eyebrows when Radó identified himself as an American and seemed a little too eager to cast off his Old World identity. Then the Europeans started unpacking their bags in New York. In 1939, Kubie's and Radó's New York Institute listed a teaching faculty of twenty-seven; a year later the faculty had added nineteen new members. The arrival of the traumatized, displaced Europeans would take a few years before its full impact was felt, but an early sign of strife came in the person of Paul Federn.

Federn's acidic manner was legendary in Vienna, and it had earned him the animosity of a generation of students. He prided himself on his absolute loyalty to Freud, and he was in that sense an unreconstructed old Freudian. After arriving in New York, Federn joined the New York Society, and the strain between him and Radó began almost immediately.

Radó had been invited to deliver a presentation to the New York Academy of Medicine and the New York Neurological Society on 2 May 1939. Given the audience, Radó spoke on a broad subject: the analytic treatment of neuroses. Before this medical crowd, he did not mince words: Freud's turn to signal anxiety was vital, but further clarification had been impeded by his death drive, "the highly speculative hypothesis" that was "so vague and remote as to be of questionable value." Radó suggested that more recently analysts had tried to tease out the metaphysics from the facts in their work on the ego, and he illustrated this with his own theory of emergency control, based on the work of Cannon.[11]

Radó's lecture was cheered by his allies from the New York Institute. George Daniels congratulated him and suggested analysts in general hoped to remake psychoanalysis in a similar way. They looked to biology to clear away "vestiges of outworn theories of instincts." *Outworn theory of instincts?* David Levy commented that the last ten years of American psychoanalysis pointed in the direction that Radó was going, as a reaction "against au-

---

10. S. Radó, "Scientific Aspects of Training in Psychoanalysis," in *Psychoanalysis of Behavior* (New York: Grune and Stratton, 1956 [1938]), 126.

11. S. Radó, "Psychoanalytic Conception and Treatment of the Neuroses," *Archives of Neurology and Psychiatry* 42 (1939): 1195–98.

thoritarianism in psychoanalysis." "The stage of obeisance to Freud" had given way to a freer utilization of his doctrine. *Obeisance to Freud?* As exemplars, Levy proudly pointed to research done by Franz Alexander, Abram Kardiner, and Karen Horney.

There was only one discussant left. Paul Federn, the bearded patriarch and standard-bearer who had come to America carrying the minutes of the Vienna Psychoanalytic Society in his bags. Federn was outraged by what he had heard. What happened next was hotly disputed, but for those who had seen Federn preside over meetings of the Vienna society, it was not surprising. Federn took the floor as he had so many times in Vienna to denounce supposedly new findings. His accent was so thick that the stenographer could not follow much of what he said. Her notes indicate that Federn scolded Radó for departing from drive theory, and accused him of leaving both Freud and the unconscious behind. Radó replied that Federn had completely misunderstood him, and the idea that he was ignoring the unconscious was astounding, but Radó did not reject the accusation that he was moving beyond Freud. Instead, he defended the legitimacy of replacing psychoanalytic theories that "can be neither verified nor refuted because they are beyond the available means of investigation" with theories that fell into the range of scientific method.[12]

Months later, Radó received the page proofs from the soon-to-be-published transcript of the meeting. To his dismay, he found that Federn's discussion now included a full-scale denunciation of Radó as a heretic. Federn was to have said:

> A few years ago, Radó broadened the meaning and importance of masochism in a rather infantile way. Now he thinks he has discovered that there is no sadomasochistic phase and that there are no different components to the sexual drive. It would not be of intrinsic merit to watch the details of his desertion of Freud. I have watched similar desertions in the cases of Adler, Jung and Rank. Radó is the chief teacher in the New York Psychoanalytical [sic] Institute, however and since he is trying to draw that school behind him, he must be opposed.[13]

In the transcript, no reply to this diatribe appeared from the accused because, in Radó's recollection, Federn had never uttered those words at the

---

12. See the transcript of the proceedings along with a letter from the secretary of the New York Neurological Society, Clarence Hare, to Lawrence Kubie, 20 March 1940, David Levy Papers.

13. Ibid.

meeting. Certain that Federn had doctored the transcript, Radó accused his adversary of behaving unethically. Lawrence Kubie tried to intercede, at first denying that any alterations were made. David Levy jumped into the fray on Radó's side. Finally, it came out that the befuddled stenographer, unable to make heads or tails of her notes, had asked "Dr. Fedor" to write up his response. Federn had freely obliged.

It was a nasty little quarrel and a harbinger of things to come. Radó, Levy, Kardiner, and Karen Horney wanted to sustain an open, pluralistic psychoanalysis that was built on pragmatism and a suspicion of metaphysical European theory. As Federn discovered, they all supported discarding Freudian drive theory and hoped to resituate psychoanalysis by dissolving its ties to unconscious libido. Some Americans like Kardiner, Horney, and Harry Stack Sullivan would look to the social environment to make a new sociology of character. Others like Radó and Alexander turned toward new physiological findings to ground their efforts. Then suddenly while they were busily reframing their own views of psychoanalysis, they were confronted by a group of Viennese led by Paul Federn, who begged to differ.

The tension in the New York Psychoanalytic Society became electric. David Levy feared that the American commitment to a scientific psychoanalysis would be compromised by the newcomers. He wrote to Kubie:

> The old-timers from Vienna are a good example of the danger of starting with holy writ. . . . [T]hey never ask themselves the question, "What is the truth?" They ask rather, "Does he agree with Freud?" implying "There is no truth but Freud." And that is why the discussions are so little grounded in empiricism, so thoroughly dialectic.[14]

Kubie asked Levy to be patient and went on to suggest that this attitude was in part loyalty to Freud, but was also characteristic of "the refugee who doesn't want to feel that everything that he has had and everything he knows had been swept away and superseded by something better."[15]

Patience wore thin. Kubie began to act in a more highhanded manner, prompting one analyst to suggest he had become a "little Hitler."[16] As it became clear that Kubie had misrepresented Federn's actions in the conflict with Radó, David Levy became furious. Normally dapper and unruffled, Kubie replied by accusing Levy of "vilifying Federn."[17] Levy had already ac-

---

14. David Levy to Lawrence Kubie, 14 November 1939, David Levy Papers.
15. Lawrence Kubie to David Levy, 17 November 1939, David Levy Papers.
16. Adolph Stern to Lawrence Kubie, undated, circa fall of 1939, David Levy Papers.
17. Lawrence Kubie to David Levy, 2 May 1940, David Levy Papers.

cused Kubie of stacking teaching appointments with those deemed orthodox; soon he found that his own course on child analysis had been handed over to the Viennese analyst Bertha Bornstein.[18]

Meanwhile, the New York Psychoanalytic Society had added not just Federn but also Ludwig Jekels, Johan H. W. Van Ophuijsen, Annie Reich, and a group of guest lecturers including Edith Jacobson, Ernst and Marianne Kris, and Heinz Hartmann. Hermann Nunberg attended meetings at the society, though he had been denied membership for refusing to pledge that he would not endorse lay analysis.[19] As one member recalled, in 1939 one heard far more German spoken at the New York society meetings than English.[20] The society that had once recruited Radó to bring weight to their fledgling institute now had at its disposal a depth of experience. Kubie decided that it was no longer necessary to follow Radó into a fight with the Viennese. In December 1940, he orchestrated the removal of Sándor Radó as the Educational Director, an action justified by Kubie's claim that "we have come to disagree with him on certain theoretical issues."[21]

Kubie knew that Radó was now fuming "like Achilles in his tent." Kardiner and Levy were also bitter about the way Kubie had allowed the newcomers to move in. Exacerbating the tension, Karen Horney began to push for radical revisions that rocked the society. She had forged her identity in a Berlin psychoanalytic community where freedom from a slavish fawning before Freud had been a matter of pride. After following Alexander to Chicago, she came to New York in 1934 and joined the society there. In 1937, she published *The Neurotic Personality of Our Time*, in which she argued that cultural forces gave the form of a neurosis. She knew that some would ask whether this cultural emphasis was still psychoanalysis:

> If one believes that it [psychoanalysis] is constituted entirely by the sum total of theories propounded by Freud, then what is presented here is not psychoanalysis. If, however, one believes that the essentials of psychoanalysis lie in certain basic trends of thought concerning the role of unconscious processes and the way they find expression, and in a form of therapeutic treatment that brings these processes to awareness, then what I present is psychoanalysis.[22]

---

18. David Levy to Lawrence Kubie, 13 October 1939, David Levy Papers.
19. Author's interview with Henry Nunberg, M.D., 27 July 2006.
20. J. A. P. Millet, "Psychoanalysis in the United States," in *Psychoanalytic Pioneers*, ed. F. Alexander, S. Eisenstein, and M. Grotjahn (New York: Basic Books, 1966), 557.
21. Lawrence Kubie to Samuel Atkin, 11 December 1940, David Levy Papers.
22. K. Horney, *The Neurotic Personality of Our Time* (New York: W.W. Norton, 1937), ix.

Like the transplanted Berliners, many Americans would have signed on to that declaration in 1937. Then two years later, Horney published *New Ways in Psychoanalysis*, a book-length critique of psychoanalytic fundamentals.[23] The book was unabashedly radical: Horney rejected libido theory, the Oedipal complex, the childhood origins of neurosis, the notion of a repetition-compulsion, and transference; she did not accept the super-ego, ego, and id, not to mention a host of other minor theories. For Horney, personality and neurosis were due to environmental influences that disturbed a child's relation to self and other. The New York Society asked Horney to present her new theories before a scientific meeting. During the meeting, Horney was accused of hiding the extremity of her ideas and was vigorously upbraided. An enraged Abram Kardiner wrote Kubie to protest the attacks that he had allowed during the meeting, including repeated claims that Horney's theories were due to her own neurosis. "Is this science or a racket?" Kardiner fumed. "I was under the illusion that I was a member of a scientific society and not a club."[24]

As reviews came in, Horney found little support elsewhere. One damning critique was written by Otto Fenichel. Though he shared Horney's distaste for orthodox Freudians, Fenichel could not countenance Horney's rejection of inner drives, which he believed eviscerated one of the central assertions of psychoanalytic theory. In times like these, he counseled his *Rundbriefe* (private round-robin letters) colleagues, the task was to save psychoanalysis from dissolution. Fenichel assailed Horney's book. After all that she rejected, he asked, what was left?[25] Another crushing review came from Horney's former Berlin ally, Franz Alexander, who spent over thirty pages decimating her arguments. Horney created a cartoonish, one-dimensional Freud, only then to present her own one-dimensional antithesis, he wrote. Between libido and culture, one empty word replaced another. Psychoanalysis had to attend to both biology and environment, the present and the past, family and culture. In arguing against a straw man, Horney had created a theory riddled with the opposite of errors—not truths, but different errors.[26]

At the New York society, the once fiery radical and now fiery conservative Fritz Wittels emerged as the most vocal critic of Horney. After resign-

---

23. K. Horney, *New Ways in Psychoanalysis* (New York: W.W. Norton, 1939).
24. Abram Kardiner to Lawrence Kubie, 24 October 1939, David Levy Papers.
25. O. Fenichel, review of K. Horney, *New Ways in Psychoanalysis*, in *Psychoanalytic Quarterly* 9 (1940): 114–21.
26. F. Alexander, "Psychoanalysis Revised," *Psychoanalytic Quarterly* 9 (1940): 1–36.

ing from the Vienna society in 1910, Wittels had made his way back into Freud's good graces in 1927. Immigrating to New York, he joined the society and took up the fight against heretics like Horney. In 1940 he wrote Kubie, saying: "The issue is Freud or no Freud." Horney's students made "fools of us by insisting on what they call democratic methods in a scientific body." What if some internist claimed microbes did not cause malaria and his colleagues voted on this view? Horney, Wittels demanded, should recant or resign.[27]

Kubie was in a difficult position. Before the arrival of the Europeans, he had fashioned himself a standard-bearer of science in psychoanalysis. He had supported Radó, Horney, Kardiner, Levy, and others as they quietly worked to reinvent psychoanalytic theory for America. He told Wittels: "I am basically opposed to any form of a 'purge' in a scientific organization." Yet Kubie agreed that such freedom did not bring with it the right to indoctrinate students. Horney's followers complained of intimidation in the classrooms. Some of them signed a petition which stated that the advancement of the science of psychoanalysis had been grossly impeded by the Education Committee.[28]

In June 1941, Horney was demoted to lecturer, and her training privileges were revoked. Having in essence been fired, she quit. Horney, four other faculty members, and fourteen students resigned from the society to form the Association for the Advancement of Psychoanalysis and the American Institute for Psychoanalysis. Horney left with Sándor Ferenczi's former student Clara Thompson, and elsewhere the two found allies, including the homegrown American analyst Harry Stack Sullivan of Washington, D.C. Under the mentorship of Adolf Meyer and William Alanson White, Sullivan had developed an interpersonal theory that left sexual drives and the technique of transference interpretation behind. Instead, he focused on the pathologies of human relationships. With the former Frankfurt school analyst Eric Fromm, Sullivan supported Horney's new group. They all hoped to advance psychoanalysis by creating a pragmatic, unesoteric field stabilized by social science. However, while these analysts were for lay analysis, Horney was firmly against it, creating a schism within the schism—again replete with rhetoric on academic freedom. In the end,

---

27. Fritz Wittels to Lawrence Kubie, 13 March 1940, David Levy Papers.

28. Gregory Zilboorg to David Levy, 6 December 1940, David Levy Papers. The undated students' petition, entitled "Resolutions Submitted to the New York Psychoanalytic Society," was enclosed in a letter dated 25 March 1941 from Bernard S. Robbins to David Levy, David Levy Papers.

Thompson, Fromm, and Sullivan split from Horney and established the William Alanson White Institute in 1942.

The departure of Horney and her allies did not end the accusations of dogmatism and heresy in the New York society. Disgruntled analysts like Radó, Levy, Daniels, and Kardiner, who had once been the core faculty of the New York Institute, plotted their own secession. Radó and Levy looked to Alexander for assistance to set up a psychoanalytic center within a medical school, and thereby concretely establish a link between medicine and psychoanalysis. With the aid of Adolph Meyer, Radó and his associates opened a new analytic center at Columbia University that began to train candidates in 1945 and was accepted by the IPA in 1949. Before long, accusations arose that the leader of the institute, Sándor Radó, had formed a school around his own teachings, in the name of scientific freedom, of course.[29]

After 1945, the stage was set. The Viennese émigrés became orthodox Freudians opposed to the former Berliners and Americans who came to be known as neo-Freudians. That the latter were called "neo-Freudian" was in itself a defeat. Horney, Radó, and Kardiner wanted to be part of a psychoanalytic science and did not want to be forever shadowed by the ghost of the man they sought to move beyond. Decades later, after delivering a paper, Sándor Radó was asked a question from the audience about Freud's views. Wearily he replied: "For thirty years Radó gives lectures by Radó. For thirty years Radó gets questions about Freud."[30]

Not only in New York, but in Washington, Philadelphia, Chicago, Los Angeles, and elsewhere, orthodox Freudians were pitted against neo-Freudians.[31] In New York, Lawrence Kubie would be cast off. The new leader of the New York society had impeccable Viennese credentials and could trace his analytic lineage to Freud, for he had been one of the Professor's last training cases. Heinz Hartmann served as director of education, then president of the New York society, and president of the IPA. With his old colleagues from Vienna and Paris, Ernst Kris and Rudolph Lowenstein, Hartmann set the theoretical agenda for American ego psychology for the

---

29. David Levy to Franz Alexander, 31 March 1942; Franz Alexander to David Levy, 16 April 1942, David Levy Papers. On the founding of the Columbia Center, see C. Tomlinson, "Sandor Rado and Adolf Meyer: A Nodal Point in American Psychiatry and Psychoanalysis," *International Journal of Psycho-Analysis* 77 (1996): 963–82.

30. Personal communication from Theodore Shapiro, 2005.

31. See, for example, Hale's account of psychoanalysis in Los Angeles where there was a schism in 1950; Nathan G. Hale Jr., *The Rise and Crisis of Psychoanalysis in the United States: Freud and the Americans, 1917–1985* (New York: Oxford University Press, 1995), 147–56.

following three decades. His emphasis on adaptation cohered nicely with American values of self-reliance, and his hope to link psychoanalysis to academic psychology would be taken up by allies, such as David Rapaport. He could also count on the support of the heir to the Freud legacy, Anna Freud in London.

Against the neo-Freudians, Hartmann also had the support of Otto Fenichel and the underground community of leftist analysts. Without openly pushing for a Marxist psychoanalytic sociology in America, Fenichel, who was privately dismissive of Hartmann's ego psychology, concluded that the greater peril lay in the reactionary interpersonal and cultural work of Horney and Kardiner, and the driveless model of Radó, all of which abandoned the radical propositions of Freudian sexuality. He advised his *Rundbriefe* colleagues that the only choice was siding with the orthodox for now.[32] As his epistolary community began to flag in 1945, Fenichel terminated the circular letter and began a grueling medical internship so as to get an American medical license. He died before he finished it.

A coalition of ego psychologists and orthodox Freudians controlled the American Psychoanalytic Association by 1946. Four years earlier, the New York society first proposed a resolution that gave authority to the association to grant certification and diplomas for psychoanalysts. The New York group also tried to get passed an amendment that banned any secessions without prior approval from the association, a proposal that seemed to misunderstand the nature of a secession. After World War II, spurred by the refugees who now dominated the New York society, the American Psychoanalytic Association transformed itself from a loosely knit federation into a central power that policed standards throughout the country. The association enforced its standards on teaching and training and no longer yielded authority on these matters to local societies. The Hartmann era in American psychoanalysis had begun.[33]

And so, Sigmund Freud's 1909 visit to Clark University helped encourage the growth of the earliest American brand of Freudianism—eclectic, pragmatic, empirical, and less "philosophical." Two decades later, this still fledgling, marginalized community was greatly bolstered by the arrival of some of the most prestigious figures from the freethinking Berlin psychoanalytic community, who quickly assimilated and became powerful figures.

32. J. Reichmayr and E. Mühlleitner, eds., *Otto Fenichel 119 Rundbriefe*, vol. 2: *Amerika (1938–1945)* (Frankfurt am Main: Stroemfeld Verlag, 1998), 1613.
33. M. S. Bergmann, "The Hartmann Era and Its Contribution to Psychoanalytic Technique," in *The Hartmann Era*, ed. M. S. Bergmann (New York: Other Press, 2000), 1–78.

A rather distinct form of psychoanalysis began to grow until the *Anschluss*, when these Americans found themselves side by side with a large contingent of dispossessed Viennese analysts. The ensuing battle—Vienna versus Berlin, Old World versus New World, Freudian versus psychoanalytic scientist—would define American psychoanalysis for the next forty years.

FIVE

Another Dimension of the Émigré Experience: From Central Europe to the United States via Turkey

HALE USAK-SAHIN

In the Baltimore area during the World War II era, three emigrant women physicians from Central Europe—Ruth Wilmanns Lidz, Edith Weigert,[1] and Frieda Fromm-Reichmann—associated with each other. They all felt the influence of Adolf Meyer of Johns Hopkins Hospital, who had come from German-speaking Switzerland and had been at the Clark conference of 1909. The three women all practiced psychoanalysis, but they had a special interest in patients who were psychotic rather than the usual neurotic analysands. All were prominent in the United States in the decades after the war as each one gave her own special twist to psychoanalytic practice. In addition, Ruth Wilmanns Lidz and Edith Weigert came to the United States via Turkey.

In tracing the experiences of those two women who were in Turkey, especially of Ruth Wilmanns Lidz, I would like to illustrate how Freud's ideas were received in different cultures in very different ways in the second quarter of the twentieth century—Europe, Turkey, and America—as these women ultimately became part of professional psychoanalysis in the United States in the continuing aftermath of Freud's 1909 visit.

Here, as in other histories, the connecting link between Central Europe, Turkey, and the U.S. was the escape of European physicians and psychoanalysts from National Socialism. Through "historical fortune,"[2] the reforms of Istanbul University in the year 1933 coincided with the emigration of

---

1. Edith Weigert did not use her maiden name, Vowinckel, professionally.
2. Arin Namal, "Die kurze Tätigkeit des österreichischen Hals-Nasen-Ohren-Spezialisten Prof. Dr. Erich Ruttin an der Universität Istanbul in den Jahren 1934 und 1935," *Wiener Klinische Wochenschrift* 115 (2003): 432–37.

many refugees from National Socialism. Hence, Turkey became a stopover for some of them on their way to other countries, especially to the U.S.[3] And so it was for Edith Weigert, who had already qualified as a psychoanalyst in Germany, and for Ruth Wilmanns Lidz, who became a psychoanalyst after she arrived in the U.S. In this respect, the impact of forced emigration on the lives and work of these professional women from Weimar Germany will also be a strand in this paper.

Perspectives from Central Europe

On 11 April 1927, the first clinic concerned with the psychoanalytic treatment of psychoses in Central Europe, Schloss Tegel, opened its doors in Berlin.[4] The beginning and fall of the progressive clinic Schloss Tegel took place in the Weimar Republic (1918-1933), an important era for the social status of women, in particular of academic ones. Grossmann describes the living and working conditions of women doctors in those times after World War I, when they began to try to negotiate between traditional and modern role patterns or, as she says, between "maternity and modernity." Women doctors in Weimar Germany worked mainly in Social Democratic health centers, with ambitions to assist proletarian women with sexuality, family limitation, contraception, and abortion. They also carried these modern lifestyles into their own lives and were very satisfied in bringing together family, mostly with help of governesses and domestic help, and work. So they were special women with modern identities, because they were able to work, and work as professionals in German society.[5]

---

3. Major accounts include Kemal Bozay, *Exil Türkei: Ein Forschungsbeitrag zur deutschsprachigen Emigration in der Türkei (1933-1945)* (Münster: LIT Verlag, 2001); Cem Dalaman, "Die Türkei in ihrer Modernisierungsphase als Fluchtland für deutsche Exilanten" (Inaugural-Dissertation, Freie Universität Berlin, 1998); Fritz Neumark, *Zuflucht am Bosporus: Deutsche Gelehrte, Politiker und Künstler in der Emigration 1933-1953* (Frankfurt: Knecht Verlag, 1980); Horst Widmann, *Exil und Bildungshilfe: Die deutschsprachige akademische Emigration in die Türkei nach 1933* (Bern: Herbert und Peter Lang Verlag, 1973); Stanford Shaw, *Turkey and the Holocaust: Turkey's Role in Rescuing Turkish and European Jewry from Nazi Persecution, 1933-1945* (New York: New York University Press, 1993).

4. Edith Weigert described the patients there as "people who were at least borderline and some of them were manic depressive, others schizophrenics." Edith Weigert, interview on 13 June 1973, p. 7 of transcript, in Maren Holmes, "Leben und Werk der Psychiaterin und Psychoanalytikerin Dr. med. Edith Weigert-Vowinckel (1894-1982)" (M.A. thesis, Freie Universität Berlin, 2006), 39.

5. Atina Grossmann, "German Women Doctors from Berlin to New York: Maternity and Modernity in Weimar and in Exile," *Feminist Studies* 19 (1993): 65-88.

One such woman was Edith Weigert, born on 6 February 1894 in Düsseldorf as the daughter of seriously ill parents. She decided already as a young girl to become a doctor and save her parents and other patients from their suffering.[6] She began to study medicine at the end of the 1910s, when it was new for women to be present in universities. Edith Weigert and her friend Edith Jacobson kept solidly together when they were humiliated by the male students who thought that medicine was a science exclusively for men.[7] After finishing her medical studies in 1924, she began her analysis with Carl Müller Braunschweig at the Berlin Psychoanalytic Institute. She finished her psychoanalytic training in 1929 and became at the same year an assistant to Ernst Simmel in Schloss Tegel. Forty years later, in the introduction of her selected papers, *The Courage to Love*, she described the clinic as follows:

> In Simmel's open-ward hospital the patients were separated from home base. They were treated with daily psychoanalysis stirring up conflicts which mobilized asocial and antisocial impulses. There were neither the restraints nor the personnel which, in mental institutions with closed wards, prevent patients from acting out dangerous impulses.[8]

Despite many achievements, Schloss Tegel went into insolvency only four years later and had to close its doors in August 1931, due to the world economic crisis and the lack of public funds. That incident was a great reverse in clinical psychoanalytical treatment of psychoses, at least in Central Europe.

Another woman who shared similar experiences in prewar times was Ruth Wilmanns Lidz. She was born in Germany on 18 June 1910, the oldest child of Karl Wilmanns, a well-known psychiatrist of the "Heidelberg school."[9] In her autobiography she recalled telling her father about her

---

6. Autobiography of Edith Weigert, unpublished ms., p. 3, in Holmes, "Leben und Werk," 14.

7. See Robert A. Cohen, "Edith V. Weigert 1894–1982: Obituary," *Psychiatry: Journal for the Study of Interpersonal Processes* 45 (1982): 271ff.

8. Edith Weigert, *The Courage to Love: Selected Papers of Edith Weigert* (New Haven, CT: Yale University Press, 1970), x.

9. Karl Wilmanns (1873–1945), a student of Emil Kraepelin, worked with psychotic patients and did research on schizophrenia from the beginning of the 1920s. He had been appointed professor and director of the psychiatric university clinic of Heidelberg in 1918. Leo Hermle, "Karl Wilmanns (1873–1945)—biobibliographische Betrachtung einer psychiatrischen Ära," *Fortschritte der Neurologie und Psychiatrie* 56 (1988): 107. His scientific interest was mainly in the asocial behavior of people of the "lower" classes, but he also worked with psychotic patients, and from 1925 onward he did research on schizophrenia. Seven years later he

future wishes: studying medicine, getting married, and having children. Thereupon Karl Wilmanns had answered her: "Well, you will need the power of an elephant."[10] Like Weigert, from childhood on she had a special interest in mental diseases, in particular schizophrenia. During World War I, the Wilmanns family lived in a small house on the grounds of the Psychiatric Clinic of Lake Constance. Thus, as a little girl, Ruth had the opportunity to be in contact with psychotic patients, and she found their behavior sometimes very puzzling:

> The position of my father allowed me to acquire experience in dealing with patients and to learn about their impressions. He asked me sometimes to go for a walk with convalescent patients. In such talks they told me about their parents and siblings. I found their stories often quite strange, but they influenced me in my later work with the families of schizophrenic patients.[11]

The coming to power of National Socialists ended the careers of distinguished European psychoanalysts and of pioneer women physicians of Weimar Germany, who were for the most part Jewish or married to Jewish men.[12] They had to escape to various countries around the world, and they experienced the pain of losing relatives, their homeland, and their social status. According to Grossmann "the harsh days of emigration were the first time that they actually had to concern themselves with domestic drudgery."[13] They all experienced a "sudden crack" in their biographies,

---

edited a book on schizophrenia of nearly eight hundred pages, which then became a standard work: Karl Wilmanns, ed., *Die Schizophrenie: Handbuch der Geisteskrankheiten* (Berlin: Springer Verlag, 1932).

10. Ruth Wilmanns Lidz, "Ein erfülltes Leben," in *Psychoanalyse in Selbstdarstellungen II*, ed. Ludger M. Hermanns (Tübingen: edition diskord, 1994), 281.

11. Ruth Wilmanns Lidz, "Von Heidelberg nach Johns Hopkins," in *Emeriti erinnern sich: Rückblicke auf die Lehre und Forschung in Heidelberg: Die Medizinischen Fakultäten*, ed. Otto M. Marx and Annett Moses (Weinheim: I. VCH Verlagsgesellschaft, 1993), 258.

12. "In terms of the aggregate, neither the overall number of persecuted Jewish women doctors in Germany, Austria, and the occupied countries, nor the number of those who emigrated, has been identified. There are some estimates, though, which can be summarised in the following way. At the end of the Weimar Republic, around 3,400 women worked as medical doctors in Germany, and they formed seven per cent of the medical profession. There is some evidence that the number of Jews among the first women to enter the medical profession in the period of the Empire was very high. . . . The estimates for women doctors thereafter being persecuted as 'non-Aryan' or Jewish differ widely between 600 and 900, and these figures do not yet include Austria or any of the occupied countries." Anna von Villiez, "The Emigration of Women Doctors from Germany under National Socialism," *Social History of Medicine* 22 (2009): 558.

13. Grossman, "German Women Doctors," 80.

especially in their professional careers.[14] Although all emigrant women suffered from the psychic aftermath of emigration, some had a successful work history and life in their new homelands. For others, the experience led to a bitter end in serious mental disease or even suicide.

In June 1933, the father of Ruth Wilmanns Lidz was dismissed because of saying in a lecture to medical students that Adolf Hitler's temporary blindness, following an air raid in World War I, was a hysterical reaction rather than an organic problem.[15] Moreover, according to National Socialist doctrine, the mother of Ruth Wilmanns Lidz was graded as three-quarters Jewish, and so Ruth was classified as a Jew by 37.5 percent. Van Villiez observes that many women did not consider themselves as Jewish until the National Socialists declared them to be "Non Aryans."[16] Also, Ruth "knew somehow that [her] grandfather Victor Meyer was of Eastern Jewish background but had never thought further" about it.[17] Thus, the young woman was the daughter of a political enemy as well as of a partly Jewish mother. She recalled the humiliation she suffered during that time:

> To be thirty-seven and a half percent meant that I could not marry a German, but could work. In fact, people avoided me. . . . One day, as I was on the way to a lecture at the Voßstraße, an assistant from the Krehlsche Clinic tried to run me down with his car, screaming "vermin" out of the window.[18]

Her parents were in a life-threatening situation and found a hideout in a retirement home for Catholic priests, run by an order of nuns who worked as nurses at Karl Wilmanns's clinic, and therefore they could hardly care for their children in those fatal times. A neighbor's son, despite his being a Nazi himself, warned Ruth that the future would be getting worse and that she should leave the country as soon as she could. So she interrupted

---

14. Von Viliez, "The Emigration of Women Doctors," 556. Atina Grossmann, "New Women in Exile: German Women Doctors and the Emigration," in *Between Sorrow and Strength: Women Refugees of the Nazi Period*, ed. Sibylle Quack (Cambridge: Cambridge University Press, 1995), 215.

15. Hermle, "Karl Wilmanns," 56, 108. "When the Gestapo searched his home, saying that they were looking for evidence he called his dog Hitler, which he said he wouldn't do to his dog, they were actually looking to see if he had a copy of the medical record that documented the hysterical blindness. He didn't, but he had heard of the hysteria from a colleague in Munich who had had Hitler as a patient in a military hospital during World War I." Victor Lidz, grandson of Karl Wilmanns, personal communication, 2 June 2010.

16. Von Viliez, "The Emigration of Women Doctors," 555.

17. Ruth Wilmanns Lidz, "Unpublished Autobiography for Her Family" (private ownership of Victor Lidz, quoted with permission), 5.

18. Wilmanns Lidz, "Ein erfülltes Leben," 284–85.

her medical studies[19] in Heidelberg,[20] and when she was offered the opportunity of learning Swedish massage and physiotherapy in Stockholm, she took the night train to Sweden in August 1933. Although the young woman had to interrupt her medical studies, she thought that she would stand a good chance in her first exile country, with her three years of study in medicine. After initial difficulties of being very hungry until she received pay after two weeks, because she had been limited to 10 marks when leaving Germany, she had a good time in Sweden. Some nine months later, she obtained a training certificate for massage, kinesiatrics, and electrotherapy. Ruth Wilmanns then began to think about ways to finish her medical studies, and so she moved to Basel in Switzerland to live with the family of her uncle and write her doctoral dissertation. In 1935, she received her medical degree at the University of Basel with a thesis entitled "How Can a Person Come to Terms with the Amputation of a Limb?"[21] Seeking an appointment in Switzerland was not realistic because it would be limited to one year, and Swiss citizens had preference. Oscar Forel, the son of August Forel, Eugen Bleuler's successor at the Burghölzli, offered her an unofficial position and a temporary home in a clinic for affluent patients, where she could gather experience with psychotic patients. Then she was offered various posts abroad, including in Bangkok, Bombay, and Istanbul, since the case of her father had become public.

That same year, 1935, Edith Weigert was also forced to emigrate to Turkey with her Jewish husband, Oscar Weigert, and their two-year-old son, Wolfgang.[22] The founder of the Turkish Republic, Mustafa Kemal Atatürk, offered Oscar Weigert an appointment in Ankara as a consultant at the Turkish Department of Trade and Industry during the reform process of 1933.[23] Like many professional women in exile who stood back to enable their husbands to work in their former occupations, Weigert spent three

19. The course of her studies: Summer Term (ST) 1929: Heidelberg; Winter Term (WT) 1929/30: Munich; WT 1930/31: Heidelberg; WT 1931/32: Munich; ST 1932: Heidelberg; WT 1932/33: Innsbruck; ST 1933: Heidelberg; 1933/1934: Dr. Kjellbers Institute Stockholm; WT and ST 1935: Basel; 6 June 1935, doctoral examination at the University of Basel.

20. She had been refused permission to register again as a student at the University of Heidelberg because of the 37.5 percent, according to Victor Lidz.

21. Ruth Wilmanns, *Wie findet sich der Mensch mit der Amputation eines Gliedes ab?* (Inaugural-Dissertation, University of Basel, Leipzig: Druck der Spamer A.-G., 1935).

22. Wolfgang Weigert was born on 20 November 1932 in Berlin and died on 30 September 2009 in Sandy Spring, Maryland. He had a private practice in psychiatry and psychoanalysis in Chevy Chase for more than thirty years. Wolfgang Weigert graduated in 1973 from Washington Center for Psychoanalysis, where he studied adult and child psychoanalysis. He had two children, David Weigert of Silver Spring and Robin Weigert of Los Angeles.

23. Holmes, "Leben und Werk," 61.

years of her life in this very different culture under harsh circumstances and "dedicated [herself] to [their] son."[24]

Perspectives from Turkey

In Turkey, in outbuildings of mosques, so-called *bimarhane* (asylums) had been built in which, in addition to the sick and neglected, psychotic patients known as *deli* (insane) were also accommodated. Because the Quran describes them as persons in need of care, the *deli* were not ostracized under the Ottoman regime but were considered extraordinary creations of Allah. Different methods of treatment were tried out to free these "poor people" from their disease. It was believed that the psychotic state could be ended by inducing panic and fear. Patients were often "cured" with "shock treatments" while being confined in dark rooms of prayer homes (*tekke*). According to Erkoç, at the beginning of the twentieth century, the greater number of Turkish psychiatrists still believed that mental diseases were caused by forces of evil.[25]

In 1909, the year when Sigmund Freud gave his lectures at Clark University, the first volume of a psychiatric textbook, *Tababet-i Ruhiye*, appeared in Turkey. It was written in the Ottoman language—which is written in Arabic script and sounds different from modern Turkish—by Mazhar Osman Uzman (1884–1951), the founder of modern psychiatry in Turkey. In 1908 he had gone to Germany in order to study with Theodor Ziehen in Berlin and Emil Kraepelin in Munich. All his life Osman Uzman attended numerous congresses in Central Europe, especially in Germany. He wanted to replace what he called the "superstitious healing movement" in Turkey by introducing modern European psychiatry.[26] Therefore he sent many of his students and employees abroad and arranged for foreign psychiatrists to come to Turkey to establish modern psychiatry in his home country.[27] In his works, the tradition of the German psychiatric school of the turn of the

---

24. Von Villiez, "The Emigration of Women Doctors," 563–64. Edith Weigert, interview on 13 June 1973, p. 11 of transcript, in Holmes, "Leben und Werk," 60.
25. Şahap Erkoç and Olcay Yazıcı, *Mazhar Osman ve Dönemi: Mecnunları, Mekanları, Dostları* (İstanbul: Argos İletişim Hizmetleri Reklamcılık ve Ticaret A.Ş., 2006), 3.
26. Mazhar Osman Uzman, *Tababet-i Ruhiye* (İstanbul: Faskül I. Kader Basımevi, 1941), 90.
27. "It was not permitted to write about insanity before the reform. A member of the Ottoman ruling class, the insane Hamid the Second, censored all publications that contained terms such as craziness, love delirium, or institutionalization, because they reminded him of his brother, who was incapable of governing." Osman Uzman, *Tababet-i Ruhiye*, 3, foreword to the second edition. This refers to the Ottoman sultan Abdülhamid the Second (1842–1918), and his assumed psychiatrically ill brother Murad the Fifth.

last century is clearly discernible. In general, his early writings show a hostile, and his later ones an ambivalent, attitude toward psychoanalysis.[28]

In the third edition of *Tababet-i Ruhiye* (1941), Osman Uzman also discussed psychoanalysis and described its theory and its most important definitions. There he acknowledged the achievements of psychoanalysis, especially in the interpretations of dreams, but he criticized its "pansexualism" and the exclusively psychological explanation of psychic diseases. He wrote: "Neither do we glorify Freudianism as a new school nor do we want to disdain it, as was done in some congresses in Germany."[29] Osman Uzman in 1933 was appointed ordinary professor at the Clinic for Psychiatry at Istanbul University. Organic psychiatry on the German model was effectively established in Turkey, excluding psychoanalytic viewpoints in training and treatment programs.

Occasionally signs of interest in psychoanalysis appeared among Turkish intellectuals. In 1927, for example, a translation of Sigmund Freud's lectures at Clark University into the Ottoman language was done by the psychologist Mustafa Şekip Tunç. A second edition of his book appeared in modern Turkish in 1931.[30]

Most importantly, in 1925, a psychiatrist, Izeddin A. Şadan, began working at the Toptaşı Bimarhanesi, an asylum in Üsküdar/Istanbul, under the direction of Osman Uzman.[31] Şadan worked according to the model of organically oriented psychiatry until he read about emerging developments

28. Şahap Erkoç, personal communication, 28 April 2010.

29. He also mentioned that psychoanalytic theories, in particular the concept of libido, had already been known by the Turks in ancient times. As an example, he mentioned the Turkish doctor Ibn Sina (Avicenna). Osman Uzman, *Tababet-i-Ruhiye*, 399, 48ff. When Ibn Sina observed symptoms like insomnia, anorexia, manic-depressive states, and psychotic thought disorders, he examined first of all the mood of the *mecnun* (people with love delirium; also a synonym for general insanity like *deli*). Thereby he applied methods similar to the association tests of C. G. Jung. "When Ibn Sina was called for the treatment of a young relative of a king ... who had lost weight and could neither eat nor sleep, he measured his pulse. After that he ordered a servant to speak loudly the names of parts of the city while checking the pulse of the prince. He noticed that his pulse rose when he heard certain names. He repeated the same procedure with the names of streets, houses, and the persons who lived inside. When the name of a certain person was mentioned, his pulse noticeably quickened. Thus the remedy for his illness was identified: after being brought together [with that girl] his melancholic state disappeared." Osman Uzman, *Tababet-i-Ruhiye*, 49–50, abbreviated translation.

30. S. Freud, *Froydizm: Psikanalize dair beş ders*, trans. Mustafa Şekip Tunç (İstanbul: Muallim Ahmet Halit Kitaphanesi, 1931). Probably the first Turkish translation of a work of Sigmund Freud.

31. Izeddin A. Şadan was born in 1893 as the son of a high-ranking official in Istanbul and received a very good education. See Betül Yalciner and Lütfü Hanoğlu, *İç bahçe: Toptaşı'ndan Bakırköye akıl hastanesi* (İstanbul: Okyanus Yayın, 2001), 35ff. He began his medical studies in 1919 at the *Mekteb-i Tıbbiye-i Şahane*, which had been established as the first medical faculty of

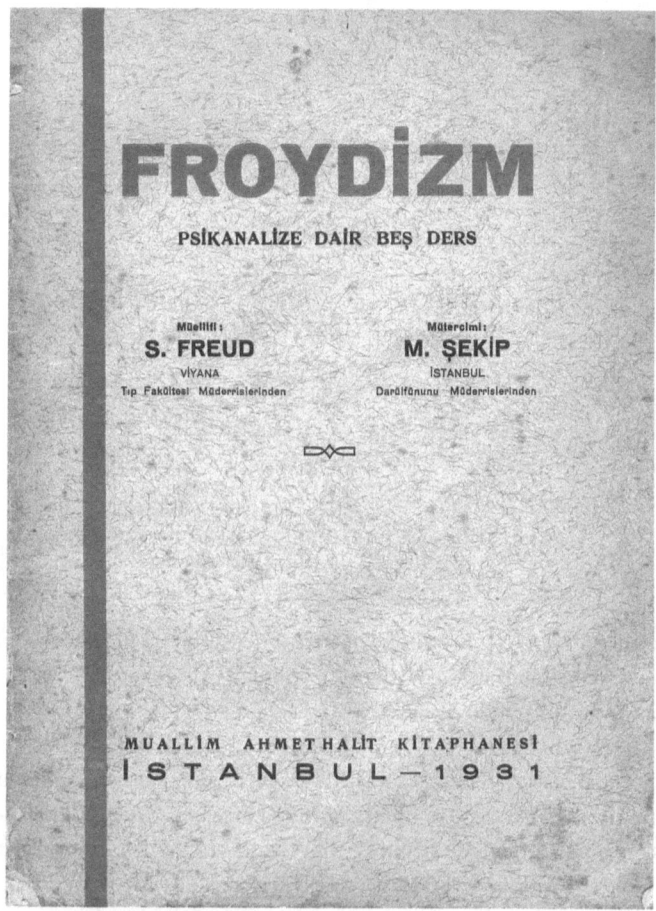

5.1. Turkish translation of Sigmund Freud's five lectures at Clark University. Cover of the second edition of the first translation of a psychoanalytic work into Turkish, *Froydizm: Psikanalize dair beş ders* (Istanbul: Muallim Ahmet Halit Kitaphanesi, 1931). Private collection of the author.

in psychopathology and psychoanalysis in the English journal the *Lancet*, and developed an interest in this new school. At the Toptaşı Bimarhanesi, however, this new theory was not particularly welcome:

> At the Toptaşı neither Brill, nor Freud, nor Bleuler, nor Jung was mentioned. . . . Once I told . . . [Mazhar Osman Uzman] about Bleuler, and he

---

the Ottoman Empire in 1827 under the regime of Mahmut the Second. Şadan wanted to specialize in psychiatry and neurology even before beginning his academic studies.

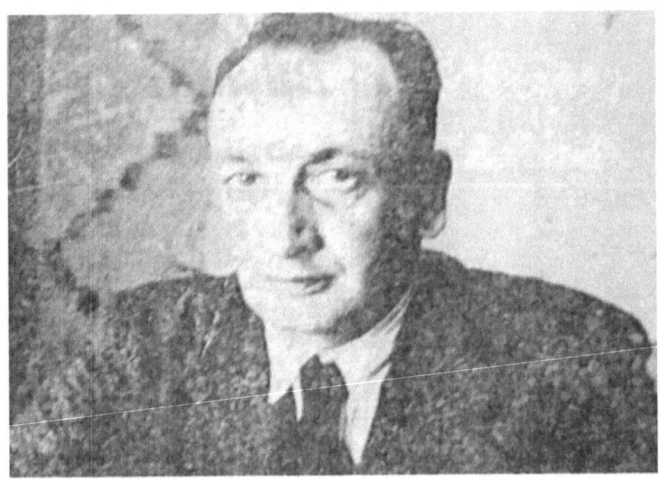

5.2. Izeddin A. Şadan, the analysand of Edith Weigert and the pioneer of psychoanalysis in Turkey, 1936. Reprinted from *Acıksöz*, 20 July 1936, page 5. Private collection of the author.

answered by saying [sarcastically]: "very interesting." The doctors at the Toptaşı followed the views of Kraepelin, with the belief that they understood him, although they did not.[32]

Soon the controversy alienated Şadan from his colleagues, who excluded him from their community. In his *hatırat* (memoirs), Şadan wrote about a turning point in his life after he had read the book *Traite theorique et pratique de psychanalyse* by Ernest Jones.[33] The method of free association and new perspectives on the psychoses impressed him. The "second experience" derived also from Jones. Şadan recounted how for the first time he read about the relation between paranoia and homosexuality. He even observed this connection, as described by Jones, in one of his patients and presented the case in a lecture, whereupon his colleagues attacked him vehemently.[34]

In July 1927, Şadan came into conflict with Osman Uzman concerning his working schedule and thereupon resigned from his job. In the same year, he went to Paris to work as an assistant of Joseph Rogues de Fursac.

32. Izzedin A. Şadan, "Hatırat," in *Istanbul Bakırköy Akıl ve Sinir Hastalıkları Hastanesi Yıllığı: Bakırköy'de 50 Yıl* (İstanbul, 1977), 133.

33. The French translation of the third edition of Ernest Jones, *Papers on Psychoanalysis* (London: Ballière, Tindall & Cox, 1923). I am grateful to Ernst Falzeder for this clue.

34. Şadan, "Hatırat," 133.

After his return from France three years later, Şadan began to publish many psychoanalytic articles in different Turkish journals and newspapers. He also translated several works by C. G. Jung, Ernest Jones, and Abraham Brill into Turkish.[35] His writings could be regarded as the first original works on psychoanalysis in Turkey.

From the 1930s on, Şadan actually got in touch with Sigmund Freud and sought his assistance in translating some of his works — for example, the *Three Essays on Sexuality* — into Turkish. In a letter of 12 August 1938, he called Freud his "Illustrious Master" and expressed sorrow about the latter's forced emigration to London. Their correspondence continued until Freud's death.[36]

According to Erkoç, the life of Şadan can be divided into two parts, a psychoanalytic period that lasted until the early 1950s, and then his turning away from psychoanalysis and joining nationalistic Turkish circles.[37] Şadan's later distance from psychoanalysis could be explained by his "strange" personality. According to the memoirs of the historian Altan Deliorman, Şadan had "paranoid traits" and was very capricious. He never married, had no children, and lived in a dark and humid flat. Yalçıner and Hanoğlu wrote that Şadan never had a practice and lived from his patrimony.[38] His "family" was the *Marmara Kıraathanesi*, a café in Beyazıt/Istanbul, where the intellectuals spent their spare time. The strange character of Şadan fascinated many patrons of the café, and they called him not "the doctor of the insane" (*deli doktoru*), but "the insane doctor" (*deli doktor*).[39]

In the "Korrespondenzblatt" of the *Internationale Zeitschrift für Psychoanalyse und Imago* for 1939, there is a note that "a [Turkish] psychiatrist, who is at present in training analysis, has achieved a thorough theoretical education and [has] translated several works of Freud into Turkish."[40] The only psychoanalyst then in Turkey among the emigrants was Edith Weigert.[41]

---

35. See Levent Kayaalp, "L'histoire d'un rendez-vous manqué: L'exemple de la Turquie," *Topique: L'Esprit du temps* 89 (2004): 124–25.

36. Izeddin A. Şadan to Sigmund Freud, 12 August 1938, Library of Congress, Sigmund Freud Papers, Box 30.

37. Şahap Erkoç, personal communication, 8 May 2009. From the second half of the twentieth century on, his writings were published in nationalistic Turkish journals, for example, in the journal *Orkun*.

38. Yalcıner and Hanoğlu, *İç bahçe*, 45.

39. Altan Deliorman, *Hatırat Kitaplığı: Türk Yurdunun Bilgeleri* (İstanbul: Timaş Yayınları, 2009), 222ff.; Altan Deliorman, personal communication, 5 May 2009.

40. *Internationale Zeitschrift für Psychoanalyse und Imago* 24 (1939): 230.

41. Her addresses in Turkey are registered in the "Korrespondenzblatt" in the *Internationale Zeitschrift für Psychoanalyse* as follows: Belvü-Palas-Oteli, Ankara (1935); Atatürk-Bulvar 54, Ankara-Yenischir (1936); Kizil Irmak Sokak, Nihat, Pasa Apartmani, Ankara-Yenischir (1937).

She did not take up formal employment there but obtained from Atatürk a special permit to practice psychoanalysis.[42] The report in the "Korrespondenzblatt" stated that "Mrs. Edith Weigert-Vowinckel is like a training center, and she arouses the interest of Turkish doctors in psychoanalysis."[43] Although she had declared in an interview that she could not practice in Turkey, she attributed this to difficulties in working with the local population. In the interview, Weigert recalled that she had a Turkish psychiatrist in analysis, but she did not refer to him by name: "We conducted this analysis in French because that was the only language in which we could meet." Her analysand must have been Şadan, because he lived at the same time as Edith Weigert in Ankara, spoke French, and translated several psychoanalytic works into Turkish.[44]

As the only psychoanalyst in Turkey,[45] Weigert felt very lonely in her country of exile. In an interview with Volkan and Itzkowitz, she stated that there were no social contacts between the emigrants who lived in Çankaya, a district in Ankara, and the resident Turks.[46] Many other emigrants recounted in their memoirs that the contact between them and the homegrown Turks were few, and they were in communication almost exclusively with professional colleagues. Only a few could adapt to the culture, and many of them had difficulties in learning Turkish.[47] Furthermore, their contacts with the international scientific community were also limited, and so for a large number of the emigrants, Turkey was just a stopover on their way to another country such as the U.S.

---

42. Vamık D. Volkan and Norman Itzowitz, *Ölümsüz Atatürk* (İstanbul: Bağlam Yayıncılık, 2007), 385.

43. *Internationale Zeitschrift für Psychoanalyse* 23 (1937): 186.

44. Weigert, interview on 13 June 1973, p. 10 in transcript, in Holmes, "Leben und Werk," 62. "I recall that when I spoke with Edith Weigert I got the impression that İzeddin Şadan did not undergo a proper psychoanalytic process. Reading the Turkish translation of his paper and parts of his memoirs I came to the conclusion that İzeddin Şadan's approach to psychoanalysis was highly intellectualized." Vamık D. Volkan, "Psychoanalysis, Turkey and the IPA," in *100 Years of IPA: The Centenary History of the International Psychoanalytical Association, 1910–2010—Evolution and Change*, ed. Peter Loewenberg and Nellie L. Thompson (London: IPA Publications, Karnac Books, 2011).

45. Nikolaj J. Ossipow, a Russian psychoanalyst and the first psychoanalyst who was forced to leave his homeland, also spent time in Turkey in the beginning of the 1920s. He had to escape from the Bolsheviks. Eugenia Fischer et al., eds., *Sigmund Freud and Nikolaj J. Ossipow: Briefwechsel 1921–1929* (Frankfurt: Brandes & Apsel, 2009).

46. Edith Weigert interview on 29 May 1974, in Volkan and Itzkowitz, *Ölümsüz Atatürk*, 385.

47. Thomas Herr, "Ein deutscher Sozialdemokrat an der Peripherie: Ernst Reuter im türkischen Exil 1935–1946," in *Die Emigration der Wissenschaften nach 1933: Disziplingeschichtliche Studie*, ed. Herbert A. Strauss (München: K. G. Saur Verlag, 1991), 215.

In general, the social situation of emigrants in Turkey in the 1930s depended in particular on their gender and on their social status in their homelands.[48] Male professors who had been called to positions at the Istanbul University and who earned much more money than their Turkish colleagues were also in a more privileged situation than were female emigrants and obtained leading positions.[49] In the years 1933 to 1934, the directors of the Medical Faculty of the Istanbul University were almost entirely male emigrant professors.[50] Despite Atatürk's granting rights to women in elections, education, and employment, his reforms took effect very slowly. Thus, women, especially emigrant women such as Edith Weigert and Ruth Wilmanns Lidz, experienced difficult working conditions.[51]

During her time in Turkey, Weigert wrote an anthropological work as well as an article about the theory of schizophrenia, which she would later publish in a major English-language psychoanalytic journal.[52] She sent her anthropological study entitled "Psychoanalytische Gedanken zum Kultus und Mythos der Magna Mater" ("Psychoanalytic Thoughts on the Cult and Myth of the Magna Mater") to Sigmund Freud and expected a publication in the journal *Imago*. In contrast to her expectations, Sigmund Freud criticized her text because she did not mention the Oedipus complex, castra-

---

48. The exact number of the emigrants in Turkey is not definitely established. The total number of the German-speaking emigrants until the end of World War II is estimated to be between 400,000 (Arslan, *Beiträge deutscher Wissenschaftler*, 86) and 500,000 persons (Strauss, *Emigration der Wissenschaften*, 10). According to Erichsen, from about 1,200 to 1,500 emigrant scholars from German Universities emigrated after 1933 to Turkey. She then relativizes the number, "because there are unexplained references to potential emigrants in the personal files at the Istanbul University." The main body of the emigrant scholars between 1933 and 1944 were employed at Istanbul University. A small number were in academic institutions in Ankara, which affiliated from 1946 to form the Ankara University. Regine Erichsen, "Die Emigration deutschsprachiger Naturwissenschaftler von 1933 bis 1945 in die Türkei in ihrem sozial- und wissenschaftshistorischen Wirkungszusammenhang," in Strauss, *Die Emigration der Wissenschaften nach 1933*, 96. Arslan, *Beiträge deutscher Wissenschaftler*, 87, determines the number of emigrated German scholars in Turkey between 1933 and 1944 to be 700 to 800 persons, among whom 208 persons are known by name. In the *Biografisches Handbuch der deutschsprachigen Emigration nach 1933*, there are in total 134 German-speaking emigrants in Turkey registered. Werner Röder and Herbert A. Strauss, *Biographisches Handbuch der deutschsprachigen Emigration nach 1933* (München: K. G. Saur Verlag, 1999), 121ff.

49. Sertan Batur, "Institutionalisierung der Psychologie an der Universität Istanbul" (M.A. thesis, University of Vienna); http://othes.univie.ac.at/10733/1/Institutionalisierung.PDF, 21.

50. Cf. Arslan, *Beiträge deutscher Wissenschaftler*, 88ff.

51. Regine Erichsen, "Das türkische Exil als Geschichte von Frauen und ihr Beitrag zum Wissenschaftstransfer in die Türkei von 1933 bis 1945," *Berichte zur Wissenschaftsgeschichte* 28 (2005): 337–53, describes the harsh conditions emigrant Austrian and German women experienced in Turkey.

52. Edith Weigert-Vowinckel, "A Contribution to the Theory of Schizophrenia," *International Journal of Psychoanalysis* 17 (1936): 190–201.

tion anxiety, and his work on totem and taboo, and so he did not support the publication of the article. As a kind of an apology, Weigert mentioned in her reply the disadvantageous scientific conditions for psychoanalytic work in Turkish exile:

> True, I am working here alone under conditions that are not amenable to exchange of opinions with scholars in my own field. My reason for wishing to be published by the psychoanalytic publishers is because I am afraid of being excluded from the scientific discussion of the psa. collective work. I consider this discussion essential to my whole research, even though at the moment my emigration status makes participation difficult.[53]

The absence of a psychoanalytic community demoralized Weigert. For her, Turkey was indeed only a stopover on her way to the U.S., where psychoanalysis had already gained ground. After her husband had finished his work in 1938, and her son had reached school age, "it was a natural way for [them] to go."[54] She became a major figure in the American psychoanalytic community, which had by then been joined by many other refugees.

Ruth Wilmanns Lidz also emigrated to Turkey in 1935, but to Istanbul, not Ankara. She was a young doctor, not trained in psychoanalysis, and her time in Turkey contributed mainly to her decision to specialize in psychiatry and later in psychoanalysis. According to her son, Victor Lidz, his mother's job in Turkey was arranged by Philipp Schwartz, a German emigrant pathologist at Istanbul University.[55] According to the records at the Guraba Clinic,[56] Ruth Wilmanns arrived in Istanbul on 15 December 1935 and began her job at the local department of otolaryngology the following day.[57]

Her circumstances seemed very strange to the young woman in the new country. She was afraid of the Turkish patients, who were sitting on the floor of the hospital. At first she could not speak with anybody in her mother tongue until she got in touch with an Austrian nurse, who explained the

---

53. Letter of 16 October 1937, in Holmes, "Leben und Werk," in English in the original, 66. The Papers of Sigmund Freud, Box 43, Folder 20, Weigert, Edith 1937–1939, Library of Congress.

54. Edith Weigert, interview on 13 June 1973, p. 12 in transcript, in Holmes, *Leben und Werk*, 69.

55. Victor Lidz, personal communication, 28 February 2009.

56. File of "Frl. Ruth Wilmanns," dated 16 December 1935. Archives of the Guraba Clinic in Istanbul. Today the clinic is known under the name of Bezm-I-Âlem Vâlide Sultan-Vakıf Gureba Hastanesi. Her file is also at the archive of the Medical Faculty of Istanbul University.

57. In her unpublished autobiography, 14, Ruth Wilmanns wrote that she arrived in Istanbul in November 1935.

new professional environment to her. Her "room" was a big hall built for approximately ten beds. The "bath" was at the end of the corridor and was encircled by a metallic wall. A little hole on the ground was the toilet, and the cleaning was done with water instead of toilet paper. According to her own words, her supervisor regarded her as his property. He did not allow her to take her meals together with the male doctors in the dining room. Although Wilmanns Lidz was a graduate physician during her exile in Turkey and should have worked according to her contract with the Guraba Clinic as a "research assistant," she in fact worked there as a nurse.[58] She felt like a "gofer girl" and had to do all the "dirty work" that the male doctors did not want to do:

> I remember one case well: A young man from the countryside had a big tumor on a cheek which was full of worms. One of the doctors had spoken with him and had checked him up and I had to clean him before an operation could be considered. It took a lot of time to do that.[59]

Outside of work, too, it was difficult for this young woman to adapt to the culture. In a Turkish bath she had the following experience:

> I first went to the Hamam—the Turkish bath—where an attendant woman threw a blue hair remover paste on my legs and pubic area without even asking. I later learned to stop her by saying, "I am European" in Turkish.[60]

She worked seven days a week, from seven o'clock in the morning until eight in the evening. Now and then she could convince her superior to grant her a free Sunday afternoon, and she enjoyed those occasions. She spent her spare time with a Turkish internist who had studied in France and with a Greek family, and she often went to the Bosporus for swimming. She thought that it was while swimming in the Bosporus that she might have contracted hepatitis, and she fell seriously ill. Her boss did not allow her to rest or take time off, although she was visibly yellow in her face. She became very depressed and lost much of her vitality.[61] She also

---

58. Ruth Wilmanns Lidz, "Von Heidelberg nach Johns Hopkins," 263. Wilmanns Lidz, unpublished autobiography, 15. In the records of the archive she is described as a nurse and not a physician.
59. Wilmanns Lidz, "Ein erfülltes Leben," 290.
60. Wilmanns Lidz, unpublished autobiography, 15.
61. Victor Lidz, personal communication, 8 December 2008. Her father told Max Müller, a psychiatrist from Switzerland, that his daughter was, after her arrival at their home in Germany, "very changed, depressed, discouraged, and no more in the possession of her previous vitality

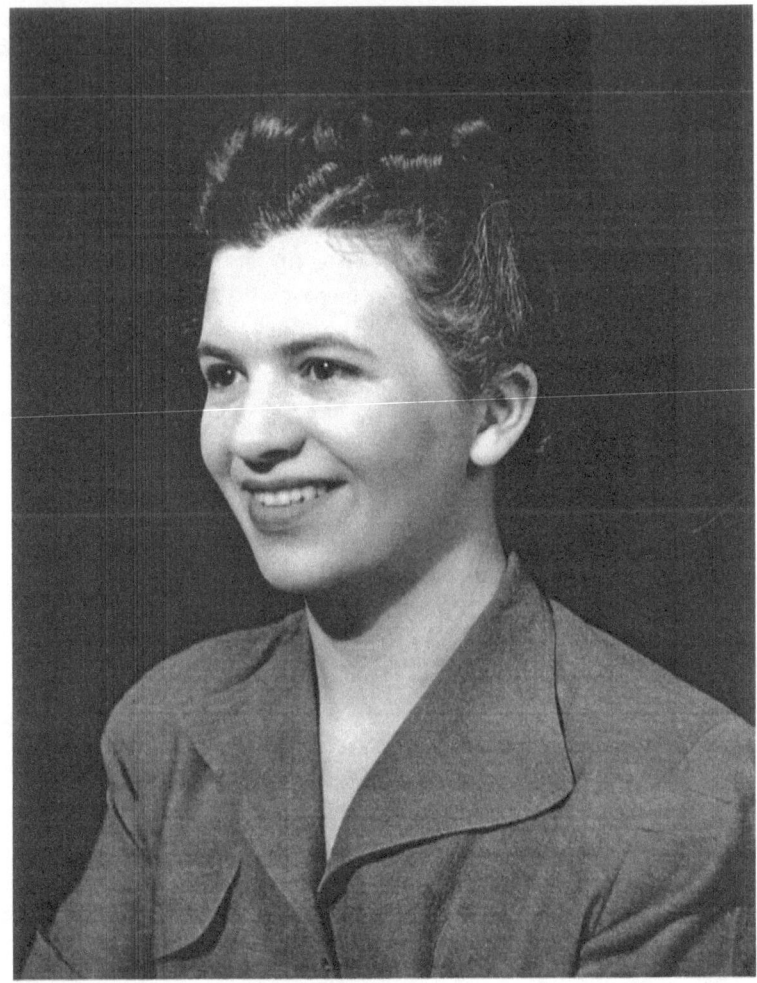

5.3. Ruth Wilmanns Lidz as a young woman in her twenties. Generously furnished by her son, Victor Lidz.

had problems in eating and wanted to return by all means to Switzerland. In her diary, she never complained about her hard work but wrote that a female doctor had no social role in Turkey. In one of her autobiographical essays, Wilmanns Lidz wrote that "in retrospect . . . it [was] probably not

---

and her recklessness." Max Müller, *Erinnerungen: Erlebte Psychiatriegeschichte 1920–1960* (Berlin: Springer Verlag, 1982), 206.

as bad as it appeared to me then, as I was young and in a very uncertain situation."⁶²

In her mid-twenties, Wilmanns Lidz wanted to specialize in reconstructive surgery.⁶³ She came to a different decision in Turkey, however. One day she had to bring her superior something from the library, and she discovered an article in an Austrian journal from February 1934 about the insulin shock treatment of schizophrenic patients, written by Manfred Sakel.⁶⁴ She read about this treatment and considered the possibility of emigrating to the U.S. if she were to learn this method. As she later explained, prior to this she had never thought about emigration to the U.S. because she remembered Americans as being "loud, beer drinking and, thus, uncivilized people, who in the summer came as tourists to Heidelberg."⁶⁵ In the end, she decided to write to Adolf Meyer at the Johns Hopkins Hospital and ask him if she could get a job there if she were to learn the insulin treatment and establish it at his clinic.

As she had a one-year contract with the Guraba Clinic, there was a problem with the termination.⁶⁶ She did not want to follow the advice from a Turkish friend just to leave Turkey. "Was there a way to get out of the contract without leaving a black mark on my record?"⁶⁷ She also asked a German-Jewish friend who had lived in Turkey for a long time and who knew the mentality very well⁶⁸ how she should act:

---

62. Victor Lidz, personal communication, 28 February 2009. Wilmanns Lidz, "Von Heidelberg nach Johns Hopkins," 264.

63. "[Her] wish grew out of seeing the injuries of World War I soldiers in Germany. However, her father discouraged this ambition, saying that too many patients for reconstructive surgery were paranoid and dangerous and therefore it was not a good field for a woman physician. In other respects, however, he clearly encouraged her desire to be a physician, I think, from an early age. Certainly it was not every bourgeois German girl whose parents installed a laboratory, with benches, Bunsen burner, chemicals, microscope, etc. for her in their new house, as her father did when they built the large house on the Bergstrasse. At any rate, the ambition to be a surgeon may have made the position in otolaryngology at the Guraba attractive. I know she was proud of the surgery she was able to do there, although she was allowed to do only simple procedures. One day's entry in her diary noted that she had done her first tonsillectomy by herself." Victor Lidz, personal communication, 2 June 2010.

64. Manfred Sakel, "Schizophreniebehandlung mittels Insulin-Hypoglykämie sowie hypoglykämischer Schocks," *Wiener Medizinische Wochenschrift* 84 (1934): 1211–14, 1265–69, 1299–301, 1326–27, 1353–55, 1383–85, 1401–4.

65. Wilmanns Lidz, "Ein erfülltes Leben," 291.

66. Records about the yearlong contract in the file "Frl. Ruth Wilmanns" at the archive of the Guraba Clinic.

67. Wilmanns Lidz, unpublished autobiography, 18.

68. He is with the utmost probability Dr. Kurt Adler, with whom she had an intimate relationship, according to her diary. Victor Lidz, personal communication, 28 February 2009.

He answered: "Let me think about it, tomorrow you will get an answer." The following day he said to me: "Ruth, are you a good actress?" I was puzzled and shocked. He explained to me that in the dean's office I should put the contract on his desk—he would sign it automatically. Hearing my plan he would say, "But what about your contract?" I could then smile and say: "Thank you, you just signed me out of it." And that is precisely how it happened. Obviously the Turks sign things in a certain way automatically![69]

Adolf Meyer replied promptly to her request and offered her a job at the Phipps Clinic of Johns Hopkins Hospital for 150 dollars a month, provided that she would establish the insulin method there. Ruth Wilmanns left Turkey on 6 September 1936 and boarded a ship to Italy.[70] From there, she took a train to Switzerland, where she "worked with great interest in Münsingen," learning the insulin treatment at the clinic there, headed by Max Müller, and then arranged for her emigration to the U.S.[71]

Perspectives from the United States

According to Grossmann, in the United States, many of the emigrant women physicians turned to socially oriented work because the licensing and financial requirements were not so strict. Social work, psychotherapy, and psychoanalysis were regarded there, as in Germany, as "womanly" and "caring."[72] Nevertheless, the American living and working conditions were very difficult for "the new women" from Weimar Germany. Only a few women were allowed to study and earn a chance for a position. In addition, women were restricted to very conservative role patterns. Wilmanns Lidz recounted in her unpublished autobiography how in America during World War II even professional women had to be careful about their personal lives. One colleague advised her to answer all questions about sexuality in the "personal studies" that they had to give Adolf Meyer with "no." An unmarried woman who already had sexual experiences or had given birth to a child was regarded as mentally ill even in medical circles.[73] Swiss-

---

69. Wilmanns Lidz, "Ein erfülltes Leben," 292.
70. The records at the Guraba Clinic and at the Medical Faculty of the Istanbul University end with the document of 13 February 1936.
71. Wilmanns Lidz, "Ein erfülltes Leben," 292.
72. Grossman, "German Women Doctors," 86.
73. Wilmanns Lidz, unpublished autobiography, 22. According to psychoanalyst Else Pappenheim, who had also emigrated to America and worked at the Johns Hopkins Hospital, only a very small percentage of psychiatrists were females in the U.S. before World War II.

born Adolf Meyer (1866–1950) also had conservative attitudes regarding the behavioral patterns of women, but he appointed many female immigrants at Johns Hopkins Hospital.[74]

Meyer had emigrated to the U.S. in 1892, at the age of 26, and for the first ten years worked as a neurologist and pathologist.[75] Due to his medical training in the Swiss tradition of the turn of the last century, he was at the time mainly interested in the organic aspects of mental disorders. As can be seen from his concept of "psychobiology," however, he then slowly moved away from pure somaticism and began to integrate psychological viewpoints into his thinking. In 1902 he became director of the Pathological Institute of the New York State Hospital, one of the most important psychiatric teaching and research centers in America. It was there, with continuing ties to medical developments in his native Switzerland, that he developed his approach to psychiatry.[76] As Skues notes in his paper above, Meyer also gave a lecture at Clark in 1909. On that occasion, Meyer spoke on "The Dynamic Interpretation of Dementia Praecox." In his address, Meyer emphasized patients' failures to adapt to their environment and occasionally also used psychoanalytic terms, such as "wish-fulfillment" and "complexes."[77]

In 1913, at the age of 44, he became professor of psychiatry at Johns

---

Pappenheim recalled that few women were allowed to study at the university in America, and that only a few got positions: "I was appalled at the general opinions about women. We experienced some set-backs. . . . At each party, first we ate together, and then the men separated from the women. Unthinkable in Vienna!" Else Pappenheim, interview with Nancy Chodorow, 27 August 1980, in *Else Pappenheim: Hölderlin, Feuchtersleben, Freud: Beiträge zur Geschichte der Psychoanalyse, der Psychiatrie und Neurologie*, ed. Bernhard Handlbauer (Graz-Wien: Nausner & Nausner, 2004), 82.

74. For more information about the life and work of Adolf Meyer, see Ruth Leys and Rand B. Evans, *Defining American Psychology: The Correspondence between Adolf Meyer and Edward Bradford Titchener* (Baltimore: Johns Hopkins University Press, 1990); Ruth Leys, "Types of One: Adolf Meyer's Life Chart and the Representation of Individuality," *Representations* 34 (1991): 1–28; Ruth Leys, "Meyer, Watson, and the Dangers of Behaviorism," *Journal of the History of the Behavioral Sciences* 20 (1984): 128–49; Ruth Leys, "Meyer, Jung, and the Limits of Association," *Bulletin of the History of Medicine* 59 (1985), 345–60; Ruth Leys, "Meyer's Dealings with Ernest Jones: A Chapter in the History of the American Response to Psychoanalysis," *Journal of the History of the Behavioral Sciences* 17 (1981): 445–65.

75. In the U.S., beginning a psychiatric career as a pathologist was not unusual at the time. See Uwe Henrik Peters, "Adolf Meyer und die Beziehung zwischen deutscher und amerikanischer Psychiatrie," *Fortschritte der Neurologie und Psychiatrie* 58 (1990): 333.

76. Nathan G. Hale Jr., *Freud and the Americans: The Beginnings of Psychoanalysis in the United States, 1876–1917* (New York: Oxford University Press, 1971), 160.

77. Adolf Meyer, "The Dynamic Interpretation of Dementia Praecox," *American Journal of Psychology* 21 (1910): 385–403.

Hopkins and at the same time director of the Henry Phipps Clinic there.[78] For many of his students, their stay at Johns Hopkins became a turning point in their lives, not least because they became acquainted with psychoanalysis. Without ever becoming a Freudian, Adolf Meyer integrated psychoanalytic theories into his dynamic psychiatry and influenced his students in finding their way to psychoanalysis, as happened for Wilmanns Lidz.

A remote relative of Wilmanns Lidz provided her an affidavit, and so she arrived in New York on 17 February 1937. She spent two days with Mr. E., a nephew of a woman who had worked in the psychiatric clinic in Heidelberg for many years: "He helped me get a train ticket to Baltimore ($3.75) and we sent a wire to Dr. Meyer to tell him when I was coming."[79] Once there, she immediately ran into difficulties because of her poor command of English:

> On arrival in Baltimore there seemed to be nobody at the station expecting me. I had no idea that February 22 was Washington's Birthday and therefore a holiday. Dr. Meyer didn't even get that wire until the next day. Being on my own, I took a cab and tried to explain to the cabdriver in French that I wanted to go to Johns Hopkins Hospital. Some place in Europe, people had told me that since Baltimore was in the south of the United States, people would be speaking French there. Needless to say, the cabbie looked at me as if I were nuts, but eventually he understood Johns Hopkins Hospital and took me there to the Broadway entrance.[80]

The next day she had an appointment with Meyer, and at the end of their meeting, he told her that she had to take English lessons. Mrs. Meyer arranged for a woman to give her lessons in conversation. Because Wilmanns Lidz's grammatical knowledge was better than that of her teacher, she soon gave the lessons up. It was very important for her not to be an outsider, as she had been in Turkey. She wanted to participate in the social and cultural life in the "New World." She was aware of the fact that to be able to do so she had to learn the new language as soon as possible. Due to her skills in other languages, she succeeded in a short time in communicating

---

78. One year after his talk at Clark University, in 1910, Meyer became the first director of the Phipps Clinic. The clinic did not begin operation until April 1913.
79. Wilmanns Lidz, unpublished autobiography, 20.
80. Ibid., 21.

in English. Her son states that in only a few months his mother could communicate with her patients and colleagues very well.[81]

Wilmanns Lidz liked her new workplace at the Phipps Clinic very much, and it completely changed her life. She became acquainted with reports of patients in case conferences, studied elaborate anamneses, and saw how patients were closely observed in therapeutic sessions. Meyer's treatment method, to regard the patient as a whole and to integrate the family into the therapy, greatly inspired her and had a decisive influence over her later therapeutic practice as a psychoanalyst.[82] Although she wrote in her reminiscences enthusiastically about her new professional environment, Wilmanns Lidz then still seemed to have difficulties in adapting: "I am attached to European, i.e., Swiss psychiatry and can't adapt to the local conceptions!" She tried to introduce insulin therapy into the Phipps Clinic. There was a problem, however, because the patients were accommodated in single rooms, and so she could not work with them simultaneously.[83] So she asked Meyer if she could set up the therapy at Springfield State Hos-

---

81. Victor Lidz, personal communication, 23 June 2009.

82. Else Pappenheim, in *Else Pappenheim*, ed. Handlbauer, 83, remembered: "Ruth Lidz was there before me and wrote particularly nicely to me in Vienna, when I already knew that I would come to Hopkins, but when I was there, although she was very kind, she no longer spoke one word of German. Her husband, Ted Lidz, was very nice, an American. She was a bit manic, and two hundred percent American." Victor Lidz, personal communication, 2 June 2010, explains that his mother "chose to speak English but she certainly spoke some German and sprinkled her conversation with German phrases—except during the war years when she did try not to display her German origins. [Pappenheim's] characterizations are hard to believe." Ruth Wilmanns Lidz "was a controlled and reserved, though warm person. I never saw a touch of mania in her. She retained a lot of reservations, as did many German immigrants and social thinkers, about American 'materialism' and the quality of American individualism. But she did try very much to fit into her new society." Pappenheim, in *Else Pappenheim*, 83, also maintained that one brother of Ruth Wilmanns Lidz went to England and worked for Sigmund Freud and the other brother became a Nazi. This information is false. Ruth Wilmanns Lidz had only one brother, and he was definitely not a Nazi. "[Her brother who went to England] worked for Ford Motor Company, presumably Dr. Pappenheim misunderstood Ford as Freud, then for ANSCO, the British and American affiliate of Agfa, then my mother helped him to come to this country where he quickly joined the army. After the war he studied to become an optical engineer. Later he was an engineer and manager for Douglas Aircraft Corporation. He died relatively young of Alzheimer's. There was only the one brother. There were two sisters. One followed my mother to Baltimore and became a nurse there. Later she married a German immigrant accountant in New York and became a housewife, raising two children. The other sister stayed in Germany." Victor Lidz, personal communication, 2 June 2010.

83. As she wrote to Max Müller: "The time at the 'Phipps' was, regarding the insulin treatment, very depressing. . . . First of all only 4 cases and secondly all were old and disadvantageous and thirdly the doctor who tested some cases before I came, always interfered and foiled my plans." Max Müller, *Erinnerungen: Erlebte Psychiatriegeschichte*, 208.

pital with larger groups, and he gave his permission. Although she maintained her appointment at the Phipps Clinic, where she worked for one day a week, she spent the rest of her time at the state hospital. There she applied insulin to a group of about twenty schizophrenic patients. After they had fallen into a deep coma, she then gave them intravenous shots of glucose until they woke up. In 1938 and 1939, she published articles on the procedure.[84]

At Springfield State Hospital, she also met Theodore Lidz, later her husband.[85] Together they did research on possible differences between schizophrenic patients with and without insulin therapy, both at the Springfield State Hospital and at the Phipps Clinic, finding no significant differences between the two groups. What they did find, however, were pathologic traits in the families of schizophrenic patients, and they wanted to investigate this finding in detail. Meyer supported them by securing a fellowship to do research on the family environment of schizophrenic patients, based on detailed documents of the family histories at the Phipps Clinic.[86] During this time they began to turn their attention to the relationship of schizophrenic patients with their families and moved away from the organic understanding of schizophrenia.

On 20 May 1942, Theodore Lidz went to war in the South Pacific theater with the medical unit from Johns Hopkins. So their study on the families of schizophrenics was interrupted, and they could not publish their results until the late 1940s.[87] A long period of incertitude and separation from her husband led Wilmanns Lidz, who was now the mother of an infant son (Victor Lidz), to seek professional help. She made an appointment with the most senior psychoanalyst in the area, Lewis Hill, and "slipped, without a clue, into an analysis."

> After he had seen me twice, he asked me to take a place on the couch. I thought it was comfortable and was clueless about the fact that I was now in an analytic treatment. I agonized over the fact that Dr. Hill was sitting behind me so that I couldn't see him. . . . After a few months my analyst advised me

---

84. Ruth Wilmanns and Max Hayman, "Zig-Zag Method in Insulin Therapy of Schizophrenia," *New York State Journal of Medicine* 38 (1938): 1–2. Ruth Wilmanns et al., "The Insulin Treatment in Schizophrenic Patients," *American Journal of Psychiatry* 95 (1939): 793–97.

85. Ruth Wilmanns Lidz and Theodore Lidz were married in 1939.

86. Wilmanns Lidz, "Von Heidelberg nach Johns Hopkins," 269–70ff.

87. Ruth Wilmanns Lidz and Theodore Lidz, "The Family Environment of Schizophrenic Patients," *American Journal of Psychiatry* 106 (1949): 332–45. Still, this was the first such study in America.

to take courses. This amazed me, because I didn't have the faintest idea about analytical education and suddenly found myself in this situation.[88]

She had a big problem with the opinions of Hill, who insisted that her father was "the head of the family." She could not share this view and told him about the equality in her family. When he wanted to hear about her earliest memories, she told him how she had played with her excrement as a one-year-old girl, and that her nanny had told her not to do that. He was fascinated by this memory, and interpreted it as a game with the penis which she found foolish and a phantasy of her analyst. Hill's interpretation also referred to her doctoral thesis on persons who had lost a limb (in German, "Glied" both means limb and penis). Although she could accept the interpretation to some extent, she was still proud that she was a woman.[89] Her psychoanalytic training took place from autumn 1943 until 1947. In May 1947, Wilmanns Lidz became a member of the American Psychoanalytic Association.

Together with her husband, who also became a psychoanalyst, she developed psychoanalytic therapy with schizophrenic patients and their families in the U.S. Against the general claim, the Lidzes did not undertake family therapy in the usual sense. They instead saw other family members and, where appropriate, the family together to clarify questions and help arrange adequate therapy for the individual patient.[90] According to them, children in pathologic families were not able to develop any boundaries in their interactions with their parents and were confused by the parents' attempts to maintain their own psychic balance. Without developing a solid self-identity, children showed pathological reactions which in some cases could lead to schizophrenia. In their theory and practice, the Lidzes em-

88. Wilmanns Lidz, "Von Heidelberg nach Johns Hopkins," 273; Wilmanns Lidz, "Ein erfülltes Leben," 300–301.

89. Ibid., 301–2.

90. "Certainly part of their therapeutic stance was to focus on family relationships and the troubles they found in those relationships in almost all schizophrenic patients. In a sense they expanded and focused Meyer's interest in the patient's history to encompass the history of the family relationships through the patient's years of being socialized. This was essential to understanding the conflicts that blocked the patient's maturation and ability to assume adult roles in life. Late in his life, my father claimed to be one of the initiators of 'family therapy.' However, my memory of his talking about families years earlier is that he was wary of the usual family therapy—engaging the whole family in therapy—because it creates ambiguities about who is the patient and to whom the therapist owes primary duties of caring. It can draw the therapist into familial conflicts. I have no memory of my mother's ever having whole families in therapy. Another aspect of this was their feeling, I think, that engaging the whole family in therapy would be to regress the patient in a way that would be harmful for a person with schizophrenia." Victor Lidz, personal communication, 2 June 2010.

phasized the role of disturbed communication in such families and contextualized schizophrenic thinking within the family environment. They considered it essential for an effective therapy that the family be integrated and treatment not limited to the symptom-bearer.[91]

Ruth Wilmanns Lidz was also in close contact with Frieda Fromm-Reichmann, who was born on 23 October 1889 in Germany.[92] Fromm-Reichmann received her psychoanalytic training in Berlin and then moved to Heidelberg, where she began to treat psychotic patients. In order to escape the National Socialist dictatorship, she emigrated via Palestine to the U.S. in 1935. In the same year she became a training analyst at the Washington Psychoanalytic Institute and took a position at the Chestnut Lodge clinic in Rockville, Maryland, where she worked for twenty years, helping to establish its reputation as a prestigious clinic specializing in the treatment of psychoses. She developed her technique of treating deeply disturbed patients, in particular schizophrenics, and called her method "Intensive Psychotherapy" with an interpersonal approach inspired by Harry Stack Sullivan.[93]

Thereby she distanced herself from classical psychoanalytic assumptions that psychoses could not be cured by psychoanalysis. According to her, the belief that psychotic patients were not analyzable resulted only from analysts' fears that they could not work with such patients. Fromm-Reichmann also criticized traditional psychiatric views of psychoses as genetic disorders and thus incurable by psychic means. From her point of view, the needs of a patient were more important than methods out of a textbook. She abandoned rules of psychoanalytic treatment whenever it was needed.[94] For example, she renounced the couch and the standard interpretations and often asked the patients direct questions instead of listening to their free associations.[95] The main points in her technique with schizophrenic

---

91. Theodore Lidz, "Der Einfluß von Familienuntersuchungen auf die Behandlung der Schizophrenie," *Psyche: Zeitschrift für Psychoanalyse und ihre Anwendungen* 26 (1972): 169–90.

92. "[W]hen my parents decided to get married (1939), my mother brought my father to meet Frieda and obtain her approval for the marriage. In that respect, Frieda stood in for my mother's father. That story also indicates that my mother had made contact with Frieda and established at least something of a renewed relationship with her in this country—a few years at least before the supervision I remember." Victor Lidz, personal communication, 23 June 2009.

93. Holmes, "Leben und Werk," 77. Frieda Fromm-Reichmann, *Principles of Intensive Psychotherapy* (Chicago: University of Chicago Press, 1960).

94. Gail A. Hornstein, *To Redeem One Person Is to Redeem the World: The Life of Frieda Fromm-Reichmann* (New York: Other Press, 2000), 43, 48.

95. Uwe Henrik Peters, "Frieda Fromm-Reichmann und die psychoanalytisch orientierte Psychotherapie der Schizophrenie," in *Psychiatrie im Exil: Die Emigration der dynamischen Psychiatrie aus Deutschland 1933–1939* (Düsseldorf: Kupka Verlag, 1992), 182.

patients were to emphasize the transference more broadly than in classical psychoanalysis, with more flexible interpretation, and to regard oedipal facts as relatively unimportant, thus alleviating patient's fears and guilt feelings. Wilmanns Lidz was impressed by "her openness about what she had learned from a particular patient, her willingness to teach so frankly from her own experiences or even mistakes."[96]

Wilmanns Lidz had first met Fromm-Reichmann in 1922 as a twelve-year-old girl, when Karl Wilmanns was the chairman of the Psychiatric University Clinic in Heidelberg. In the Botanical Gardens, she and her father wanted to pick some orchids for her mother, and as they came by Fromm-Reichmann's institute, they stopped to greet her. There was no further contact until Wilmanns Lidz's emigration to America in 1937, when her father wrote her that Fromm-Reichmann lived "near Baltimore" and sent her the address of Chestnut Lodge.[97] Fromm-Reichmann had both a personal and professional influence on Wilmanns Lidz and supervised her during her analytical training at the Washington-Baltimore Psychoanalytic Institute. Ruth was very grateful because Fromm-Reichmann permitted her to bring along her three- or four-year-old son Victor, who would play in the waiting room during the supervision.[98] After World War II, when Wilmanns Lidz again went through a depressed phase, she went for therapy with Fromm-Reichmann, rather than returning to her former analyst, Lewis Hill.[99]

As far as modifications of certain psychoanalytic techniques in the treatment of schizophrenic patients were concerned, Wilmanns Lidz followed, with few exceptions, the treatment methods of Fromm-Reichmann. The key modification in her technique was that the patient no longer had to lie on the couch and free associate to an abstinent psychoanalyst about

---

96. Hornstein, *To Redeem One Person*, 46–47. Holmes, "Leben und Werk," 95. Ruth Wilmanns Lidz, "The Use of Anxiety and Hostility in the Treatment of Schizophrenic Patients," in *Psychoanalysis and Psychosis*, ed. Ann-Louise S. Silver (New York: International Universities Press, 1989), 208. In English in the original.

97. Wilmanns Lidz, "The Use of Anxiety," 207.

98. "I was 3 or 4 years old at the time and remember being put to nap on the backseat of the car while my mother drove to Chestnut Lodge along with another young doctor who also had supervision with Frieda. I made puzzles on the floor of the waiting room while first the other doctor and then my mother had their hours of supervision. Then we drove back and I was told to sleep on the backseat. Frieda always had some kind words for me in between the supervisory sessions!" Victor Lidz, personal communication, 23 June 2009.

99. "Hill also became my father's analyst. Although he was regarded as a senior and leading analyst in Baltimore, I don't know why my father went to him when my mother's experience with him had not been very fruitful of new personal insight. Neither of my parents later spoke of their analyses as very helpful, certainly not in the way that a number of other people I know speak of their analyses." Victor Lidz, personal communication, 2 June 2010.

his or her early childhood, which, in her view, would only lead to further regression. Instead, Wilmanns Lidz "emphasized having the patient sit up, talking directly to the therapist, giving frequent supportive feedback to the patient, focusing on immediate interpersonal relationships of the patient, talking about the feelings that the patient was experiencing in the therapeutic session, and generally supporting the patients' reality testing and functioning. She viewed the patients' difficulties in psychodynamic terms, but worked with patients in ways that helped them to overcome their regressive tendencies rather than encouraging regression as a way to get to unconscious issues."[100]

All of the strands of this story came together in the United States. Weigert was also close to both Frieda Fromm-Reichmann and Ruth Wilmanns Lidz, and she also gained a major role in American psychoanalytic circles shortly after her emigration to the United States. In 1938, Weigert became a member of the Washington-Baltimore Psychoanalytic Society, and in the same year she obtained, with a recommendation from Fromm-Reichmann, an appointment at the Sheppard and Enoch Pratt Hospital, which, like Chestnut Lodge, specialized in treating psychoses with psychoanalytic methods. There, like Wilmanns Lidz at Johns Hopkins Hospital, she experimented with the insulin method. She was interested in the psychoanalytic effects of that treatment and came to the conclusion that all artificial treatment methods of psychoses should be avoided except psychotherapy.[101] In the beginning of the 1940s, she left her appointment at the Sheppard and Enoch Pratt Hospital and established a private practice. As Victor Lidz reports:

> Yes, my mother and Edith Weigert knew each other well. My mother looked on Dr. Weigert as a wise and helpful senior colleague. . . . After my mother left her academic position at Johns Hopkins Hospital around the end of World War II, she shared offices with several other psychiatrists in Baltimore. I believe that Dr. Weigert was the senior member of the several psychiatrists there. They shared a receptionist-secretary and a waiting room. Each of them had a private office off of the waiting room. It was not a group practice, but just several individual physicians who managed costs by sharing the rent and salary for the receptionist-secretary.[102]

---

100. Victor Lidz, personal communication, 17 August 2009.
101. Holmes, "Leben und Werk," 81–82.
102. Victor Lidz, personal communication, 23 February 2009.

Another Dimension of the Émigré Experience / 151

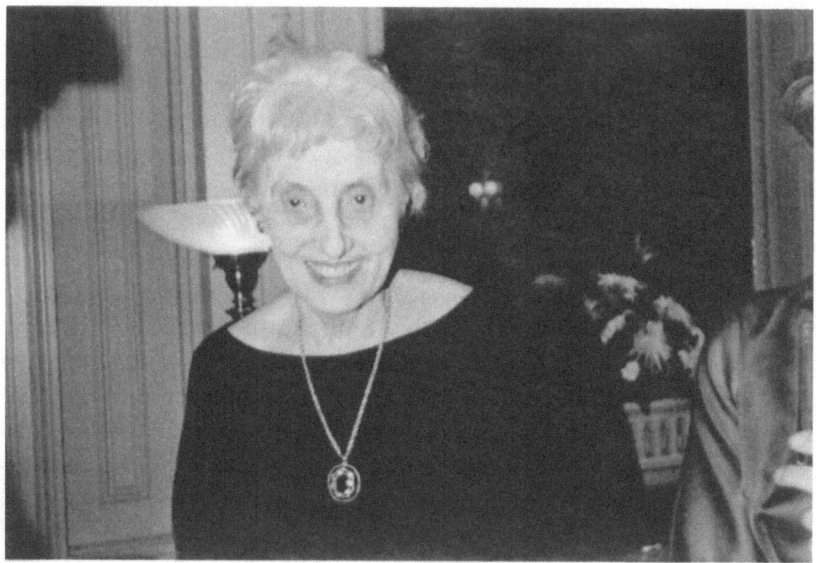

5.4. Edith Weigert as an eminent psychoanalyst in the United States. Generously furnished by her grandson, David Weigert.

In 1944, Weigert became the president of the Washington-Baltimore Psychoanalytic Society, and after the schism two years later, like Frieda Fromm-Reichmann, she chose to stay in the Washington group that was not orthodox Freudian and developed new methods in treating patients.

She also gained support from Fromm-Reichmann, in both her professional and personal life. Holmes, who had interviewed relatives and friends of Weigert, reports that the struggles of her emigration experiences had an impact on her life.[103] She suffered in the beginning of her life in America from episodes of depression, and Frieda Fromm-Reichmann, who herself was adversely affected by feelings of guilt as someone who had not perished in the Holocaust, helped her to survive these episodes of depression.[104]

As we have seen in the biographies of these three women who escaped from National Socialism and emigrated via the Middle East to the United States, they all experienced the severe consequences of a forced emigration. Like so many female colleagues, they had to break away from their families and their status of emancipated woman in Weimar Germany. Weigert and

---

103. Holmes, "Leben und Werk," 73.
104. Peters, "Frieda Fromm-Reichman," 186.

Wilmanns Lidz experienced the harsh conditions of the culture in Turkey. On their arrival in America they also had to contend with low social status as women, even though they held professional degrees. Nevertheless, their challenges in American society led to solidarity among them, and they continued their psychoanalytic work on psychoses, which they began in their homelands, and made important contributions in that field in the U.S.

Conclusion

Although the Burghölzli was a leading center for psychoanalytic research on schizophrenia in Central Europe, the break between Freud and Bleuler and Jung led to a diminution of effective research. Also the bankruptcy of the clinic Schloss Tegel discouraged developing therapies for psychotic patients. In addition, National Socialism put an abrupt end to the development of psychoanalysis, including the psychoanalytic theory and treatment of schizophrenia.

Through the forced migration of European psychoanalysts to the U.S., psychoanalysis developed within the cultural setting of America. In this study we have followed three European doctors as they emigrated and established themselves in American medicine and psychoanalysis: Edith Weigert, Ruth Wilmanns Lidz, and Frieda Fromm-Reichmann. All had in common an interest in psychoanalysis and, distinctively, in the psychotic rather than the usual neurotic patient. Their ways of arriving in the U.S. varied greatly. I have focused on two examples that are of special interest because they involved experiences with a country and culture that has hitherto hardly been studied in this context, namely, Turkey.

There, in the first half of the twentieth century, organic psychiatry, not psychoanalysis, flourished. This could be explained by the fact that Turkish psychiatrists preferred to adopt from the West an organic concept of mental diseases rather than psychoanalytic theories. They could accept an organic concept rather than a psychological explanation, which seemed to them alien and therefore was of little explanatory value in their own culture. In short, at that time, psychoanalytic concepts were unacceptable for most Turkish psychiatrists—not least because Islamic beliefs about the etiology and the "healing" of mental illnesses continued to exist in the population.

In contrast to the resistance of psychiatrists in Turkey and political hostility in Central Europe, the aftermath of Sigmund Freud's visit to the U.S. created openings for three women working on the psychoanalytic approaches to mental illness. Moreover, they received assistance from Adolf Meyer, who implicitly integrated psychoanalytic ideas into his dynamic psychiatry and into the treatment of psychoses. Indeed, the later work of Meyer's direct student Wilmanns Lidz can be seen as an example of the rippling impact of Sigmund Freud's visit to America on later generations of psychiatrists.

Acknowledgments

I am immensely grateful to Victor Lidz for permission to publish materials about his mother, and for his willingness to explain her background to me. Many thanks to David Weigert, who gave me permission to publish a photograph of his grandmother Edith Weigert and told me about her personal and professional background. For helpful suggestions and references I thank Ann-Louise Silver, Vamık D. Volkan, Şahap Erkoç, Altan Deliorman, Tevfika Tunaboylu Ikiz, Peter Wilmanns, Maren Holmes, Selvihan and Serpil Akkaya, and Sertan Batur. Many thanks to Laryn McLernon for assisting me with English translations. Thanks to my colleagues and friends Arin Sharif-Nassab, Clemens Drechsel, Yvonne Egger-Habib, and to Karl Fallend, the adviser of my doctoral thesis, "Psychoanalyse in der Türkei: Eine historische und aktuelle Spurensuche," for their constructive comments on earlier drafts of my paper. I am grateful to my whole family, especially to my brother-in-law Erman Usak for his hospitality and to my husband, Tolga Usak, for accompanying me during my research in Turkey.

I offer my sincere thanks to the archives of the Guraba Clinic Istanbul; Medical Faculty of the Istanbul University—Mehmet Bilgin Saydam and Talat Parman; Robert College—Tulu Derbi; Türk Tarih Kurumu Ankara; the Freud Museum in London—Michael Molnar; Library of Congress Washington—Harold P. Blum; Archives of the University of Innsbruck—Peter Goller; the Municipal Archive, Innsbruck; the State Archive, Basel—Hermann Wichers; the Johns Hopkins Medical Archives—Marjorie Kehoe. Sincere thanks to the facilities of the Leopold-Franzens-University, Innsbruck, for financial support: Fakultäten Servicestelle—Vice Rector Margret Friedrich, Büro für Internationale Beziehungen—Elisabeth Watzdorf, Studienabteilung—Maria Schiessling, and Vizerektorat für Forschung—Barbara Aufschnaiter, Kirsten Valeruz, and Rector Tilmann Märk. Special thanks go to Ernst Falzeder for the revision of my manuscript, assisting me with English translations, and his constructive comments. Finally I would like to thank John Burnham, who edited my paper and supported me in all issues.

PART TWO

After World War II: The Fate of Freud's Legacy in American Culture

INTRODUCTION TO PART II

A Shift in Perspective

The encounter of Ruth Wilmanns Lidz and Edith Weigert with Turkish culture furnishes a link with Part II, which begins with Dorothy Ross's essay on the relationship of psychoanalysis to modernism. The Turks in the 1930s were working to make their country "modern," but intellectual and cultural elements and elites necessary to sustain modernism (as opposed to modernity) were not yet in place. What Wilmanns Lidz and Weigert found in Turkey compares not only with Europe but with a third national setting, America. The comparison serves to suggest the cultural infrastructure that was in place in the United States to receive and develop the ideas and expectations of various kinds of carriers of Central European psychoanalysis.

In Part II, the account of each of our authors begins at the point when Freud's visibility was rising to a peak in American society and culture, the 1940s to the 1960s. The authors of the chapters in Part I have already provided a narrative of how Freud and psychoanalysis could reach that high point. In the 1920s and 1930s, psychoanalysis spread among special parts of the population, frequently in forms that Freud and other purists disdained. By the 1940s, often under émigré leadership, a new institutional structure had come into existence, and George Makari has shown how it launched the era of orthodox ego psychology. Together, these developments created a sense that there was a stable and powerful psychoanalytic movement in the United States, centered not only in New York, Boston, and Washington-Baltimore, but in Chicago, Detroit, Los Angeles, San Francisco, and Topeka, Kansas.

The émigrés, whatever their own frustrations, had surprisingly substantial social effects throughout the country. Many émigrés and their American contemporaries lived and worked well into the second half of the twentieth century. One explanation for the impact of émigré analysts, beyond their intellectual power in mutually enlightening discussions, was their willingness to take leadership roles. Moreover, as historian H. Stuart Hughes, who was sometimes an eyewitness, recalled: "The native-born were deferential to a fault: uncertain of the rigor of their own training, they were only too happy to let the Viennese and the Berliners tell them what to do. . . . The difficulty here was that the newcomers did most of the talking."[1]

The most obvious new element that mid-century émigré and other ego psychology psychoanalysts introduced to the United States was a substantial emphasis on theory. It is only fair to point out that it was not just in psychoanalysis that European émigrés brought to empirically and experimentally inclined Americans a much keener appreciation of abstract scientific theory. Physicists, for example, under a parallel stimulus from European arrivals, also showed a remarkably expanded interest in theory.[2] For psychoanalysis, world-class theoretical work attracted a number of very bright people, the kind of people who would mix with and influence other members of the intellectual elite.

Moreover, alongside the "orthodox" analyst core were many neo-Freudians whose influence was substantial from the World War II period to long after the 1960s. Altogether, commentators during the years just after World War II agreed that Freudianism, in however accurate or garbled a form, was penetrating into popular venues as well as among physicians and other intellectuals. As the eminent, but definitely not sympathetic, psychologist O. Hobart Mowrer recalled: "Anyone who reached adulthood prior to 1950 knows how perversely Freudian theory and practice dominated not only in the specific field of psychotherapy, but also education, jurisprudence, religion, child rearing, and art and literature, and social philosophy."[3]

Our authors in Part II focus, not on the implicit narrative of the psychoanalysts, but on developments in the culture outside of psychoanaly-

---

1. H. Stuart Hughes, "Social Theory in a New Context," in *The Muses Flee Hitler: Cultural Transfer and Adaptation*, ed. Jarrell C. Jackman and Carla M. Borden (Washington, DC: Smithsonian Institution Press, 1983), 116–17.

2. Stanley Coben, "The Scientific Establishment and the Transmission of Quantum Mechanics to the United States, 1919–32," *American Historical Review* 76 (1971): 442–66. Among other major works on the émigré intellectuals are H. Stuart Hughes, *The Sea Change: The Migration of Social Thought, 1930–1965* (New York: Harper and Row, 1975); Lewis A. Coser, *Refugee Scholars in America: Their Impact and Their Experiences* (New Haven, CT: Yale University Press, 1984); Anthony Heilbut, *Exiled in Paradise: German Refugee Artists and Intellectuals in America, from the 1930s to the Present* (Boston: Beacon Press, 1983); and Uwe Henrik Peters, *Psychiatrie im Exil: Die Emigration der dynamischen Psychiatrie aus Deutschland, 1933–1939* (Düsseldorf: Kupka Verlag, 1992).

3. O. Hobart Mowrer, quoted in Marty Jezer, *The Dark Ages: Life in the United States, 1945–1960* (Boston: South End Press, 1982), 232.

sis, looking from the context rather than the inside of the psychoanalytic movement. Each author, in a different way, first explores intellectual and social factors in American culture before examining how psychoanalytic thinking played into the cultural changes that began before World War II but evolved in a stronger or weaker form to the end of the century. All of these accounts then proceed to some extent into the ultimate decline in both technical psychoanalysis and in the status of overtly Freudian thinking among intellectuals in general.

Because psychoanalysis had been so closely connected to psychiatry and medicine in the United States, when psychiatry and medicine changed in the 1960s–1980s and after, the primary carriers of Freudian ideas were deeply affected. On the intellectual and theoretical levels, neuroscientists offered vivid somatic, not psychoanalytic, explanations of mental events. Medicine became tied more and more to machines and pills, and less and less to the doctor-patient relationship. Not only was psychiatry as a medical specialty deeply affected by commercial and economic forces, but powerful social trends tended to reduce patients to mere consumers of medical goods and services. Institute-trained psychoanalysts, who had dominated postwar psychiatry, lost out in substantial measure to dispensers of medications and to "counseling services."[4]

By the last decades of the twentieth century, the counselors, and particularly a rapidly growing number of clinical psychologists, did sometimes use psychoanalytic ideas and techniques, but, typically, in only a piecemeal way. Moreover, these professionals did not serve as a fountainhead of cultural and intellectual excitement in any way comparable to the ego psychologists (who were mostly MDs) or even some of their successors such as the Kohutians. Nor did the academics who worked in such specialized fields as literature, film studies, and interdisciplinary humanities where psychoanalytic thinking still carried weight. It was rather during the 1940s, 1950s, and early 1960s when a group of public intellectuals announced Freud to be a preeminent thinker of the modern world, that Freud's ideas exerted the greatest influence on American culture. Our Part II authors therefore turn their inquiry to this intelligentsia who served as indicators as well as leaders of cultural change.[5]

---

4. John C. Burnham, "Psychology and Counseling: Convergence into a Profession," in *The Professions in American History*, ed. Nathan Hatch (Notre Dame, IN: University of Notre Dame Press, 1988), 181–98; Jonathan Engel, *American Therapy: The Rise of Psychotherapy in the United States* (New York: Gotham Books, 2008).

5. See, for example, Hugh Wilford, *The New York Intellectuals: From Vanguard to Institution* (Manchester: Manchester University Press, 1995).

Dorothy Ross introduces the major intellectual carrier of Freud's legacy, modernism. Psychoanalysis, she points out, was indeed a modernist invention, and the high point of modernism in the United States coincided with the high point of the influence of Freud's ideas. She anatomizes the streams and levels of modernism through which psychoanalysis entered American culture, showing how the two worked in concert. Ross defines modernism as the "complex of ideas" that continued, first, the romantics' revolt against the authority and hypocrisy of nineteenth-century bourgeois society and, second, the romantics' exploration of the self. It was because of these intellectual currents that psychoanalysis, like modernism generally, contained both Dionysian and Apollonian possibilities, respect for the power of human nature's instinctual resources and also its capacity for civilization.

Ross explains the fate of psychoanalytic thinking by linking it to the retreat of the Apollonian modernists in the face of the radical cultural politics of the 1960s and the advent of postmodernism in the 1970s. At the same time, feminist and countercultural thinkers who had absorbed radical modernist values often found Freud not modernist enough. The result, as Ross explains, was that among intellectuals psychoanalysis no longer carried nearly the authority it had earlier.

Louis Menand then introduces a second major theme in the mid-century American cultural context: anxiety. Indeed, Menand identifies anxiety as a concept that came to mark the era just after World War II. He asks the ironic question, how did anxiety become so popular? In answering that question, he finds some remarkable answers to the more general question, why did psychoanalysis become so important in mid-century American culture, and why did that popularity then diminish?

Menand finds evidence of particular ways in which psychoanalytic ideas affected and were transformed by intellectuals and educated Americans in the distinctive Cold War culture that grew out of World War II. This was indeed "the age of anxiety," a characterization widely accepted at the time of the atomic bombs, McCarthyism, and intellectual explorations. The tragic pessimism underlying the age's defining Broadway musical, *Camelot*, easily played off of the tragic elements in Freud's theoretical constructs. Menand examines particularly how waves of imported existentialism affected intellectuals and their understanding and use of Freud's ideas. The Apollonian version of Freud described by Ross drew on the anxiety and existentialism to which Menand gives center stage. Yet, as Menand will comment, in that era, psychoanalytic ways of thinking were so powerful that they even influenced the uses of the very technical material means, the tranquilizers, that in the end undermined mental medicine as it had been practiced since the late nineteenth century.

Elizabeth Lunbeck moves the story into the post-1950s decades with a revealing examination of a charismatic analytic leader who was deviant, and not deviant, as the cultural and technical territory around Freud's legacy had changed and was changing. She can show the extent to which even core practitioners Americanized psychoanalysis in the rapidly shifting culture of the late twentieth-century United States.

The pattern that Lunbeck finds in the popularization of Kohutian psychoanalysis therefore represents a new Americanizing pattern—but one in which, as Lunbeck emphasizes, Kohut was able, perhaps consciously, to draw on some styles of thinking still powerful among American thinkers—optimism, meliorism, self-improvement. What is perhaps most striking, however, is how the technical practice of psychoanalysis continued to interact with other intellectual traditions and also with identifiable new trends that became clear a generation after mid-century. Lunbeck thus provides a transition from the narrative of technical psychoanalysis to the parallel and interrelated narrative of intellectuals' use of Freudian thinking after World War II. She shows how Kohut as an analyst joined the outlook of the so-called generation of narcissism with psychoanalytic thinking.

Public intellectuals understood the timeliness of Kohut's message. But, Lunbeck still implicitly inquires, what was Freudian about it? It is true that longtime American practitioners believed that their patients seemed to have changed. It is true that analysts more and more accepted a psychiatry that was only loosely dynamic, or a psychotherapy that was both dynamic and not orthodox. Already by 1989, analyst Robert Wallerstein could look back and say that from the 1970s on, there had developed within the psychoanalytic community a distinctive psychoanalytic psychotherapy in addition to old-style orthodox psychoanalysis.[6] Lunbeck confirms the observation of analyst Otto Kernberg, writing from the inside, that Kohut opened "the road for other alternative theories to be studied and tolerated in the United States" among practicing analysts in the last four decades of the century after Freud left.[7]

---

6. Robert S. Wallerstein, "Psychoanalysis and Psychotherapy: An Historical Perspective," *International Journal of Psycho-Analysis* 70 (1989): 563–91. A later, full description of the adaptation of analysts is in T. M. Luhrmann, *Of Two Minds: The Growing Disorder in American Psychiatry* (New York: Alfred A. Knopf, 2000).

7. Otto F. Kernberg, "The Hartmann Era: Reflection on an Overview by Martin S. Bergmann," in *The Hartmann Era*, ed. Martin S. Bergmann (New York: Other Press, 2000), 154.

Jean-Christophe Agnew offers still further perspective on the complex cultural changes from the 1940s to the 1980s. He not only synthesizes but extends the intellectual narrative that Ross, Menand, and Lunbeck initiate. Agnew refers again to "the Sixties" and underlines even more strongly that the late twentieth century was a time very different from the mid-twentieth century. He identifies other ways in which intellectuals worked within a variety of high cultural contexts, such as those described by Ross, Menand, and Lunbeck, to integrate psychoanalytic thinking into high culture during the rest of the century.

To understand the fate of Freud's ideas, Agnew maintains, along with the other Part II authors, one must indeed start with the intellectuals' response to the challenge of totalitarianism and World War II. There was soon also the self-consciousness of the United States as a dominating world power. But one must, following Ross, see also the permutations and ambivalences of the intellectuals' modernism. Particularly in both Ross's and Agnew's accounts, the story, as noted above, depends importantly on the later shift when the personal became political. A whole range of late twentieth-century thinkers moved away from overt Freudianism because they suddenly found Freud an agent of perhaps coercive conformity rather than the radical who had been so attractive to an earlier avant-garde. Yet this turning away underlines how deeply and routinely elite and other educated Americans had, on some level, absorbed at least some of Freud's teachings.

As these four final authors contend, what the intellectuals wrote did not just ripple superficially into popular thinking. By the postwar decades, Freud's ideas were deeply affecting the language, conceptual resources, and outlooks of many populations in whom American culture was embodied. Examining how intellectuals perceived and used psychoanalytic ideas in the decades before 1980, one can begin to work out how Freud's thinking continued to have an indirect but profound historical impact for another thirty years. Not least of the questions our authors raise, then, is why, in an intellectual environment that had become largely unreceptive to Freudianism, even after 2000 there were vibrant islands of fundamental interest in psychoanalytic thinking in psychotherapy and in the arts and interdisciplinary studies—a still unexamined legacy of Freud.

SIX

Freud and the Vicissitudes of Modernism in the United States, 1940–1980

DOROTHY ROSS

During the period from roughly 1940 to 1980, the ideas of Sigmund Freud were accorded their greatest academic and popular respect in the United States and then, as other authors have noted, precipitously declined in prestige. These same decades also mark the peak of the intellectual authority in American culture of modernism and the turn to postmodernism. The story of Freud's influence is bound up with the vicissitudes of modernism. The humanistic intellectuals who brought Freud to prominence during the 1940s and 1950s were advocates of modernism. By 1980 the authority of modernism had splintered and weakened, exposing Freud to critique from all points on the political spectrum.

The focus of this paper is on a group of academics and public intellectuals who propagated Freud's authority from university chairs and in the highbrow press. These influential voices on Freud were cultural critics in literature and the social sciences who not only used Freud in their intellectual work but functioned as public intellectuals, announcing his importance to colleagues and the educated middle-class public: writers for *Partisan Review* like Phillip Rahv and William Barrett; academics like Lionel Trilling, H. Stuart Hughes, Philip Rieff, Norman O. Brown, Herbert Marcuse, Daniel Bell, and Frederick Crews; feminist writers Betty Friedan and Kate Millett; and psychoanalyst Erik Erikson.[1]

---

1. For a suggestive, though tendentious, analysis of the role of public intellectuals in this mid-century period, see Russell Jacoby, *The Last Intellectuals: American Culture in the Age of Academe* (New York: Basic Books, 2000 [1987]). The full story of Freud's intellectual authority would have to take account of the much larger group of humanists and social scientists who used his ideas in their specialized work but did not become advocates of his ideas. See, e.g., Robert Oliver, "Sex, Anger, and Confusion: The Use of Freudian Theory by American Historians and Anthropologists" (Ph.D. diss., Vanderbilt University, 1996). For the participation of historians and cultural critics in a wider discussion of modernism and modernity since the

The internal history of psychiatry and psychoanalysis constitutes a largely separate story. Historians, including some of the essayists in this volume, have studied the professional psychoanalytic movement in the United States, showing how the Progressive-era rise of American psychiatry, emigration of European analysts in the 1930s and 1940s, and medicalization of the profession during the 1940s and 1950s created simultaneously both a Freudian orthodoxy that was more rigid in doctrine and practice than Freud's own and a host of heterodox Americanizers and neo-Freudian critics. The rise and decline of psychoanalysis within psychiatry roughly paralleled the trajectory of Freud's authority among intellectuals, reaching a peak in the 1950s and early 1960s and declining thereafter with the resurgence of biological psychiatry.[2] The humanist advocates of Freud were aware of professional opinions in medicine. They initially often spoke of psychoanalysis as a science, and the increasing questioning of its scientific credentials in the 1970s undoubtedly influenced them. But the intellectuals who made Freud into a leading intellectual voice of the twentieth century had their own reasons for admiring or dismissing Freudian ideas.

Those reasons centered on modernism. "Modernism" is a term of many meanings—it is sometimes used to refer to the whole body of ideas that are characteristic of modern industrial, bureaucratic society. "Modernism" is used here in a more restricted sense, to denote a set of ideas and works of art that came to full expression in Europe in the late nineteenth and early twentieth centuries and that revolved around the exploration of subjectivity. If we divide modern culture into two broad stems with roots in the Enlightenment, one branching off toward objective truth in nature, the other toward romanticism, modernism follows from the subjective direction taken by romanticism.[3]

---

mid-twentieth century, see Dorothy Ross, "American Modernities: Past and Present," *American Historical Review* 116 (2011): 702–14.

2. The classic account of psychoanalysis in the United States is Nathan G. Hale Jr.'s two volumes, *Freud and the Americans: The Beginnings of Psychoanalysis in the United States, 1876–1917* (New York: Oxford University Press, 1971) and *The Rise and Crisis of Psychoanalysis in the United States: Freud and the Americans, 1917–1985* (New York: Oxford University Press, 1995). The second volume pays some attention to popularization, but not to this intellectual class. For the European history of psychoanalysis as theory and practice, with an epilogue that carries the story to the 1940s United States, see George Makari, *Revolution in Mind: The Creation of Psychoanalysis* (New York: HarperCollins, 2008). For the turn away from psychoanalysis in American psychiatry, see Elizabeth Lunbeck, "Psychiatry," in *The Cambridge History of Science*, vol. 7: *The Modern Social Sciences*, ed. Theodore M. Porter and Dorothy Ross (Cambridge: Cambridge University Press, 2003), 663–77.

3. Among a large literature, see Charles Taylor, *Sources of the Self: The Making of Modern Identity* (Cambridge, MA: Harvard University Press, 1989), chap. 24; Matei Calinescu, *Five Faces*

The two stems often intertwined—few modern writers or artists could not claim a heritage from both—but their thrust was different. Modernists, like the romantics before them, placed themselves in opposition to a modern world of mechanism, instrumental reason, and mass society. But unlike the romantics, they looked for meaning and value in a cosmos devoid of God and an amoral inner and outer nature demystified by Darwinian biology. Turning inward, they found resources that could be refashioned and set to the Apollonian or Dionysian ends of order or release, paths marked out by the preeminent modernist philosopher, Friedrich Nietzsche. If Apollo represented the "form-giving force," a combination of reason and passion that gave shape to the self, to civilization, and to the world, Dionysus represented the ceaseless creative and destructive energies within self and nature that clamored for release. In their effort to construct meaning, modernists relied on both, but differed—as Nietzsche did himself over the course of his lifetime—in the emphasis they gave to Apollonian or Dionysian goals.[4] In the process, they transformed alienation, the sickness of modern man, into an heroic stance of the intellectual and artist. But modernism spoke in no single voice, creating over the course of the twentieth century a multitude of ever-new formulations. Postmodernism is the latest offshoot of the modernist impulse and, despite its rejection of important modernist premises and strategies, remains grounded in their shared core problems of subjectivity and the determinations of the self.[5]

Freud's chief advocates at mid-century were modernist intellectuals. Although he was always recognized as equally a man of the Enlightenment, Freud was presented by them as a central figure in modernism.[6] His advo-

---

of Modernity: Modernism/Avant-Garde/Decadence/Kitsch/Postmodernism (Durham, NC: Duke University Press, 1987); Astradur Eysteinsson, *The Concept of Modernism* (Ithaca, NY: Cornell University Press, 1990); Raymond Williams, *The Politics of Modernism: Against the New Conformists* (London: Verso, 1989); David Hollinger, "The Knower and the Artificer, with Postscript," in *Modernist Impulses in the Human Sciences 1870–1930*, ed. Dorothy Ross (Baltimore: Johns Hopkins University Press, 1994), 26–53.

4. See Walter Kaufmann, *Nietzsche: Philosopher, Psychologist, Antichrist*, 3d ed. (New York: Vintage Books, 1968 [1950]), esp. 128–31.

5. On the complex relationship between modernism and postmodernism, see Allan Megill, *Prophets of Extremity: Nietzsche, Heidegger, Foucault, Derrida* (Berkeley: University of California Press, 1985); David Harvey, *The Condition of Postmodernity* (Oxford: Basil Blackwell, 1989); John McGowan, *Postmodernism and Its Critics* (Ithaca, NY: Cornell University Press, 1991).

6. Contemporary intellectual historians agree. The classic account of Freud as modernist is in Carl E. Schorske, *Fin-de-Siècle Vienna: Politics and Culture* (New York: Knopf, 1980). Among recent treatments of Freud as modernist, see John Brenkman, "Freud the Modernist," in *The Mind of Modernism: Medicine, Psychology, and the Cultural Arts in Europe and America, 1886–1940*, ed. Mark S. Micale (Stanford, CA: Stanford University Press, 2004), 172–96; John E. Toews, "Refashioning the Masculine Subject in Early Modernism: Narratives of Self-Dissolution and

cates were also members of a liberal intellectual class that was consolidating a central role in American culture during the 1940s, 1950s, and early 1960s, in part by establishing the high authority of modernism. "To speak of modern literature is to speak of that peculiar social grouping, the intelligentsia, to whom it belongs," Phillip Rahv wrote. Formed by assimilating Jews and disaffected Protestants around the ideal of a secular, cosmopolitan culture, the intellectual class was anchored at mid-century in university departments in the humanities and social sciences and in respected journals of opinion.[7]

Members of this class had much to gain from embracing modernism. Modernism spoke to their uneasy relationship with American society. It supported their secular, cosmopolitan ideal and promised to transform the still quasi-Protestant university culture in the humanities, a promise of special benefit to Jewish intellectuals. It spoke with particular force to the literary scholars establishing themselves in the universities who in these decades created the high modernist canon and a "mystique" around its works and authors: T. S. Eliot, D. H. Lawrence, James Joyce, Franz Kafka, and Thomas Mann, to name a few. Modernism provided literary scholars with a body of works that claimed to speak to the deepest problems of the modern world and a body of difficult works that required their critical skills, creating a platform for heroic performance to match that of their subjects. Most importantly, modernism legitimated the salient political attitudes of these intellectuals, as they turned inward, away from their destroyed Marxist hopes of the 1930s to wartime nationalism and a chastened Cold War liberalism.[8]

Self-Construction in Psychoanalysis and Literature, 1900–1914," in ibid., 298–335; John E. Toews, "Historicizing Psychoanalysis: Freud in His Time and for Our Time," *Journal of Modern History* 63 (1991): 504–45.

7. David Hollinger analyzes the formation of this class around a cosmopolitan ideal but does not link them to Freud. See his "Ethnic Diversity, Cosmopolitanism, and the Emergence of the American Liberal Intelligentsia," in Hollinger, *In the American Province: Studies in the History and Historiography of Ideas* (Baltimore: Johns Hopkins University Press, 1985), 56–73. For analysis of the core group of "New York intellectuals," see Daniel Bell, "The 'Intelligentsia' in American Society" (1976), in Bell, *The Winding Passage: Essays and Sociological Journeys, 1960–1980* (Cambridge, MA: Abt Books, 1980), and Alexander Bloom, *Prodigal Sons: The New York Intellectuals and Their World* (New York: Oxford University Press, 1986). Rahv is quoted in James B. Gilbert, *Writers and Partisans: A History of Literary Radicalism in America* (New York: John Wiley, 1968), 188.

8. Hollinger, "Ethnic Diversity, Cosmopolitanism"; David A. Hollinger, "Jewish Intellectuals and the De-Christianization of American Public Culture in the Twentieth Century," in Hollinger, *Science, Jews, and Secular Culture: Studies in Mid-Twentieth-Century American Intellectual History* (Princeton, NJ: Princeton University Press, 1996), 17–41; David A. Hollinger, "The Canon and Its Keepers: Modernism and Mid-Twentieth-Century American Intellectuals,"

Freud's mid-century advocates produced a number of different views of Freud and psychoanalysis, each shaped by different understandings of modernism and different political aims, the most influential being the Apollonian Freud of Trilling and Rieff, the domesticated Freud of Erikson, and the Dionysian Freud of Marcuse and Brown. Their chief rivals for public notice were the neo-Freudians, represented here by Erich Fromm, who criticized Freud and abandoned his central tenets even as he claimed Freud's paternity and declared his greatness. It was not however the conflicts among these views of Freud that precipitated his decline in intellectual stature, so much as the ways in which the radicalism of the 1960s forced the reconsideration of modernism. When modernism was appropriated by a radical political and cultural left, the intellectual class splintered, weakening the authority of modernism and opening the way for a retreat from Freudian ideas. Modernism was the lens that refracted changing political and cultural anxieties into changing estimates of Freudian ideas.

The first American intellectuals who had circulated Freudian ideas in the 1910s and 1920s—young critics of America's superficial and Puritanical culture—largely understood Freud as a liberatory, Dionysian modernist. Psychoanalysis was one of the ideas that presided over the Greenwich Village bohemians' sexual revolution, permissive child rearing, and experimental artistic strategies.[9] These modernist dispositions sobered somewhat among intellectuals affected by World War I and altered substantially among the larger numbers influenced by Marxism during the 1930s. Left intellectuals who were attracted to both Marxism and literature but repelled by dictatorial Stalinist rule found in modernism a justification for the alienated stance and authentic voice of the artist and intellectual. Philip Rahv and William Phillips re-founded the *Partisan Review* in 1937 around that modernist program. Already aware of Freud, they began to study his work seriously in 1939.[10]

By 1942 Rahv considered "the growth of psychological science and, particularly, of psychoanalysis" one of the major means by which literature was recovering "its inwardness." William Barrett in the 1947 *Partisan Review*

---

in Hollinger, *In the American Province*, 74–91; Gilbert, *Writers and Partisans*; and Schorske, *Fin-de-Siècle Vienna*, xxiii–xxv. For specific attention to the Jewish component of this intellectual constellation, see also Bell, "The 'Intelligentsia,'" and Bloom, *Prodigal Sons*.

9. For early twentieth-century modernists and Freud, see Hale, *The Rise and Crisis of Psychoanalysis*, chap. 4; Malcolm Cowley, *Exile's Return: A Literary Saga of the Nineteen-Twenties* (New York: Viking Press, 1951 [1934]), esp. 52–65.

10. Gilbert, *Writers and Partisans*, esp. 218.

linked psychoanalysis to the reigning modernist philosophy, existentialism, and the central modernist value, authenticity. "Modern man has lost the religious sanctions which had once surrounded his life at every moment with a recognizable test capable of telling him whether he was living 'in the truth' or not." Freud had shown that the problem was psychological, that we are "creatures of . . . divided and self-alienated consciousness." Only Freud can tell us "how we are to live truthfully," Barrett asserted, "how authenticity is to be achieved either in art or life."[11]

The leading literary champion of Freud was a cosmopolitan Jewish intellectual, professor of English at Columbia university, and an influential framer of the modernist canon, Lionel Trilling.[12] Trilling engaged with modernist literature as a college student in the 1920s, but he started out the 1930s as a Marxist unsympathetic to Freud. By 1940, now a member of the *Partisan Review* board, he declared psychoanalysis "one of the culminations of the Romanticist literature of the 19th century" and a crucial influence on modern art and literature.[13]

Trilling's 1940 essay "Freud and Literature" already presented the tragic account of Freud's ideas that was to exert wide influence during the 1940s and '50s. According to Trilling, Freud showed man to have "a kind of hell within him from which rise everlastingly the impulses which threaten his civilization." This "night side" was not Freud's dominant note, however. The Apollonian Freud—the guardian of civilization—worked to bring the irrational under control of the rational: "The idea of the reality principle and the idea of the death instinct form the crown of Freud's broader speculation on the life of man." Trilling was drawn to the late Freud whose vision was darkened by World War I. Although Trilling praised Freud for making "poetry indigenous to the very constitution of the mind," it was

---

11. Philip Rahv, "On the Decline of Naturalism," *Partisan Review* 9 (1942): 483-93, esp. 492; William Barrett, "Writers and Madness," *Partisan Review* 14 (1947): 5-22, esp. 7. For a survey of existentialist themes and influences in twentieth-century American culture, see George Cotkin, *Existential America* (Baltimore: Johns Hopkins University Press, 2003).

12. For an overview of Trilling's career, see Mark Krupnick, *Lionel Trilling and the Fate of Cultural Criticism* (Evanston, IL: Northwestern University Press, 1986); for a recent account that focuses on Trilling's anticommunism, see Michael Kimmage, *The Conservative Turn: Lionel Trilling, Whittaker Chambers, and the Lessons of Anti-Communism* (Cambridge, MA: Harvard University Press, 2009). It is noteworthy that in the authoritative bibliography of Trilling's work, the number of separate works that cite Freud (30) exceed those for Matthew Arnold (21), the subject of Trilling's first book and his touchstone for the remainder of his career, or for any other modernist writer. See Thomas M. Leitch, *Lionel Trilling: An Annotated Bibliography* (New York, Garland, 1993).

13. Lionel Trilling, "Freud and Literature" (1940), in *The Liberal Imagination* (New York: Viking, 1950), 34-40, esp. 35.

the somber *Civilization and Its Discontents* that he included in his curriculum of great modernist texts, not *The Interpretation of Dreams*. He praised *Beyond the Pleasure Principle* (1920), where Freud strengthened the power of the reality principle and introduced the idea of a death instinct, planting aggression at the instinctual core of the psyche. The battle between wish and reality, life and death, could never be won, Trilling said. "Everything that [Freudian man] gains he pays for in more than equal coin; compromise and the compounding with defeat constitute his best way of getting through the world." It was the "grandeur" of this "grim poetry" that Trilling admired, "its ultimate tragic courage in acquiescence to fate."[14]

Trilling and his intellectual cohort were stating Freudian ideas in an heroic modernist language: Freudian man acted out the agonistic image of the modern artist. "Is this not the essence of the modern belief about the nature of the artist," Trilling would rhetorically ask, "the man who goes down into that hell which is the historical beginning of the human soul, a beginning not outgrown . . . preferring the reality of this hell to the bland lies of the civilization that has overlaid it?"[15] The Freud who faced unblinkingly the chaos within and constructed from it the only truth available to human beings vindicated the modernist project and validated the moral seriousness of Trilling's intellectual class.

Trilling's Freud also legitimated a new political voice. In 1940 this was the anti-Stalinist voice of American left liberals disabused of their utopian hopes and anxious to reform America's simplistic optimism. By 1950, when Trilling republished the essay in *The Liberal Imagination*, the "grim poetry" of the modernist Freud could also express the combination of heady ambition and anxiety the intellectuals felt in assuming the mantle of America's world-historical role at a time of Cold War abroad and McCarthyite attack at home. American liberals, Trilling said, needed "the tough, complex psychology of Freud." He famously described the modernist virtues he wanted to graft onto liberalism as "variousness, possibility, complexity, and difficulty," but the lessons of these essays—and certainly of his Freud—were seldom "possibility." With good reason, Joseph Frank suggested a better title for the book would be "The Conservative Imagination."[16]

14. Ibid., 40–41, 52, 56–57. For Trilling's modernist curriculum, see Lionel Trilling, "On the Teaching of Modern Literature" (1961), in Trilling, *Beyond Culture: Essays on Literature and Learning* (New York: Viking, 1965), 23.
15. Ibid., 20–21.
16. Lionel Trilling, "The Function of the Little Magazine," in *The Liberal Imagination*, 99; Lionel Trilling, "Preface," in ibid., xiv–xv. On Frank, see Joseph Frank, "Lionel Trilling and the Conservative Imagination," *Sewanee Review* 64 (1956): 296–309. It is indicative of what would happen to Freud's reputation in the 1970s, below, that when Frank revisited his critique of

Trilling recommended the "tough, complex psychology of Freud" specifically against "the easy rationalistic optimism of Horney and Fromm."[17] Erich Fromm marked the border that separated the neo-Freudians from the modernist advocates of Freud. Along with Karen Horney and Harry Stack Sullivan, Fromm made Freud the baseline from which the neo-Freudians departed. In place of libido, Fromm put the drives for self-preservation and for social relatedness; in place of "biologically given nature," he put "the social process which creates man." Originally part of the radical Frankfurt school of social theorists who sought to integrate the insights of Marx and Freud, Fromm's pioneer social psychology was layered with historical utopianism and romantic optimism. In capitalist society, Fromm said, true psychological freedom could be glimpsed only in the creativity of artists and children, but the continued evolution to a planned society would develop persons who do not "repress essential parts" of themselves, who are capable of "the spontaneous activity of the total, integrated personality." Fromm was less a modernist than a utopian socialist, and he found Freud "so imbued with the spirit of his culture that he could not go beyond certain limits which were set by it." The neo-Freudians' Freud, mired in a retrograde culture, was not a modernist hero.[18]

Fromm's optimistic view of human possibility in the future went hand in hand, however, with fears of the deepening shadow of Nazism, fears the American modernists shared. Fromm's *Escape from Freedom*, reprinted twenty-two times during the twenty years after its publication in 1941, analyzed "those dynamic factors in the character structure of modern man, which made him want to give up freedom in Fascist countries and which so widely prevail in millions of our own people." Feeling isolated, anxious, and powerless, modern man escaped from freedom into authoritarianism, destructiveness, or automaton conformity. Fromm laid out for mid-century readers what would become widespread fears of conformity during the 1950s, fears not just of foreign totalitarianism but of a "soft," cultural, totalitarianism at home.[19]

Trilling in 1978, he put the blame for Trilling's problematic attitudes on the influence of Freud. See Joseph Frank, "Appendix (January 1978)," *Salmagundi* 41 (Spring 1978): 46–54.

17. Trilling, "The Function of the Little Magazine," 99; Trilling also wrote a harsh review of Karen Horney's *Self-Analysis*: "The Progressive Psyche," *The Nation*, September 1942, 215–17.

18. Erich Fromm, *Escape from Freedom* (New York: Holt, Rinehart and Winston, 1941), 9, 12, 258–60.

19. Ibid., esp. 6. On fears of totalitarianism and Fromm's role in framing them, see Wilfred M. McClay, *The Masterless: Self and Society in Modern America* (Chapel Hill: University of North Carolina Press, 1994), chap. 6.

For Trilling, the social emphasis of the neo-Freudians was itself symptomatic of the conformity they opposed. As postwar consumerism and Cold War orthodoxy took hold during the 1950s, Trilling moved toward a more liberatory Freud. In 1955, he was invited to give the Freud Anniversary Lecture of the New York Psychoanalytic Society and the New York Psychoanalytic Institute. The great strength of both modern literature and Freud, he said, was that they "make us aware of . . . the high authority of the self in its quarrel with its society and its culture." Our liberal democratic culture, Trilling feared, was permeated by the view that the individual should conform to the cultural environment, a view forwarded by the holistic conception of culture being promoted by social scientists. Even orthodox psychoanalysis, he chided, has fed into the emphasis on the individual's "adjustment" to society.[20]

In that context, the dark, biological ground of human nature in which Trilling had seen man's tragic fate now began to look like

> a liberating idea. It proposes to us that culture is not all-powerful. It suggests that there is a residue of human quality beyond the reach of cultural control. . . . Somewhere in the child, somewhere in the adult, there is a hard, irreducible, stubborn core of biological urgency, and biological necessity, and biological *reason*, that culture cannot reach.

Instead of resignation, he concluded with a note of defiance. That biological core "reserves the right, which sooner or later it will exercise, to judge the culture and resist and revise it." Although commentators have rightly questioned this reduction of the self to biology, Trilling had always been attracted to the Dionysian instinctual life he also feared. The heroic modernist self he constructed could stand acquiescent toward fate or defiant toward culture.[21]

Trilling attributed to Freud himself the grandeur and courage that he celebrated in his idea of the self. This was already implicit in his 1940 essay

---

20. Lionel Trilling, "Freud: Within and Beyond Culture," in Trilling, *Beyond Culture*, 89–118, esp. 103–10. This is a slightly revised version of the original, *Freud and the Crisis of Our Culture* (Boston: Beacon Press, 1955). In the original, Trilling elaborated on his quarrel with American culture (50–53), and also declared that his college students of 1955 responded to the great modernist and Freudian texts as fresh, strange, and momentous, just as he had himself thirty years before (10). For a very different judgment of his students just six years later, see below.

21. Trilling, "Freud: Within and Beyond Culture," 113, 115. For a sensitive analysis of the personal sources of Trilling's ambivalence, see Louis Menand, "Regrets Only: Lionel Trilling and His Discontents," *New Yorker*, 29 September 2008.

and became more explicit through the 1950s. Freud, Trilling told the psychoanalysts, was a "great personality." He had found in nineteenth-century science "that ethos of heroism which he always looked for in men, in groups, and in himself." Trilling himself likened Freud's ambition to that of the great poets, for like them, "Fame was the spur to Freud's clear spirit, to his desire to make clear what was darkly seen." He had a "masculine character," Trilling suggested, "the ability to dare and endure, to know and not to fear reality." Trilling did not construct this portrait of Freud as modernist hero out of thin air. Freud many times disclosed his wish for artistic genius, his self-image as an heroic "conquistador" of new lands, and his attitude of stoic acceptance of fate. But Trilling drew out these themes in a modernist language that conferred authority on the man as well as his ideas.[22]

The respect that Trilling bestowed on Freud during the 1950s was widespread in intellectual and academic communities. Among the intellectuals and professionals who gathered in a symposium to mark the centenary of Freud's birth in 1956, all acknowledged Freud's central importance. The historian Benjamin Nelson, who worshipfully introduced the published volume, took pride in the "free world" liberty that allowed Freud's ascendancy, underlining the Cold War context in which the conference occurred, and noted that all the participants preferred Freud to the neo-Freudians. Almost all of the humanist intellectuals who participated associated Freud with the great modernist writers and thinkers, sometimes specifically with the existentialists, the modernists who had "discovered existential anxiety as a constitutive element of human life." It was an Apollonian Freud, often a heroic one, whom they described as forging the conceptual tools necessary to deal with modernity's unease. The chief reservations were registered by the representatives of religion, who praised Freud's recognition of something like original sin but criticized his failure to appreciate spirituality, and by the representatives of academic psychology, who found much to

---

22. Trilling, "Freud: Within and Beyond Culture," 89, 91, 100, 102. For a similar American focus on the modernist thinker as hero, see Jennifer Ratner-Rosenhagen, "Conventional Iconoclasm: The Cultural Work of the Nietzsche Image in Twentieth-Century America," *Journal of American History* 93 (2006): 728–54. On Freud's attitudes toward his own accomplishments, see Ernest Jones, *The Life and Work of Sigmund Freud*, vol. 1: *The Formative Years and the Great Discoveries, 1856–1900* (New York: Basic Books, 1953), 35, 195–97, 348; vol. 2: *Years of Maturity 1901–1919* (New York: Basic Books, 1955), 2, 19, 183, 224–46, 344, 346–47. Trilling's heroic portrait echoes and augments that of Jones; see Trilling, "Introduction," vii–xviii, in Ernest Jones, *The Life and Work of Sigmund Freud*, ed. and abr. by Lionel Trilling and Steven Marcus (New York: Basic Books, 1961).

praise but pointedly denied his theories the title of "science." The literary critic Alfred Kazin alone among the conference participants located Freud's greatness in his Dionysian strain—his "insistence on individual fulfillment, satisfaction and happiness," his sanction of private passions and the importance of sex.[23]

The heroic Apollonian Freud was also much in view in H. Stuart Hughes's influential history of European social thought between 1890 and 1930, *Consciousness and Society*, published in 1958. Hughes made Freud "obviously the towering figure of the era." It was an era of both scientific reason and a plunge into the irrational. In Hughes's formulation, the agon of the modernist hero was to hold on to the Enlightenment, even while facing the full force of the irrational. Freud passed the first test: he sloughed off his original positivism without succumbing to a substitute faith. But like Leonardo, Hughes said, he was "torn by two impulses: the passion for scientific knowledge and the passion for creating works of art." In the end, Hughes regretted, the speculative artist "finally gained the upper hand." Max Weber ended as the hero of the volume—alone he precariously bridged the intellectual chasms of the age. Still, it was the Oedipus complex—"one of the most brilliant discoveries in the history of the human mind"—that Hughes used to analyze Weber's divided self.[24]

The crowning testament to Freud's 1950s intellectual authority was delivered by Philip Rieff's *Freud: The Mind of the Moralist* in 1959. Taking Freud as the pivotal and now dominant thinker of the twentieth century, Rieff, a social theorist, set out to assess the moral consequences of the Freudian ascendancy in strikingly modernist terms. Throughout the text, he placed Freud along with Nietzsche at the culmination of the romantic/modernist line. Freud spoke from and to the core modernist problem

---

23. *Freud and the 20th Century*, ed. Benjamin Nelson (New York: Meridian Books, 1957): on Nelson, 5, 6; on existentialism, 7–8, 133; on religious reservations, essays by Will Herberg, Jacques Maritain, and Reinhold Niebuhr; on scientific reservations, essays by Gardner Murphy and Jerome Bruner; on Kazin, 15, 17. For the incorporation of Trilling's view of modernism and Freud into literary criticism more generally, see Richard Ellmann and Charles Feidelson Jr., eds., *The Modern Tradition: Backgrounds of Modern Literature* (New York: Oxford University Press, 1965), esp. preface, pt. 5.

24. H. Stuart Hughes, *Consciousness and Society: The Reorientation of European Social Thought, 1890–1930* (New York: Knopf, 1958), 19, 32, 127–29, 334–35, 431. Another important text for social scientists was Dennis H. Wrong's widely cited article "The Oversocialized Conception of Man in Modern Sociology" (1961), which urged that sociologists follow the insights of Freud rather than the oversocialized formulations of the neo-Freudians. Wrong, who counted himself among the "New York Intellectuals," wrote the essay after rereading Freud and reading the "brilliant" texts of Marcuse, Brown, and Rieff cited below. See Dennis H. Wrong, *The Oversocialized Conception of Man* (New Brunswick, NJ: Transaction, 1999), x–xii, 1, 31–54, esp. 49.

of how to affirm the self in "a purposeless and meaningless universe." He taught modern man "how to live without belief." Freud's analytic therapy provided him the only means available to achieve a kind of authenticity, to assure himself "that he is himself alone and not merely acting out various roles."[25]

Rieff's Freud, like Trilling's, was an Apollonian voice of civilization and a defender of the modernist individual. As against the neo-Freudian Americanizers Fromm and Horney, Rieff echoed Trilling: "Freud's instinctualism [gave] an admirable sharpness to his estimate of human nature [and] kept some part of character safe from society."[26] Rieff's Freud was a modern hero, but not a tragic hero facing an implacable fate. Despite his "dark vision of the embattled self," Freud allowed for "the comic solvent, therapy," Rieff argued. Freud himself was practical and a meliorist. His self-analysis owed more to his "detached," "dispassionate" attitude than to his daring. Rieff was more uncertain about the "psychological man" being created by the Freudian era. While this new modal type had the existentialist's freedom to choose himself, such heroic notes were few and far between.[27]

Rieff produced, in fact, a chorus of discordant notes. The Freudian ideas hailed at the start of the book looked far less attractive by the end. What appeared in Trilling as stoic and heroic resignation was labeled by Rieff as "the managerial virtues of prudence and compromise." While Freud was not an advocate of "adjustment," his prudence was close to it, Rieff said, producing a self-centered "indifference to politics." Rieff made the Freudian "psychological man" the heir of capitalism's "economic man," with his calculating mentality and recognition of scarcity: "he is anti-heroic, shrewd, carefully counting his satisfactions and dissatisfactions." Psychoanalytic "technics" threatened to invade and conquer "the last enemy—man's inner life." Here was a psychoanalysis that compounded, rather than cured, the alienation of the modern individual.

For Rieff, the fault lay deep in modernity: democracy made Freud's insights the property of the ordinary middle class, creating a "democratic tyranny of psychologizing." The turn inward to interiority was presented less as an affirmative move than as the result of "the individual's failure to find anything else to affirm except the self." Rieff repeatedly acknowledged Freud's own greatness, but his conservative responses to the modern

25. Philip Rieff, *Freud: The Mind of the Moralist* (Garden City: Doubleday, 1961 [1959]), xxii–xxiii, 71, 96–101, 162, 334.
26. Ibid., 35–39, 122, 372, esp. 35.
27. Ibid., xxiii, 60, 67–69, 71–72, 240, 389.

democratic world revealed an ambivalence about the moral consequences of psychoanalysis that would soon deepen to implicate Freud.[28]

While Trilling and Rieff were setting out an Apollonian Freud that opposed the neo-Freudians' Americanized version, Erik Erikson was using neo-Freudian insights to domesticate both modernism and Freud. I mean "domesticate" in all its senses: to bring the foreign within the ambit of the native, to bring the wild into the sphere of the home, and to tame. Erikson was influenced by Fromm's theory of how individual character is formed by "the social process," but he always claimed to be a loyal Freudian. Standing somewhere between the neo-Freudians and the ego psychology developing within mainstream psychoanalysis, Erikson anchored his explication of individual development in Freud's libido theory, and then linked the psychosexual stages of development that Freud defined to psychosocial changes, "a succession of potentialities for significant interaction" with parents and the environment. In the resonant prose of his *Childhood and Society* (1950), psychoanalytic ideas reached an audience that would have shied away from Freud's more reductionist language of body parts.[29]

Erikson never claimed to be a modernist. He made the construction of a stable psychosocial identity the center of his theory. Adolescence brought the accrued instinctual and social capacities together in a firm identity, Erikson argued, upon which was built, in further stages, an adult life of meaningful love and work. Erikson thus gave the self a core of continuity over time and anchored it within rather than outside society: affirmation of the self—identity—could be achieved only within the roles society provided. Although himself an immigrant to the United States in 1933, probably half-Jewish by birth, Erikson separated himself from the refugee identity of the German intellectuals who emigrated to America during the 1930s. He responded to political upheaval and its crisis mentality with a studied assertion of the possibilities offered by modernity in the United States.[30]

Yet with his education in German romanticism and his artistic proclivities, Erikson also inscribed a measure of modernist values in his develop-

---

28. Ibid., 79, 278, 280, 362, 390–92.

29. Erik H. Erikson, *Childhood and Society* (New York: W. W. Norton, 1963 [1950]), esp. 67 and parts 1 and 3; Erik H. Erikson, *Identity and the Life Cycle* (New York: International Universities Press, 1959). On Erikson, see Lawrence J. Friedman, *Identity's Architect: A Biography of Erik H. Erikson* (Cambridge, MA: Harvard University Press, 1999).

30. On Erikson's American assimilationist stance, see Friedman, *Identity's Architect*, esp. 103–4, 143–47.

mental theory and middle-class life. The heroism the Apollonians admired appeared in Erikson's account of the difficulty of achieving balance and mutuality. Development was a lifelong endeavor, a cumulative achievement of traditional virtues, but also a series of struggles never fully surmounted. Then, too, Erikson offered the possibility of an authentic self, an identity that drew on the person's deepest wishes and intuitions as well as the social world. Authenticity was really the theme of Erikson's second book of the decade, *Young Man Luther*, the story of a youth determined to find his own way of "meaning it." And if alienation was not a mark of authenticity for Erikson, he did insert a youthful period of alienation into the healthy life-cycle. Nor did he take the society as given. Using a language of liberal reform, he criticized the "mechanical" character of life in modernity, particularly in America, and enjoined society to provide its members meaningful roles.[31]

The Dionysian prize was Freud's "utopia of genitality." It implied, Erikson wrote, "mutuality of orgasm / with a loved partner / of the other sex / with whom one is able and willing to share a mutual trust / and with whom one is able and willing to regulate the cycles of work, procreation, recreation / so as to secure to the offspring, too, all the stages of a satisfactory development." That "utopia" now reads like a caricature of 1950s domesticity. But it promised, to those who accepted its challenges and limits, the experience of sexual freedom: "orgastic potency" and "the climactic turmoil of orgasm, a supreme experience of the mutual regulation of two beings." Erikson's Freudian version of psychological development tamed modernist experience and brought it within the ambit of the respectable middle class, at the same time widening and humanizing the bourgeois values he brought with him from Europe and found in America. He found his largest audience during the 1960s, when young people who were sympathetic to the modernist cultural ethos welcomed his message of an available authenticity within middle-class life.[32]

A third modernist version of Freudian ideas to appear in the 1950s took

---

31. Ibid., chap. 1; Erikson, *Childhood and Society*, 190, 273–74, 306–25, 412. On authenticity, see Erikson's *Young Man Luther: A Study in Psychoanalysis and History* (New York: W. W. Norton, 1958), esp. 209–10, and Friedman, *Identity's Architect*, 271–77. The "judiciousness" he urged in conclusion was not Apollonian "maturity" but closer to his friend Margaret Mead's disengagement from doctrinaire commitments. Erikson's cosmopolitan is a positive version of Rieff's detached psychological man; he is tolerant because he hangs loose: Erikson, *Childhood and Society*, 416–17; Margaret Mead, *Coming of Age in Samoa* (New York: HarperCollins, 2001 [1928]), chap. 14.

32. Erikson, *Childhood and Society*, 92, 265–66; Friedman, *Identity's Architect*, 237–41, 303–23.

Dionysian possibilities far more seriously. Herbert Marcuse's *Eros and Civilization* and Norman O. Brown's *Life Against Death* made Freud the central figure in the understanding of modernity and its radical future. Marcuse, a refugee from Nazi fascism, and Brown, an American classicist, both turned to psychology to restore lost political hopes. Cognizant of Freud's late work and the radical critique of modernity it implied, they believed the new technologies of mass destruction made Freud's death instinct plausible and a total escape from modern technological society urgent. Taking their cue from the early Freud, who had put libido at the center of psychic development, they looked to Eros for salvation.[33]

Marcuse found a "hidden trend in psychoanalysis": by exposing the essential antagonism between civilization and happiness, Freud upheld "the tabooed aspiration of humanity." For the individual, Marcuse said, psychoanalysis restores "the forbidden images and impulses of childhood [that] tell the truth that reason denies." A Frankfurt school social philosopher steeped in Marx, he argued that the advance of science and technology was abolishing want and, with it, the necessity of repression. The logic of history opened the way for escape from modernity's mechanical rationality into the aesthetic dimension of life. The death instinct presented no insuperable obstacle; the problem rather was "the systematic constraints which civilization places on the life instincts, and . . . their consequent inability to 'bind' aggression effectively." With Eros in command, the aesthetic exploration of "pleasure, sensuousness, beauty, truth, art, and freedom"—hitherto only the domain of geniuses and Bohemians—would restore the body's polymorphous perversity and create a new order as a "realm of play." Modernity could be remade to accord with the modernists' aesthetic vision.[34]

Brown's book gained attention for both its radical theory and striking psychoanalytic observations on Western literature. Like Marcuse, he too expected a new affluence in society, but he relied largely on the change of consciousness psychoanalysis produced. For Brown it was primarily fear of death, recognition of being a body, that led to the repression of polymorphous perversity and to technological efforts to conquer nature. By recovering the memory of the original infantile fusion of subject and object,

---

33. Herbert Marcuse, *Eros and Civilization: A Philosophical Inquiry into Freud* (Boston: Beacon Press, 1955), and Norman O. Brown, *Life Against Death: The Psychoanalytical Meaning of History* (Middletown, CT: Wesleyan University Press, 1959), esp. xvii–xviii. On Marcuse, and secondarily on Brown, see Paul A. Robinson, *The Freudian Left: Wilhelm Reich, Geza Roheim, Herbert Marcuse* (New York: Harper & Row, 1969), and Richard King, *The Party of Eros: Radical Social Thought and the Realm of Freedom* (Chapel Hill: University of North Carolina Press, 1972).

34. Marcuse, *Eros and Civilization*, esp. 18–20, 172, 222–23, 272.

life and death, one could recover the dialectical consciousness that would unite all dualisms and banish repression. Without repression, a body fully satisfied would no longer fear death.[35]

During the 1950s, then, modernists valorized Freud himself and the significance of his ideas even as they set out very different conceptions of the intellectual, cultural, and political implications of his work. For a time, the multiple adaptations of Freud seemed only to multiply his presence in the culture and enrich his meaning. Differences did not overwhelm the common admiration for Freud and his ideas. In 1959, for example, no doubt finding kinship with their acceptance of the death instinct and their disdain for neo-Freudian revisionism, Trilling praised Marcuse's *Eros and Civilization* and especially Brown's *Life Against Death*. Despite what Trilling called his own "thoroughly anti-Utopian mind," he was content to read Brown, he said, as he read Blake—for its intellectual pleasures, "with all practical objections suppressed." If these writers had reservations about Erikson's heterodox Freudianism during the 1950s, they did not express them publicly, and Erikson was included among the mixed group of admirers at the 1956 centenary of Freud's birth, where only the neo-Freudians were excluded. And even the neo-Freudians couched their criticism of Freud's theories within a frame acknowledging the fundamental character of his discoveries and the greatness of the man. When the neo-Freudian David Riesman published his 1946 lectures on Freud in 1954, he apologized for their overly critical tone: it had been meant to counter a University of Chicago audience "too inclined to swallow him whole." Fromm in his 1959 *Sigmund Freud's Mission*, though unsparing in his criticism, considered Freud, if not a hero, a "truly great man" and wrote that he could not imagine a future world without Freud's ideas.[36]

Why then did the intellectual tide turn against Freud? Certainly the attacks on him and psychoanalysis that would increasingly prevail were not new. Even in Trilling's 1955 speech to the psychoanalysts—a speech that can be taken as one high point of Freud's intellectual authority—Trilling felt the need to answer the criticisms of Freud that would later gain trac-

---

35. Brown, *Life Against Death*, esp. parts 3 and 6.
36. Lionel Trilling, "Paradise Reached For," *Mid-Century* (Fall 1959): 16–21, esp. 21; Marcuse, "Epilogue: Critique of New-Freudian Revisionism," in *Eros and Civilization*; Brown, *Life Against Death*, 203–4; David Riesman, *Individualism Reconsidered* (Glencoe, IL: Free Press, 1954), 306; Erich Fromm, *Sigmund Freud's Mission: An Analysis of His Personality and Influence* (New York: Harper & Row, 1959), esp. 1, 117–20.

tion: Freud was too radical, too reactionary, too personally ambitious, too speculative rather than scientific, too much the male chauvinist; his acolytes were too dogmatic.[37] What occurred later was not new misgivings about Freud and psychoanalysis so much as a changed climate of opinion in which long-standing misgivings took on new weight.

Just as the rising authority of modernism advanced Freud's ideas and valorized Freud himself, so changes in the evaluation of modernism reflected back on Freud. When cultural and political radicalism exploded during the 1960s, modernism began to look different. By the 1960s and 1970s, student radicalism, the antiwar movement, the emergence of feminism, rapidly changing sexual mores, and the rise of a "New Left" and counterculture dramatically shifted perspectives. Modernism was not the only source of the new attitudes, but the young radicals announced their debt to Marcuse and Brown, and desires for authenticity and loosening sexual norms were easily linked to the modernist insights they had explored in college.[38] As cultural and political radicalism unfolded, critics across the political spectrum found reasons to question the implications of modernism.

To the Apollonians, it now seemed that modernism had succeeded all too well. Trilling mapped their disillusion with modernism in the 1960s, as he had charted its rise in the 1940s and 1950s. A defining moment for Trilling may well have been the Phi Beta Kappa address by Norman O. Brown at Columbia University in 1960, where, as Trilling remembered it, Brown "spoke of the 'blessing' and the 'supernatural powers' which he desired to attain and which . . . came only with madness." Brown surely did not mean "literal insanity," Trilling said, only a "metaphorical insanity," but Trilling was no longer able to overlook these intellectual extremisms and suppress "all practical objections."[39]

The following year he publicly wondered whether it was appropriate to

---

37. Trilling, "Freud: Within and Beyond Culture," 91, 98–101, 109, 113.

38. For a comprehensive view of the 1960s, see Howard Brick, *Age of Contradiction: American Thought and Culture in the 1960s* (New York: Twayne, 1998). On the modernist values of youth radicalism, see Morris Dickstein, *Gates of Eden: American Culture in the Sixties* (New York: Basic Books, 1977): "It was not modernism that was responsible for the alienation of the young in the sixties, but modernism contributed to the cultural form and the utopian content which that dissidence took on" (267). See also James Miller, *"Democracy Is in the Streets": From Port Huron to the Streets of Chicago* (New York: Simon and Schuster, 1987), and Doug Rossinow, *The Politics of Authenticity: Liberalism, Christianity, and the New Left in America* (New York: Columbia University Press, 1998).

39. Lionel Trilling, *Sincerity and Authenticity* (Cambridge, MA: Harvard University Press, 1972), 169; Louis Menand, "Introduction," to Sigmund Freud, *Civilization and Its Discontents* (New York: W. W. Norton, 2005 [1930]), 26.

teach modern literature to college students. Making these shocking texts the subject of dutiful papers and tests blunted their power to call into question the deepest levels of the self. Yet contrariwise, Trilling feared that the intended message of these texts—that one ought to free oneself from the middle class—was in fact getting through to these middle-class students. Was that a message we teachers should be sending, he asked? When a student inquired in class how to "generalize" from Mann's *Magic Mountain* "to young people at large," Trilling drew the line he had tried to draw in his own life: the ideas in the course had reference only to "the private life . . . [they] touched the public life only in some indirect or tangential way." Even bringing them before a class, he now feared, encouraged their entry into "the practical sphere."[40]

By 1965, when he republished the essay in *Beyond Culture*, the public consequences of modernist ideas were plainly visible. Trilling was now certain that the adversary culture promulgated by modernist literature and entrenched in the universities and a sizable portion of the middle class had become dangerous. Look what has become, he warned, of the ideas of "sex, violence, madness, and art itself." He was forced to the conclusion—"which, indeed, rather surprises me"—that "art does not always tell the truth or the best kind of truth."[41]

Trilling took his final measure of modernism in 1972 in a historical study of authenticity, the modernist ideal that he believed had become an absolute—and unthinking—demand of the adversarial American culture. He praised again the Freud whose late work had planted *in*authenticity deep within the psyche, where it stood firm against "all hopes of achieving happiness through the radical revision of social life." It was the Apollonian Freud and Nietzsche who had proved themselves the genuine modernists. Their acceptance of negation, their patrician stance of "simultaneous commitment and detachment," sustained a true authenticity, "the authenticity of human existence that formerly had been ratified by God." Trilling thus read out of modernism the Dionysian turn it had taken in American culture, but kept hold of Freud and Freudianism.[42]

Many of the postwar Apollonian celebrants of Freud, however, began to hold Freud's ideas at least partly responsible for the new cultural radicalism, even while exempting Freud himself from indictment. Their conservative response to the radicalism of the 1960s turned them against modern-

---

40. Trilling, "On the Teaching of Modern Literature," esp. 28.
41. Trilling, "Preface," *Beyond Culture*, xvi–xviii.
42. Trilling, *Sincerity and Authenticity*, 5, 147–51, 156–59.

ism, and Freud suffered in the process. Daniel Bell, like Trilling, read the Dionysian strain out of modernism, but his was a deeper and more influential indictment that linked the radical turn of the 1960s to postmodernism. If modernism began in the estimable bourgeois values of individuality and self-awareness, Bell said, it had gone on to produce an "unyielding rage" against rationality, morality, and the limits of existence. The triumph of modernism ended in a new stage of Western history and a new "postmodern mood," a compound in which only impulse, pleasure, and emotion were valued, in which all boundaries were erased, and "acting out" rather than aesthetic creation was the highest form of human being. Bell made the Dionysian Freudians prime exemplars of the new postmodern mood: they had "pressed the logic of modernism toward its most radical theoretical conclusions" and "sounded a note" taken up by "the cultural mass" and "the porno-pop culture of the day."[43]

If we ignore Bell's alarmist gloss, his intuition that postmodernism was built upon core modernist insights remains useful: postmoderns extended the modernist critique of rationality into an unsettling exploration of how language and culture formed subjectivity itself. Rejecting the modernists' elitist historical narrative with its avant-garde stance, they explored a more relaxed experience of modernity's hedonistic consumer culture. Precisely these features, of course, excited Bell's fears. The alarmist gloss was crucial to the growing reaction against modernism. Bell was careful to exempt Freud himself. Psychoanalysis was for Freud a "half-way house," a "compromise" between instinct and reality; he made clear that "life has to consist of boundaries and balance." Still, Freud had forged "intellectual bridges to the postmodern ideas."[44]

Freud figured more centrally in the debacle Rieff now feared. In his 1966 *The Triumph of the Therapeutic*, Rieff returned to the "psychological man" he had forecast earlier, this time with a conservative social theory that explained his deep ambivalence. Culture, Rieff said, was "a design of motives directing the self outward, toward those communal purposes in which alone the self can be realized and satisfied." It survived "by the power of its institutions to bind and loose men in the conduct of their affairs with

43. Daniel Bell, "Beyond Modernism, Beyond Self," in *Art, Politics, and Will: Essays in Honor of Lionel Trilling*, ed. Quentin Anderson, Stephen Donadio, and Steven Marcus (New York: Basic Books, 1977), 220, 231–32, 245, 248. Bell's essay expanded the cultural analysis he set out in *The Cultural Contradictions of Capitalism* (New York: Basic Books, 1976). For a favorable discussion of the Dionysian Freudians' transitional position between modernism and postmodernism, see Marianne DeKoven, *Utopia Limited: The Sixties and the Emergence of the Postmodern* (Durham, NC: Duke University Press, 2004).

44. Bell, "Beyond Modernism, Beyond Self," 231, 234, 236.

reasons which sink . . . deep." It necessarily issued moral decrees. Christian culture had long provided the communal purposes and the decrees to bind men to them, but Christian culture was now replaced by the therapeutic culture of the "psychologizers"—inheritors of the dualistic modernist tradition, "which pits human nature against social order." Its goal was only individual happiness, its horizon only management of the self. How, Rieff asked, can such a culture be a worthy one?[45]

Rieff went out of his way to reiterate his esteem for Freud's genius. Freud "has systematized our unbelief; his is the most inspiring anti-creed yet offered a post-religious culture." But at the same time, Rieff noted, Freud "prepared the way for the post-Freudians" by emphasizing the instinctual price that civilization exacts. And it was precisely "unbelief" that Rieff saw as the problem. Psychoanalysis created only a "negative community": it set people free to concentrate further upon the self. Rieff's only recourse was to separate Freud himself from his ideas: "The exemplary cast of Freud's mind and character is more enduring than the particulars of his doctrine. In culture it is always the example that survives; the person is the immortal idea. Psychoanalysis was the perfect vehicle for Freud's intellectual character." Given Rieff's premises, he could not convincingly claim that psychoanalysis was the perfect vehicle for ours. By the late 1970s, facing what he called an "erotocratic culture" given over wholly to "remissiveness," Rieff condemned Freud for not grounding repression securely and for denying a sacred order of belief to enforce it. "There derives from Freud's mind more than any other that fresh symbolic action, repressing the repressive, from which this century has taken its direction."[46]

By the late 1970s, then, the conservative political and cultural reaction was well under way, a shift undoubtedly encouraged by the more precarious condition of the United States economically and as a world power. Many of the architects of Freud's intellectual authority in the 1950s who had praised him for Apollonian modernist virtues had retreated from a modernism tainted with the radicalism of the sixties and had tarnished Freud with the vices of modernism and its postmodern successors. The shift withdrew from Freud's ideas what had been a high cultural imprima-

---

45. Philip Rieff, *The Triumph of the Therapeutic: Uses of Faith After Freud* (Wilmington, DE: ISI Books, 2006 [1966]), esp. 1–3, 51, 223. For an excellent account of Rieff's conservative trajectory, see Kenneth S. Piver, "Philip Rieff: The Critic of Psychoanalysis as Cultural Theorist," in *Discovering the History of Psychiatry*, ed. Mark S. Micale and Roy Porter (New York: Oxford University Press, 1994), 191–215.

46. Rieff, *The Triumph of the Therapeutic*, 25, 32, 37, 72. Philip Rieff, "Epilogue: One Step Further," in Rieff, *Freud: The Mind of a Moralist*, 3d ed. (Chicago: University of Chicago Press, 1979), 368, 376, 381–83, 396.

tur, and without that imprimatur, the criticisms of Freud could multiply and be more easily heard.

Frederick Crews provides an example of how the recoil from Freud among humanist intellectuals gathered steam during the 1970s. A graduate student in English when the modernist canon was becoming institutionalized, Crews could take its ascendancy for granted; his disciplinary concerns revolved around how to pursue the critical craft. Sympathetic to radicalism and "first drawn to Freud by his promise of a Faustian key to knowledge," Crews identified with the Freudians and set himself against the New Critics and theorists who urged that criticism focus only on the text itself or formalist categories. Both camps proclaimed modernist values, whether the Freudians' exploration of subjectivity or the New Critics' purist demand that the text not be made to "mean" anything beyond itself. The New Critics claimed as well, however, that by containing interpretation they could achieve a kind of objectivity. Crews initially was not moved by the charge that "psychological speculation" was "unscientific," but urged critics to follow "intuition" and look below surface "evidence." His 1966 study of Nathaniel Hawthorne showed Hawthorne to be, like Freud himself, a "self-examining neurotic," whose characters followed "perfectly . . . the logic of psychoanalysis." In 1969 he still argued for "us Freudians" and chose "the capacity to be moved" over "the quest for total certainty."[47]

Apparently the rise of countercultural radicalism and the New Left led him to reconsider. What he called the Freudians' closed system of thought and the students' radical Freudianism, with its "blend of libidinal anarchism and 'existential' self-absorption," now made Freudian ideas seem a serious threat to "free institutions." By 1975, psychoanalysis also seemed a threat to the literary discipline. Crews complained that Freud's closed theoretical system destroyed the richness of literature, but in the end it was certainty that claimed his allegiance. With reference to Ricoeur's "epistemology of suspicion," he argued that "the epistemology in which Freudianism squarely resides" is premised on a subjectivity that makes "any definite statements about literature [impossible]."

If psychological needs governed the author, so too did they govern the reader and literary critic. Crews called up the specter of a university class on

---

47. Frederick Crews, *The Sins of the Fathers: Hawthorne's Psychological Themes* (Oxford: Oxford University Press, 1966), 5–6, 260–61. On Crews's attitudes during the early 1960s, see Frederick Crews, *Out of My System: Psychoanalysis, Ideology, and Critical Method* (New York: Oxford, 1975), chaps. 1–5, esp. xiv, 35–36, 60–61, 80–83. On the New Critics and the literary discipline, see Gerald Graff, *Professing Literature: An Institutional History* (Chicago: University of Chicago Press, 1987), chaps. 9, 11–12.

poetry turned into an "encounter" session that "permits all readers to trade associations to the poem on a relaxed and equal basis." Following the logic of Freud's epistemology, there was no longer an objective poem to analyze, only every reader's poem, and no longer a hierarchy of analysts. Rehearsing the epistemological debates that would occupy the humanities as postmodern theories gained ground during the 1980s, Crews concluded that Karl Popper's philosophy of science, with its social theory of validation, was necessary to save his own and his discipline's claim to authority.[48]

Crews followed out this new quest for certainty all the way to the culture wars. By 1980 he was ready to publish a scathing critique of psychoanalysis in the neoconservative *Commentary* magazine. Likening psychoanalysis to mesmerism or phrenology, he declared both its psychological theory and therapeutic effectiveness wholly unproven by empirical evidence or logic. The critique focused almost entirely on the failure of psychoanalysis to meet empirical and rational standards of truth.[49] By the 1970s, of course, Crews could cite a considerable body of critical studies by psychiatrists and academic psychologists questioning the scientific basis of psychoanalytic ideas and the effectiveness of its therapy. Surveying a spate of critiques of Freud that appeared around 1980—Frank Sulloway, Jeffrey Masson, and Adolf Grünbaum—Paul Robinson noted their "obliviousness to the linguistic turn in intellectual affairs" and their "uninflected positivist views" and suggested that the anti-Freudian mood was part of the 1980s "broad-scale revolt against the culture of modernism." Robinson is surely correct that the anti-Freudian mood was linked to a revolt against the culture of modernism, "a revolt against the uncertainties and ambiguities that the modernist legacy burdened us with, above all the sense that the self is unreliable, indeed largely unknowable."[50]

Crews is an example of a humanist intellectual who was well aware of the epistemological implications of the postmodern turn and attacked Freud because of them. He made sure to associate Freud with Nietzsche and Heidegger and with the postmodern European theorists who had begun to excite conservative fears: "Continental thinkers, from Jürgen Habermas and Paul Ricoeur to Jacques Derrida and Jacques Lacan and the late Roland Barthes, who for the moment strike literary commentators as most advanced," he noted disparagingly, "are all Freudians in their way."[51] By

48. Crews, *Out of My System*, chaps. 6 and 9, esp. 129, 177–81.
49. Frederick Crews, "Analysis Terminable," *Commentary* 70 (July 1980): 25–34.
50. Paul Robinson, *Freud and His Critics* (Berkeley: University of California Press, 1993), 3, 15–17.
51. Crews, "Analysis Terminable," 25.

1980 Freud's modernism excited the opprobrium of a younger generation of intellectuals recoiling not only from the political and cultural turmoil of the 1960s but also from the deeper political and cultural uncertainties introduced by postmodernism during the 1970s.

By no means did all the criticism of Freud come from those moving rightwards away from modernism. One of the most potent challenges to Freud's intellectual authority in the public arena came from new feminist scholars. Betty Friedan began that attack in *The Feminine Mystique* of 1963. The right of women to self-realization on the same terms that society grants to men is grounded in American individualism, but it has been fueled and inflected by different cultural traditions at different times. During the 1910s and 1920s, both Freud and modernism were central to the first wave of the modern feminist movement, with Freud generally seen as an ally in women's sexual liberation. Leading the second wave into new territory, Friedan like the male Freudians traced a path from the left politics of the 1930s to psychoanalysis and like them demanded self-realization in the modernist idiom of existentialism: "in the end, a woman, as a man, has the power to choose, and to make her own heaven or hell."[52]

Friedan equally used the idiom of Eriksonian identity: Erikson, a "brilliant psychoanalyst," had diagnosed the identity crisis facing young men today. She proclaimed "this same identity crisis in women." Her hallmark of healthy identity for women was the same one Erikson had prescribed for men alone—"creative work of [one's] own that contributes to the human community." In its central faith that it was possible to construct an authentic self through socially meaningful work, Friedan's was a domesticated modernism. So was her belief that "self-realization . . . is inextricably linked to [the highest sexual fulfillment]." Quoting the humanist psychologist Abraham Maslow, she claimed that only the fully realized woman could enjoy "the sexual pleasures . . . in their most intense and ecstatic per-

---

52. On the connections between feminism, modernism, and Freud, see Christine Stansell, *American Moderns: Bohemian New York and the Creation of a New Century* (New York: Metropolitan Books, 2000); Mari Jo Buhle, *Feminism and Its Discontents: A Century of Struggle with Psychoanalysis* (Cambridge, MA: Harvard University Press, 1998); Jane Gerhard, *Desiring Revolution: Second-Wave Feminism and the Rewriting of American Sexual Thought, 1920–1982* (New York: Columbia University Press, 2001). For the changing political context of Friedan's work, see Daniel Horowitz, *Betty Friedan and the Making of the Feminine Mystique: The American Left, The Cold War, and Modern Feminism* (Amherst: University of Massachusetts Press, 1998). For Friedan's existentialism, see Betty Friedan, *The Feminine Mystique* (New York: W. W. Norton, 2001 [1963]), 50–51, 64–65, 126, 429, 431, 434, 461–62, 550n, esp. 53.

fection," could appreciate "freshly and naively, the basic goods of life with awe, pleasure, wonder, and even ecstasy." Here were modernist epiphanies within a liberal framework of love and work.[53]

It was against this standard that Friedan measured Freud's own ideas and declared them wanting. Freud was the central figure in Friedan's attack on the feminine mystique. Although she stood by "the basic genius of Freud's discoveries" and gave him some credit for insisting that women had a sexual nature, she declared unequivocally that "the Feminine Mystique derived its power from Freudian thought." Freud's definition of women by their sexual biology and the meanings he attributed to it of passivity, deficiency, and "penis envy" gave "the conventional image of femininity new authority" when it otherwise might have disappeared. Even in domesticated form, modernist ideals had the power to hold Freud accountable.[54]

Friedan's critique of Freud was only one of many attacks that resonated in the 1960s and 1970s as the women's movement gained force. Kate Millett was more radical than Friedan, calling for the abolition of patriarchy, monogamous marriage, and fixed gender roles. She too declared Freud "beyond question the strongest individual counter-revolutionary force in the ideology of sexual politics." Indeed Millett found such modernist writers as D. H. Lawrence and Norman Mailer to be prime exemplars of reactionary sexual attitudes. It was only the homosexual sensibility of Jean Genet that reached the revolutionary conclusions Millett sought. Genet's brutal depictions of homosexual roles had shown that "divorced from their . . . assumed biological congruity, masculine and feminine" were merely "terms of praise and blame, authority and servitude." According to Millett, Genet had demonstrated "the utterly arbitrary and invidious nature of sex role" and thereby exposed the instability of "gender identity." As the gay liberation movement added its voice to the feminist critique of psychoanalysis, Freud increasingly appeared not as a modernist hero but as a prisoner of his Victorian culture.[55]

Freud's personal demotion was perhaps inevitable given the highly visible target his advocates had erected in the 1950s and the decline in authority of his ideas in medical and highbrow culture. His Apollonian advocates

53. Friedan, *The Feminine Mystique*, on identity: 50–51, 65, 86, 185, 429, 438, 510–11, esp. 134–36, 459; on sexuality, 438, 444–45.
54. Ibid., 166–69.
55. Kate Millett, *Sexual Politics* (Garden City, NY: Doubleday, 1970), 178, 343, 362–63. See also Buhle, *Feminism and Its Discontents*, chap. 6; Ronald Bayer, *Homosexuality and American Psychiatry: The Politics of Diagnosis* (Princeton, NJ: Princeton University Press, 1987 [1981]); *Out of the Closets: Voices of Gay Liberation*, ed. Karla Jay and Allen Young (New York: New York University Press, 1992 [1972]), 141–53.

had to work hard to maintain his stature when they turned against the modernism to which his ideas were linked. By the 1970s, however, there was also a considerable body of personal criticism arrayed against Freud. The neo-Freudians had linked their criticism of his ideas to accounts of his neurotic weaknesses and cultural biases. Conflicts in the psychoanalytic camp itself produced biographical material on Freud that could be used against him. Critics unearthed evidence of Freud's male chauvinism, bourgeois evasions, equivocations about his Jewishness, and domineering jealousy toward colleagues. The evidence, moreover, was recovered from the defenses, concealments, and counter-stories Freud had woven around himself: the great truth-teller, it seemed, had not told the truth about himself.[56] If Freud's defenders past and present can conclude that he was, after all, only human, in a post-sixties culture in which the modernist ideal of authenticity heightened sensitivity to hypocrisy, the personal attacks against Freud took hold. Erikson met the same fate when Marshall Berman in 1975, writing from the New Left, accused him—this theorist of identity—of hiding his own Jewishness.[57]

During the 1970s, then, Freud no longer appeared to be the towering intellectual presence of the twentieth century, but his ideas still commanded some authority on the public stage. Feminist writers like Shulamith Firestone and Nancy Chodorow found openings for feminist theory in Freud's analysis of women as well as in a number of revisionist psychoanalytic schools. Theorists of homosexuality adapted Freud's theory of bisexuality while at the same time rejecting postwar psychoanalysts' normalizing of heterosexuality. From the cultural right, the historian Christopher Lasch followed Rieff into a scathing indictment of America's therapeutic culture, but drew on Freud's Oedipal model of the nuclear family to make his case.[58]

---

56. Riesman, *Individualism Reconsidered*, chaps. 21–22; Fromm, *Sigmund Freud's Mission*, chaps. 2–9; Elisabeth Young-Bruehl, "A History of Freud Biographies," in *Discovering the History of Psychiatry*, ed. Micale and Porter, 157–73.

57. Marshall Berman, "Life History and the Historical Moment," *New York Times Book Review*, 30 March 1975, 1–2, 22. See also Friedman, *Identity's Architect*, 429–36. Trilling was one of those who wrote Berman congratulating him on the essay: "a good and useful job you have done on Erikson! . . . I've suspected everything since *Childhood and Society*" (ibid., 434).

58. Gerhard, *Desiring Revolution*, 96–97, 167–71; Buhle, *Feminism and Its Discontents*, chaps. 6–7; Joanne Meyerowitz, "How Common Culture Shapes the Separate Lives: Sexuality, Race, and Mid-Twentieth-Century Social Constructionist Thought," *Journal of American History* 96 (2010): 1057–84. On Lasch, see Eric Miller, *Hope in a Scattering Time: A Life of Christopher Lasch* (Grand Rapids, MI: William B. Eerdmans, 2010), esp. 138–51, 226; Christopher Lasch, *Haven in a Heartless World* (New York: Basic Books, 1977), and *The Culture of Narcissism: American Life in an Age of Diminishing Expectations* (New York: W. W. Norton, 1979).

For these writers, and even more for others after 1980, Freud's corpus no longer provided the foundation on which other ideas must be built, but was reworked within other frameworks and could be selectively pillaged. In that form, his ideas have become embedded in specialized areas of academic culture. Under the aegis of the postmodern left, departments of literature, humanities, and film remain repositories of Freudian thought among American intellectuals, although it is psychoanalytic theory seen through the lens of linguistic theories. Postmodernists see in Freud's writings, Allan Megill notes, "a virtuoso pursuit of interpretation," not the guide to modern life that Freud himself proposed and that American modernist intellectuals found so compelling during the postwar decades. Still, as Erich Heller suggested in 1983, psychoanalysis "would not have been invented had it not been for the disappearance from our beliefs of any certainty concerning the nature of human being." So long as that uncertainty continues, Freud is likely to remain among the vital modernist thinkers who addressed it.[59]

In sum, the highly favorable reception of Freud's ideas during the middle decades of the twentieth century among intellectuals and their educated middle-class audience owed a great deal to the simultaneous turn of American culture toward modernism, and the rapid loss of his intellectual ascendancy during the following decades owed a great deal to the vicissitudes of modernism as its authority splintered on the cultural politics of the 1960s. Freud was presented to Americans—in several guises—as the preeminent modernist; when many of his advocates blamed modernism for student radicalism and countercultural excess, his intellectual authority began to decline. The rise of feminism and postmodernism during the 1970s accelerated the decline, as Freud was linked by some to modernist/postmodernist vices and found by others to be lacking in the modernist virtues of a liberalizing culture. Freud is an important marker of the dissolution of the modernist ascendancy at mid-century into the postmodern multiplicity and ideological polarization of the twentieth century's *fin-de-siècle*.

---

59. For revealing accounts of Freud's post-1980 influence on the humanities, see *Literature and Psychoanalysis*, ed. Edith Kurzweil and William Phillips (New York: Columbia University Press, 1983); *Psychoanalysis and Culture at the Millennium*, ed. Nancy Ginsburg and Roy Ginsburg (New Haven, CT: Yale University Press, 1999); Ernest Wallwork, *Psychoanalysis and Ethics* (New Haven, CT: Yale University Press, 1991). On postmodernism and Freud, see Megill, *Prophets of Extremity*, 321–22. Erich Heller is quoted from "Observations on Psychoanalysis and Modern Literature," in the Kurzweil and Phillips volume, 76.

SEVEN

Freud, Anxiety, and the Cold War

LOUIS MENAND

Sigmund Freud and psychoanalysis enjoyed considerable professional and social success in the United States after 1945, success that persisted for twenty years. American psychiatry was dominated by psychoanalytic theory, and Freudian concepts flourished in both sophisticated and popular cultural realms. Historical analysis of this phenomenon is complicated, for a number of reasons. For one thing, it is not obvious why psychoanalytic theory appealed to a society generally antipathetic to abstract systems and philosophical pessimism. For another, "Freudianism" in postwar America was not a unitary signifier. Like Marx, Freud enforced orthodoxy among his disciples; as did Marx's, his followers turned his system to diverse ends after his death, some of which would probably have appalled him. Finally, and most strikingly, Freudianism managed to coexist in the cultural imagination with trends in psychiatry and intellectual life with which it was partly and sometimes wholly incompatible. Somehow, for a surprisingly long period, the incompatibility did little to subvert the cultural authority of Freudian theory. Freud was regarded as a pioneer of modern thought, a scientific discoverer, and psychoanalysis was considered the theoretical foundation for psychiatric practice. Psychoanalysis went through what one historian has described as a "golden age of popularization."[1]

The purpose of this essay is to suggest that one reason for the "fit" between Freudianism and postwar American culture had to do with what might be called the Cold War discourse of anxiety. This discourse, too, was not unitary. It was an amalgam of strains in psychological, philosophical, political, and religious thought, not all of them consistent with one an-

1. Nathan Hale Jr., *The Rise and Crisis of Psychoanalysis in the United States: Freud and the Americans, 1917–1985* (New York: Oxford University Press, 1995), 276.

other. As in the case of psychoanalysis, the contradictions eventually produced some unintended consequences. For a prolonged period, though—stability being highly valued in the early Cold War years—the concept of anxiety seemed, to many people, the key to the times. Insofar as that concept could be regarded as central to Freud's thought (and the claim is debatable), Freudianism was incorporated into the era's self-understanding. As a discovery about the psyche, Freudianism validated the discourse of anxiety. As a general explanation of the contemporary condition, the discourse validated Freud.

The historiography of the Cold War is notoriously unsettled, and this has to do with an underlying controversy about whether the Cold War might have been avoided. The question seems a pointless counterfactual, except insofar as it was an issue internal to the Cold War itself: that is, arguments over whether the Cold War might have been avoided were part of the political culture of the Cold War period. One result has been an obsession with the postwar timeline. The practice is to stick a pin in the calendar at some point between Yalta, where the Allied leaders discussed the future of postwar Europe, in February 1945, and the declaration of the Truman Doctrine, when Harry Truman committed the United States to opposing internal and external threats to free societies, in March 1947, and to argue that the pin marks the moment when events tipped over into a Cold War geopolitics—with the implication that a different choice earlier on the timeline could have led to a non–Cold War outcome. Everything past that point of no turning back then belongs to what is called Cold War culture, which is endowed with a distinctive period character.

Diplomatically and militarily, there certainly was, after the announcement of the Truman Doctrine, a Cold War between the United States and its allies, and the Soviet Union and other Communist states, and that conflict persisted, in varying degrees of coldness, for more than forty years. Culturally, though, matters are never so discrete. So the first thing to say when addressing a cultural question about the Cold War period is that people in the period understood and defined themselves within discourses that were shaped before there was a Cold War. The big bang of the postwar period in Europe and the United States was not the Cold War. The big bang was the Second World War. Cold War conditions inflected existing discourses, though, and the discourse of anxiety is an example. Before the Cold War, there was anxiety. During the Cold War, there was anxiety about anxiety.

The currency of the phrase "the age of anxiety" is owed to W. H. Auden's book-length poem *The Age of Anxiety*, which was published in 1947. Auden called the poem "a baroque eclogue." The term borders on oxymoron—

baroque implies artificiality and complexity; eclogue connotes the natural and the simple—and the work is, even by Auden's standards, an eclectic mélange of formal elements. The poem is a quasi-allegory, constructed around a quest motif, and featuring four characters, who represent four aspects of the psyche identified by Carl Jung (intuition, feeling, sensation, and thought). The prosody is Anglo-Saxon alliterative meter. The style is modernist, influenced specifically by *Finnegans Wake*. And the theology is Christian existentialist. It is not, in short, a readily accessible work, and it is fair to assume that many people who bought it or referred to it never managed to finish it. As one of Auden's editors has remarked, the poem is "extraordinarily famous for a book so little read; or, extraordinarily little read for a book so famous."[2]

But its impact was swift. Jacques Barzun, reviewing *The Age of Anxiety* in *Harper's* in September 1947, proposed that "the very title roots it in our generation."[3] (Barzun was a friend of Auden's: in 1951, they would collaborate, with Lionel Trilling, in starting a book club, called The Readers' Subscription.) Auden's book won the Pulitzer Prize for Poetry in 1948, and it inspired a number of artists. Leonard Bernstein wrote a symphony based on it, *The Age of Anxiety*, which premiered in 1949. In 1950, Jerome Robbins composed a ballet (which Auden is supposed to have disliked) based on Bernstein's symphony. And in 1954, the Living Theatre Studio presented a stage version of the poem in New York City.[4]

The Age of Anxiety is a poem about the Second World War, not the Cold War. It effectively concludes a sequence that begins with "A Summer Night (Out on the lawn I lie in bed)" (1933) and includes "September 1, 1939" (1939). Auden began writing it, in New York City, in July 1944, a month after the D-Day invasion. He finished it in the fall of 1946, when relations between the United States and the Soviet Union were just beginning to slide toward confrontation. In between, Auden served as a major in the Morale Division of the U.S. Strategic Bombing Survey. His assignment was to assess the psychological impact of the Allied bombing campaign against Germany. That campaign was physically and humanly devastating, and it also seems likely that it is while he was in Germany on this mission that Auden became fully aware of the Nazi war against the Jews. The experience would have given him a horrifying picture of the destructive power of total war.

---

2. Alan Jacobs, "Introduction" to W. H. Auden, *The Age of Anxiety: A Baroque Eclogue*, ed. Alan Jacobs (Princeton, NJ: Princeton University Press, 2011), xii.

3. Jacques Barzun, "Workers in Monumental Brass," *Harper's Magazine* 195 (September 1947), quoted in Jacobs, "Introduction," 118n.

4. Jacobs, "Introduction," xli.

The poem is set on All Souls' Night, Halloween, and it opens in a New York bar. (The characters eventually move to an apartment.) There are allusions to wartime events—the radio is on, with news from the front—but the poem does not address the war directly. The premise is that wartime reduces everyone to "the anxious status of a shady character or a displaced person"; wartime is therefore, as the poem puts it, "good for the bar business."[5] It is also good for compelling people to confront spiritual and existential questions, and these questions—as the quest motif, the archaic meter, and the use of traditional genre designations all suggest—are universal.

Auden meant by anxiety what the theologian Reinhold Niebuhr meant by it in *The Nature and Destiny of Man*, published, in two volumes, in 1941 and 1943. "Being both free and bound, both limited and limitless, is anxious," Niebuhr wrote there. "Anxiety is the inevitable concomitant of the paradox of freedom and finiteness in which man is involved. Anxiety is the internal precondition of sin. It is the inevitable spiritual state of man."[6] The human condition is a paradox of radical freedom and radical unfreedom. In theological terms: my will to do good in the world is inexorably constrained by my inherent sinfulness. The full awareness of the paradox produces anxiety. Auden was a reader and admirer of Niebuhr, and he likely knew this passage. But Niebuhr derived his understanding of anxiety from a writer who was even more important for Auden than Niebuhr was, Søren Kierkegaard.

Kierkegaard's emergence in the English-speaking intellectual world was due principally to the efforts of Walter Lowrie, an Episcopal clergyman who learned Danish at the age of sixty-four in order to read Kierkegaard.[7] Lowrie translated some of Kierkegaard's works himself; he also assisted, and subvented, the work of other translators, principally David Swenson and Alexander Dru. Altogether, he helped to oversee the production of translations of thirty of Kierkegaard's books by ten translators, plus a selection from the journals, in a span of eight years. The translations began appearing in the 1930s; they were published first by Oxford University Press and then, because of a paper shortage during the war, by Princeton. Lowrie's two-volume biography of Kierkegaard came out in 1938; a one-volume edition appeared in 1942.

---

5. Auden, *Age of Anxiety*, 3.

6. Reinhold Niebuhr, *The Nature and Destiny of Man: A Christian Interpretation*, 2 vols. (New York: Charles Scribner's Sons, 1941–43), 1:182.

7. George Cotkin, *Existential America* (Baltimore: Johns Hopkins University Press, 2003), 35–87.

Lowrie's translation of *The Concept of Dread* was published in 1944—one hundred years after the book first appeared in Denmark (and the same year that Auden began work on *The Age of Anxiety*). The word that Lowrie, after extensive consultation with other translators, rendered as "dread" is *angst*. A more recent translation, by Reidar Thomte, translates the title as *The Concept of Anxiety*, though "dread" seems the stronger word, since it carries a religious connotation. Milton used the word "dread," many times, in *Paradise Lost* ("To moral ear / The voice of God is dreadful" [12:236]). He does not use the word "anxiety"—although it was in the language: John Donne, for example, used it in a sermon. And the subject of Milton's poem is the same as the subject of Kierkegaard's book: the meaning of original sin.

Auden's fascination with Kierkegaard began in 1940; he would later, in 1952, edit a popular anthology, *The Living Thoughts of Kierkegaard*. Kierkegaard was one of the thinkers who led Auden to Christianity, and *The Age of Anxiety* is a Christian poem. Kierkegaard's writing might be described as an effort to answer the question, Can one be a Christian without Christianity—that is, can one lead a life of faith without a doctrine or a congregation? For Kierkegaard, the religious stage of existence is non-communal and post-institutional. It cannot be achieved in church, since organized religion turns faith into ethics. It is a mediating institution. Attaining the religious stage requires, in Kierkegaard's well-known phrase, "the teleological suspension of the ethical."[8] The individual who sacrifices himself in the name of an ethical imperative is a tragic hero, and represents the universal. The Kierkegaardian Knight of Faith is only an individual, and "the single individual as single individual is higher than the universal, whereas the universal is in fact mediation."[9] The Knight of Faith has to reject the demands of the ethical, since those are the demands of the social and the finite, and to stand alone before God. That relation, between man and God, is dreadful because it cannot be mediated. "The single individual as the single individual stands in an absolute relation to the absolute."[10]

For Kierkegaard, the classic case of the teleological suspension of the ethical is the story of Abraham commanded to sacrifice Isaac, since obeying that command requires Abraham to violate ethical proscriptions. The Abraham story is the subject of *Fear and Trembling*, which Kierkegaard considered, along with *Sickness unto Death*, to be part of a trilogy with *The*

---

8. Søren Kierkegaard, *Fear and Trembling; Repetition*, trans. Howard V. Hong and Edna H. Hong (Princeton, NJ: Princeton University Press, 1983), 54.
9. Ibid., 82.
10. Ibid., 56.

Concept of Dread. Anxiety is the psychological condition undergone by the Knight of Faith, the state Abraham experiences when he is confronted with the recognition that if he fulfills God's command to kill Isaac, he might be, not a man of faith, but simply a murderer. That is a major ethical imperative to regard as illusory. As Kierkegaard puts it: "Anxiety is freedom's possibility, and only such anxiety is through faith absolutely educative, because it consumes all finite ends and discovers all their deceptiveness."[11]

The religious conception of *angst* was influential in American culture after the war, and its appeal did not distribute reliably along political or sociocultural lines.[12] Whittaker Chambers was a Kierkegaardian; so was the management theorist Peter Drucker. The abstract expressionists Barnett Newman and Mark Rothko were influenced by Kierkegaard, and by *Fear and Trembling* in particular. Newman made a series of "zip" paintings, between 1948 and 1950, based on the story of Abraham and Isaac. Rothko read that story as an allegory of the act of painting. The protagonist of Updike's Rabbit novels, the first of which, *Rabbit, Run*, came out in 1961, is named, rather unsubtly, Harry Angstrom. His restless self-absorption, his chronic low-level existential crisis, might be the beginning of a spiritual awareness, but he cannot transcend it. He has a skeptical relation to the ethical, which is promising, but he is trapped by other demons. In Kierkegaardian terms, he appears to be locked in the aesthetic stage. Kierkegaard played a prominent part in Paul Tillich's *The Courage to Be*, published in 1952. Tillich's title is plainly Kierkegaardian, and the book is virtually a meditation on anxiety. "Today it has become almost a truism to call our time an 'age of anxiety,'" Tillich wrote. "This holds equally for America and Europe."[13]

Anxiety plays an important part in atheistic existentialism as well, and this is a place where the wires get somewhat crossed. The teleological suspension of the ethical has different implications in a philosophical system that is based on the denial of a supernatural realm than it does in a theological argument. European existentialism had an American vogue right after the war, but it was brief. Tillich published an article on "Existential Philosophy" in 1944, in which he called it "a specifically German creation,"[14] and William Barrett's little book *What Is Existentialism?*—published in 1947

---

11. Søren Kierkegaard, *The Concept of Anxiety: A Simple Psychologically Orienting Deliberation on the Dogmatic Issue of Hereditary Sin*, trans. Reidar Thomte (Princeton, NJ: Princeton University Press, 1980), 155.

12. Cotkin, *Existential America*, 119–26.

13. Paul Tillich, *The Courage to Be*, 2d ed. (New Haven, CT: Yale University Press, 2000 [1952]), 35.

14. Paul Tillich, "Existential Philosophy," *Journal of the History of Ideas* 5 (1944): 44.

by *Partisan Review*, where Barrett was an editor—was concerned largely with the philosophy of Martin Heidegger. "That which anxiety is anxious about is 'Being-in-the-world' itself," Heidegger wrote. In Barrett's paraphrase: "Anxiety flows from the fundamental trait of man: that *he is a being whose being is characterized by the fact that he is concerned about his own being*. This separates him from all other beings in the universe."[15]

An interest in French existentialism in the United States began around the time of Stuart Gilbert's translation of Albert Camus's *L'Etranger*, published by Knopf in 1946, and Bernard Frechtman's translation of Jean-Paul Sartre's celebrated postwar lecture, delivered in France in 1945. It was published there, in 1946, as *L'Existentialisme est un humanisme*, and in the United States, by the Philosophical Library, as *Existentialism*, in 1947. (The book had a high price, suggesting that the audience was expected to be eager but small.) When Camus, Sartre, and Simone de Beauvoir visited the United States after the war, they were covered as celebrities in the press.

In atheistic existentialism, anxiety is the mark of an authentic confrontation with the recognition that there is no prior supra-personal constraint on individual freedom, a recognition that is both dreadful and liberating. In this respect, it is not, as a psychological state, different from the anxiety of the Knight of Faith, but the Sartrean version can seem to underwrite an irresponsible individualism. Outside of the French Department at Yale, Sartre had a skeptical reception among American academics. Lowrie, whose politics were markedly conservative, despised him, and the American intellectuals around *Partisan Review* lost their enthusiasm for existentialism fairly quickly after 1947, partly because of Sartre's refusal to renounce Communism and the Soviet Union. Barrett's later book *Irrational Man*, which was published in 1958 and which became the chief reference on existentialism for American readers for several decades, treated the philosophy as a slightly alien school of thought. "Existentialism was so definitely a European expression," Barrett wrote there, "that its very somberness went against the grain of our native youthfulness and optimism."[16] Still, simply the title of *L'Etranger* seemed irresistible to English-language writers: Bellow's *Dangling Man* came out in 1944, Richard Wright's novel *The Outsider* in 1953, and the British writer Colin Wilson's popular work of popular philosophy, *The Outsider*, in 1956.[17]

---

15. William Barrett, *What Is Existentialism?* (New York: Partisan Review, 1947), 31.

16. William Barrett, *Irrational Man: A Study in Existential Philosophy* (Garden City, NY: Doubleday, 1958), 10.

17. Cotkin, *Existential America*, 92–104; Ann Fulton, *Apostles of Sartre: Existentialism in America, 1945–1963* (Evanston, IL: Northwestern University Press, 1999), 20–47; William

The concomitant rise of psychoanalysis in the United States after the war was a consequence, in part, as previous essayists have noted, of the purging of European psychoanalysis by Hitler and Stalin, which produced a group of émigrés whose influence on American intellectual life was disproportionate to its size. But it was also a result of significant public investment, much of it through the offices of the National Institute of Mental Health, which was established in 1949 and was generously funded through the 1950s. Seventy percent of NIMH's initial budget was committed to subsidizing education, and between 1948 and 1976 the number of psychiatrists in the United States increased from forty-seven hundred to twenty-seven thousand.[18] Between 1946 and 1956, the number of psychiatric residency programs doubled. In 1954, 12.5 percent of medical students chose psychiatry as their specialization, an all-time high.[19]

Relatively few of these students became psychoanalysts. By 1957, there were fewer than a thousand psychoanalysts in the United States (and probably fewer than two thousand in the world); the American Psychoanalytic Association had only six hundred and ninety-five members.[20] Psychoanalytic theory had little impact in university psychology departments. But it did establish itself in medical schools. Reading the complete works of Freud in the *Standard Edition*—a work that, though it was prepared in Britain, was largely funded by the American Psychoanalytic Association—was once a common requirement.[21] Even students who went into other specialties learned about psychoanalysis as part of their training. Psychiatric practice tended to be eclectic, but most American psychiatrists employed Freudian assumptions.

The ground had been prepared for the acceptance of some of the premises of psychoanalysis by the experience of treating trauma during the Second World War. Battle trauma was a major medical problem in the war. One million soldiers suffered neuropsychiatric breakdowns; in combat divisions, hospital admissions for psychiatric conditions were two hundred fifty per one thousand soldiers.[22] In 1945, 60 percent of the patients in

---

Barrett, *The Truants: Adventures Among the Intellectuals* (Garden City: Anchor Press/Doubleday, 1982), 123–30.

18. Hale, *Rise and Crisis of Psychoanalysis*, 246.

19. Joel Paris, *The Fall of an Icon: Psychoanalysis and Academic Psychiatry* (Toronto: University of Toronto Press, 2005), 26.

20. Hale, *Rise and Crisis of Psychoanalysis*, 289.

21. Paris, *Fall of an Icon*, 49; Eli Zaretsky, *Secrets of the Soul: A Social and Cultural History of Psychoanalysis* (New York: Knopf, 2004), 295.

22. Allan V. Horwitz and Jerome C. Wakefield, *The Loss of Sadness: How Psychiatry Transformed Normal Sorrow into Depressive Disorder* (New York: Oxford University Press, 2007), 125.

Veterans' Administration hospitals were there with psychiatric diagnoses.[23] (One traumatized soldier, famous in a different postwar context, was J. D. Salinger, who fought in the Battle of the Bulge in the winter of 1944–45, where Americans suffered nearly eighty thousand casualties in three days. Seymour Glass, who commits suicide in Salinger's story "A Perfect Day for Bananafish" [1948], is a traumatized veteran, as, apparently, is Sergeant X in "For Esmé with Love and Squalor" [1950].)

Trauma is a problem in any war, but disorders need legitimation (General Patton's treatment for shell shock, slapping the afflicted solider in the face, was not legitimating), and the provision of a psychiatric diagnosis helped to legitimate trauma and stress-related disorders, such as anxiety, as medical conditions. Roy Grinker and John Spiegel's *War Neuroses* (1943, republished in 1945), written for the army, in which both men were commissioned, is essentially a handbook for physicians treating shell-shocked veterans. Grinker and Spiegel used the term "anxiety" in diagnosing the condition of traumatized soldiers. Grinker (later the first editor of the *Archives of General Psychiatry*, founded in 1959) championed narcoanalysis, a treatment that uses sodium pentothal to induce an abreaction, as the best method of treatment, and his work with narcoanalysis was reported in the *New York Times*.

Freud used abreaction to treat hysterical patients early in his career, and the problem of traumatic memory, which Freud interpreted as a form of masochism, had a crucial role in his transformation of his system after the First World War. More important, though, Grinker, Spiegel, and other psychiatrists who studied the problem concluded that everyone—not only the weak or those with latent psychiatric disorders—is vulnerable to nervous breakdown when exposed to wartime conditions. War neurosis is, in effect, a disease that anyone can catch. And, like many diseases, it is preventable (by, for example, rotating troops regularly out of high-stress situations) and treatable (by inducing an abreaction, by drugs, or by psychotherapy). The result of this legitimation was the normalization of a certain class of mental disorders as somatic responses to stress. The process of the medicalization of stress was consummated with the publication of Hans Selye's enormously influential *The Stress of Life*, in 1956.

Under these circumstances, Freudianism and existentialism must have seemed an obvious cocktail to mix. One of the first people to link Kierkegaard with Freud was the American psychologist O. H. Mowrer. In an address in Chicago to the American Association for the Advancement of Sci-

---

23. Zaretsky, *Secrets of the Soul*, 280.

ence in 1947, Mowrer remarked that Kierkegaard "anticipated Freud in an astonishing number of ways."[24] In fact, he went on to say, Kierkegaard was in some respects "more correct" than Freud, because for Freud anxiety is the enemy of the ego, but for Kierkegaard it is the sign of a positive development. It signals a leap into a higher stage of existence. One of the most striking passages in *Fear and Trembling* is the description of the Knight of Faith: the man of faith appears completely ordinary, entirely at home in finitude; he is, in appearance, indistinguishable from less developed men. Mowrer was not wrong: the Knight of Faith is like the imagined (or idealized) patient after successful psychoanalysis, an ego serenely adjusted through the process of a terrible awareness.

Ludwig Binswanger was the first prominent psychiatrist to incorporate existentialist theory into psychoanalytic practice, but the figure who did the most to popularize the connection was the American psychologist Rollo May. May was associated with the William Alanson White Institute, which was founded in 1946 by Erich Fromm and Clara Thompson, who were soon joined by Harry Stack Sullivan and others. May's *The Meaning of Anxiety*, published in 1950, also aligned Kierkegaard's concept of dread with psychodynamic theory. May asked Lowrie whether he could translate Kierkegaard's *angst* as "anxiety," rather than "dread," and Lowrie said he could. This was plainly a strategy in aid of the assimilation that May wanted to perform of existential dread to psychiatric neurosis, since *angst* was Freud's word as well, and James Strachey had translated it as "anxiety."

May's book made a move that no orthodox Freudian would have made, but that was the key move in the adaptation of psychoanalysis to the social and cultural conditions of postwar America: it historicized anxiety. May argued that anxiety is a condition of modernity, and he provided an abbreviated intellectual history, starting with Descartes and Spinoza, to account for the rise in anxiety levels he believed to have taken place. May argued that there had been a breakdown in cultural order during the nineteenth century, which he associated with a loss of faith in the power of autonomous reason. "In the nineteenth century," he wrote, "we can observe on a broad scale the occurrence of fissures in the unity of modern culture which underlie much of our contemporary anxiety."[25] And the process, he thought, was accelerating. May cited the Middletown studies by the sociologists Robert and Helen Lynd, pointing out that the Lynds identified an increase in

---

24. O. H. Mowrer, *Learning Theory and Personality Dynamics* (New York: Roland Press, 1950), 452.

25. Rollo May, *The Meaning of Anxiety*, 2d ed. (New York: W. W. Norton, 1977), 32.

anxiety between the 1920s, the period of their first Middletown study, and the 1930s, when they did their second study. May concluded that anxiety in 1950 could be understood as a response to distinctive historical conditions. And May thought that this type of anxiety, the anxiety of modernity, had been diagnosed and described both by existentialist thinkers, notably Kierkegaard, and by psychiatric theory. May was himself a disciple of Otto Rank, and he was somewhat critical of Freud. But the thrust of his book was that the anxiety of modern man is a proper object of psychiatric treatment.

The position that anxiety is a neurotic condition that is environmentally caused, that it is a disorder that is naturally a piece of modern life, is arguably the heterodoxy that was necessary to bring psychoanalysis into the mainstream of medical practice in the United States. How, after all, did Freud explain anxiety? In "Anxiety and the Instinctual Life," in the *New Introductory Lectures* of 1933, he defined it as the fear of one's own desires. "What he is afraid of," Freud says, of the anxious patient, "is evidently his own libido."[26] The formulation, though not the biology, sounds Kierkegaardian. As Kierkegaard wrote in his journal: "Dread is a desire for what one dreads."[27] But Kierkegaard was not thinking of desire for the mother. Freud was. The child feels anxiety because he fears that the punishment for acting on his desire will be castration. (For women, Freud says, the fear is of loss of love, which is somewhat less dramatic.) Earlier in his career, Freud had argued that repression of libidinal drives created anxiety. He now reversed the causal chain. It is anxiety, an irrational fear of punishment, that makes us repress our drives.

A theory that anxiety derives from a childhood fear of castration has no obvious relation to theories of anxiety that connect the condition to developments in modern thought or modern life. And it is not a theory it is easy to imagine getting much of a purchase on American culture. And so this analytic piece, although Freud was insistent on it and although it is central to his entire system, virtually disappears in the postwar appropriation of psychoanalytic theory. The standard handbook on psychoanalysis for American medical students, Otto Fenichel's *The Psychoanalytic Theory of Neurosis*, published in 1945, synthesizes orthodox Freudian accounts of neurotic disorders, as arising from conflicts among the drives, with most of the environmental and interpersonal approaches in psychoanalytic theory that Freud himself was skeptical of. "There is no 'psychology of man' in a

---

26. Sigmund Freud, *New Introductory Lectures on Psychoanalysis*, in S.E. 22:84.
27. Quoted in Søren Kierkegaard, *Kierkegaard's The Concept of Dread*, trans. Walter Lowrie (Princeton, NJ: Princeton University Press, 1944), xii.

general sense, in a vacuum, as it were, but only a psychology of man in a certain concrete society and in a certain social place within this concrete society,"[28] Fenichel wrote at the beginning of his book, and that position defines mainstream psychiatry in the postwar period. Like the members of the Frankfurt school, Fenichel really did believe there could be a Marxist Freudianism—though no one was less a Marxist than Freud. Fenichel thought that psychoanalytic theory was consistent with a historicist understanding of human development, and that Freud's account of the psyche was, willy-nilly, an account of the psyche under capitalism. Fenichel died a few months after completing *The Psychoanalytic Theory of Neurosis*, but his work belongs with the renegade Freudians of the 1950s, all of whom had a powerful, though historically bounded, influence on American intellectual culture: Wilhelm Reich, Herbert Marcuse, and Norman O. Brown.

Whether anxiety was attributed to environmental stress or to psychic conflict, the notion that it is the central symptom of neurotic disorder is everywhere in mid-century psychodynamic theory, whether the writer is strictly Freudian or not. Freud himself, in the 1917 *Introductory Lectures on Psychoanalysis*, called anxiety "a riddle whose solution would be bound to throw a flood of light on our whole mental existence."[29] Karen Horney called it the "dynamic center of neurosis."[30] Howard Liddell, in 1949, wrote that "I have come to believe that anxiety accompanies intellectual activity as its shadow and that the more we know of the nature of anxiety, the more we will know of intellect."[31] Mowrer, in 1950, called it "the absolutely central problem in neurosis and therapy."[32] The first *Diagnostic and Statistical Manual of Mental Disorders*, published in 1952 and psychoanalytic in approach, states that "the chief characteristic of [psychoneurotic] disorders is 'anxiety.'"[33]

The belief that neuroses are a normal by-product of modern existence—that to be modern just is to suffer anxiety, and that suffering anxiety is a legitimate reason to seek medical help—was crucial to the emergence of a phenomenon that would eventually contribute to the demise of psychoanalysis. This was the rise of psychopharmacology. The war, again, was behind the growth of the pharmaceutical industry. It played two distinct roles.

28. Otto Fenichel, *The Psychoanalytic Theory of Neurosis* (London: Routledge and Kegan Paul, 1946), 6.
29. Sigmund Freud, *Introductory Lectures on Psychoanalysis*, in S.E. 16:393.
30. Quoted in May, *Meaning of Anxiety*, 18.
31. Howard Liddell, "The Role of Vigilance in the Development of Animal Neurosis," in *Anxiety*, ed. P. Hoch and J. Zubin (New York: Grune and Stratton, 1949), 185.
32. Mowrer, *Learning Theory and Personality Dynamics*, 486.
33. American Psychiatric Association, *Diagnostic and Statistical Manual of Mental Disorders* (Washington, DC: American Psychiatric Association, 1952), 31.

The first was scientific. As all modern wars have, the Second World War instigated and expedited technological developments that ultimately had peacetime uses. In the case of psychopharmaceuticals, it was the search, by a Czechoslovakian émigré named Frank Berger, for an agent that would assist in the preservation of penicillin, which was a drug much in demand by the military. Berger's search led to the fortuitous discovery that the chemical mephenesin is a muscle relaxant, a finding that Berger announced in 1946. The discovery was significant because of the discovery a few years later that chlorpromazine, a truly revolutionary drug, could be used to sedate psychotics. Under the U.S. brand name Thorazine, chlorpromazine made possible the massive deinstitutionalization of the mentally ill in the 1960s.[34]

A drug closely related to mephenesin, meprobamate, was synthesized by Berger and others at Wallace Laboratories in New Jersey and sold as Miltown, a drug that has been called the first pharmaceutical blockbuster. Miltown was initially categorized as a minor tranquilizer, which suited Wallace Laboratories because of the association with Thorazine, despite the lack of a chemical similarity between the two medications. Later, Miltown was reclassified as an anxiolytic. It was an instant hit, in part because Hollywood figures quickly endorsed it. Comedians like Milton Berle worked references to Miltown into their routines. Within a year, one out of every twenty Americans had tried either Miltown or Equanil, the name under which Wyeth sold meprobamate. Within two years, a billion tablets had been manufactured, and Miltown/Equanil accounted for a third of all prescriptions by the end of the 1950s. They were eclipsed, after 1960, by Valium and Librium, which continued to maintain a huge market share in the pharmaceutical industry until the backlash caused by the Thalidomide disaster and reports of the drugs' addictive properties.[35]

David Herzberg has argued that recognition of a specific disorder associated with situations of obvious extreme stress—wartime conditions—made it easier for the manufacturers of anti-anxiety drugs such as Miltown/Equanil to identify anxiety as a legitimate disorder, particularly for high-functioning members of modern American society.[36] The view is the same as the psychodynamic view in the postwar period: the impairment of the

---

34. Elliot S. Valenstein, *Blaming the Brain: The Truth about Drugs and Mental Health* (New York: Free Press, 1998), 169.

35. Andrea Tone, *The Age of Anxiety: A History of America's Turbulent Affair with Tranquilizers* (New York: Basic Books, 2009), ix–xvii and passim.

36. David Herzberg, *Happy Pills in America: From Miltown to Prozac* (Baltimore: Johns Hopkins University Press, 2009), 32.

ego's functioning by stress is a legitimate medical disorder that can be addressed by psychiatry. Herzberg also reports that advertisements for tranquilizers regularly used the language of psychoanalysis, and that references to Freud were common in journalistic accounts of psychopharmaceuticals in the 1950s. Strangely, no disjunction between psychodynamic theories and psychopharmacological treatments seems to have been recognized. One discourse buttressed the other.

In short, the Cold War discourse of anxiety reveals itself to be a somewhat improbable amalgam of European existentialism, psychoanalytic theory, some sociology and the history of ideas, and the promotional practices of the pharmaceutical industry. Was there a spike in the rate of occurrence of anxiety symptoms themselves, or not? Was this a case of defining stress upward, or of pathologizing normal mood changes, as has more recently been claimed has happened in the cases of sadness and shyness?[37] Or was there a pandemic of anxiety-related symptoms in response to the genuinely novel circumstance of the threat of nuclear annihilation? Unsurprisingly, the authors of the discourse of anxiety tended only to gesture toward the atomic bomb, since worry about a concrete threat is objective, and can thus be defined as fear. "The emergence of the Atomic Age brought the previously inchoate and 'free-floating' anxiety of many people into sharp focus," is the way May handled the topic. He suggested that this might be interpreted as "fear of irrational death" and thus qualify as anxiety.[38] (It is not obvious why death by an atomic bomb is any more irrational than death by food poisoning or in an automobile accident.) May was dancing around Freud's warning: "In view of all that we know about the structure of the comparatively simple neuroses of everyday life," Freud had written in "Inhibitions, Symptoms, and Anxiety" in 1926, "it would seem highly improbable that a neurosis could come into being merely because of the objective presence of danger, without any participation of the deeper levels of the mental apparatus."[39] Freud was referring specifically to the analysis of traumatic neuroses at the time of the First World War. It was always crucial to the definition of anxiety that it be experienced as something that exceeds any obvious object, that it is something that has become, as it were, wired into the human condition.

In any event, the question for this paper isn't whether there was an increase in anxiety in the postwar period, but why there was a *discourse* of

37. Horwitz and Wakefield, *The Loss of Sadness*; Christopher Lane, *Shyness: How Normal Behavior Became a Sickness* (New Haven, CT: Yale University Press, 2007).
38. May, *Meaning of Anxiety*, 13, 14 n. 29.
39. Sigmund Freud, "Inhibitions, Symptoms, and Anxiety," in S.E. 20:129.

anxiety. Why, in the Cold War, did people become anxious about anxiety? The answer to this question introduces another aspect of postwar intellectual culture, the literature on totalitarianism. This was the work produced by writers such as Erich Fromm, George Orwell, Arthur Schlesinger Jr., Bruno Bettelheim, Isaiah Berlin, Arthur Koestler, and Hannah Arendt. Their writings might be characterized (though incompletely as far as Berlin and Arendt are concerned) as the psychologizing of totalitarianism. The question they asked was, How could millions of people apparently not only submit to, but be willing to die for, totalitarian regimes? It seemed obvious that since people could not be understood to do this from self-interest or other rational motives, the answers must have to do with personal and group psychology.

In the beginning of *The Meaning of Anxiety*, May took up the issue briefly. "Without going into the complex determinants of fascism, we need only note that it is born and gains its power in periods of widespread anxiety. . . . [P]eople grasp at political authoritarianism in their desperate need for relief from anxiety," he wrote.[40] May was drawing on Fromm, one of the founders of the William Alanson White Institute, and specifically on Fromm's *Escape from Freedom*, an influential analysis of fascism published in 1941. "Modern man, freed from the bonds of pre-individualistic society, which simultaneously gave him security and limited him, has not gained freedom in the positive sense of the realization of his individual self; that is, the expression of his intellectual, emotional and sensuous potentialities," Fromm wrote. "Freedom, though it has brought him independence and rationality, has made him isolated and, thereby, anxious and powerless. This isolation is unbearable and the alternatives he is confronted with are either to escape from the burden of his freedom into new dependencies and submission, or to advance to the full realization of positive freedom which is based upon the uniqueness and individuality of man."[41]

Schlesinger made a similar argument in his manifesto for postwar liberalism, *The Vital Center*, published in 1949. Schlesinger cited Kierkegaard, about whom he probably learned from Niebuhr, to support the assertion that "anxiety is the official emotion of our time."[42] Schlesinger's book, like all the writings of the literature on totalitarianism, is motivated by the question, implicit in the problem of why people are drawn to totalitarian ideologies: Could it happen here? Are there conditions within the liberal

40. May, *Meaning of Anxiety*, 12.
41. Erich Fromm, *Escape from Freedom* (New York: Holt, 1994 [1941]), x.
42. Arthur M. Schlesinger Jr., *The Vital Center: The Politics of Freedom* (Boston: Houghton Mifflin, 1949), 52.

democracies themselves that might make people—either the intellectuals or the masses, or both—susceptible to totalitarianism? Schlesinger does not conclude that since anxiety is one of the preconditions for an attraction to totalitarianism, it is therefore a danger to be eliminated. Instead, consistent with both the existentialist and the theological traditions, Schlesinger insists that in a free society, anxiety can be a strength. His book was a call to arms, a Cold War tract. "The totalitarians regard the toleration of conflict as our central weakness," he says at the end of *The Vital Center*. "So it may appear to be in an age of anxiety. But we know it to be basically our central strength."[43]

It is a balancing act—thus the "center" of Schlesinger's title. Too much anxiety makes people rush toward the self-annihilation promised by extremist ideologies; too little anxiety makes people supine and vulnerable to extremist ideologies. As May put it: "The cleavage between expectations and reality has its normal and healthy form as well as its neurotic form. This cleavage, indeed, *is present as one condition of all creative activity*. . . . [M]an's creative abilities and his susceptibility to anxiety are two sides of the same capacity, uniquely possessed by the human being, to become aware of gaps between expectations and reality."[44] Anxiety, evidently, is like cholesterol: there is the bad kind, but there is also the good kind. The tradeoff is recognizable in contemporary arguments for and against antidepressants. Some sadness is naturally selected for, and should not be medicalized, but some is pathological and a legitimate condition for intervention.

Freud played a role in the literature of totalitarianism for another reason as well, and this had to do with his concept of the death-drive as he presents it in *Civilization and Its Discontents* (1930). Freud had first elaborated that concept in *Beyond the Pleasure Principle* (1920), but he put it to extraordinary use in the later work. As often happened, he was motivated in part by the heterodoxy of a would-be disciple—in this case, Wilhelm Reich, who had joined the Communist Party and visited the Soviet Union, where he preached the necessity of sexual revolution for political revolution to be effective. Two roads that Freud did not want to go down were free love and revolution, and Reich was trouble on both counts.[45] The only political reference Freud made in *Civilization and Its Discontents* (apart from an apparent allusion, in the last sentence, added in 1931, to the success

---

43. Schlesinger, *Vital Center*, 255.
44. May, *Meaning of Anxiety*, 389–90.
45. Zaretsky, *Secrets of the Soul*, 220–24.

of the Nazi Party in the Reichstag elections) was to the folly of believing that the abolition of private property might lead to happiness. "I have no concern with any economic criticisms of the communist system," Freud explained. "I cannot inquire into whether the abolition of private property is expedient or advantageous. But I am able to recognize that the psychological premises on which the system is based are an untenable illusion. . . . Aggressiveness was not created by property."[46] This is because the death-drive is a biological feature of the organism (of all organisms, Freud believed). Civilization did not create that drive, and civilization cannot, in the end, mitigate its demands. It constitutes a built-in resistance to reform. Freud would later invoke it in analyzing patients' resistance to therapy, in "Analysis Terminable and Interminable": people don't *want* to get better.

When *Civilization and Its Discontents* came out, Lionel Trilling wrote a review for a little magazine called the *New Freeman*, dismissing the argument as absurd. But the magazine folded before the review was printed.[47] Trilling had reason to be relieved, because after the war, Freud's death-drive became the virtual centerpiece of Trilling's anticommunism and, more generally, his anti-utopianism. He invoked it in his paper "Freud and the Crisis of Our Culture," which he published as a little book in 1955, where (it was the role he assumed during the Cold War) he chastised liberals, from within liberalism, for their exaggerated faith in progress. He tried, though, to turn Freud's idea to a positive account, by suggesting that the biological resistance to efforts to shape character might be interpreted as the grounds for the possibility of independence and nonconformity. Freud, Trilling speculated, "needed to believe that there was some point at which it was possible to stand beyond the reach of culture. Perhaps his formulation of the death-instinct [Strachey's translation of *Todestrieb*] is to be interpreted as the expression of this need."[48] By the end of his career, though, having passed through the 1960s, Trilling was less optimistic. "It may be thought to stand like a lion in the path of all hopes of achieving happiness through the radical revision of social life," he wrote of the death-drive in his last book, *Sincerity and Authenticity*, in 1972.[49]

Trilling's calculated swerve from Freud was typical of the period. It was

---

46. Sigmund Freud, *Civilization and Its Discontents*, in S.E. 21:113.
47. Notes, 1970–1974, Lionel Trilling Papers, Rare Book and Manuscript Library, Columbia University, Box 5, Folder 1.
48. Lionel Trilling, *Freud and the Crisis of Our Culture* (Boston: Beacon Press, 1955), 40.
49. Lionel Trilling, *Sincerity and Authenticity* (Cambridge, MA: Harvard University Press, 1972), 151.

an effort to repurpose the Freudian system for concrete political ends, or to meet concrete historical exigencies. Freud, characteristically (for he was an extremely clever man), anticipated this response from future readers, and he addressed them in the last pages of *Civilization and Its Discontents*: "I have not the courage to rise up before my fellow-men as a prophet, and I bow to their reproach that I can offer them no consolation: for at bottom that is what they are all demanding—the wildest revolutionaries no less passionately that the most virtuous believers."[50]

The intellectual culture of the early Cold War period was driven by the "Can it happen here?" question to the extent that any extreme, ideological or affective, tended to be regarded with, well, anxiety. Social formations and cultural tendencies seemed to many postwar American intellectuals to be highly brittle, in need of continual moral and critical policing. But discourses with as many asymmetries as the discourse of anxiety tend to implode. The victim in this case, unsurprisingly, was psychoanalysis. Freud's offhand remark, to Marie Bonaparte, about the medical future of psychiatric treatment—"The hope of the future here [for treatment of neuroses] lies in organic chemistry or the access to it through endocrinology," he wrote to her in 1930—is frequently cited,[51] but it is hard to get from the assumptions and methods of Freudian psychoanalysis to those of postwar psychopharmacology and postwar sociology. With the publication of Joseph Schildkraut's amine theory of depression in 1965, Freudianism began its professional death march. With the publication of *DSM-III*, in 1980, it met that death.

Of wider significance, though, was the effect of putting questions of psychology, and mental states generally, at the center of cultural attention, as is noted by other contributors to this book. This was an effect both of the literature on totalitarianism, which tended to analyze totalitarian tendencies as arising from obscure psychological causes rather than as conscious responses to specific economic or political conditions, and of the fascination with psychotropic medications. In both cases, the principal concern was social cohesion: it was dangerous to allow certain beliefs or certain affective responses to modern life to metastasize beyond the mechanisms of control. Once the political has been made personal, though, once psychological conditions are used as an explanation for political conditions, then the personal becomes political. And when that happens, agencies of social

50. Freud, *Civilization and Its Discontents*, 145.
51. Quoted in Valenstein, *Blaming the Brain*, 11.

control begin to lose their authority, since the locus of political struggle is now in the private realm. It was the psychologizing of the situation of women, by Betty Friedan in *The Feminine Mystique* (1962), that helped inspire the women's movement. And that movement made life better for American women—made them, to borrow from Freud's original title for *Civilization and Its Discontents*, happier in culture. Human nature did not change when this happened, nor did the sky fall down.

EIGHT

Heinz Kohut's Americanization of Freud

ELIZABETH LUNBECK

Allow me to begin by highlighting the improbability of Freud's long hold on us in the United States. It is a commonplace of social criticism that the American cultural landscape has nurtured a range of distinctively optimistic mental therapies—touting self-esteem, enjoining self-help, promising self-actualization—in keeping with this country's history of abundance and plentitude that stand in stark contrast to the dour but brutally realistic pessimism of Sigmund Freud's science of psychoanalysis. Where Americans, blissfully oblivious to limits both social and psychic, cultivated the child within and frantically sought to realize their inborn potential as they chose from the cornucopia of home-grown therapies on offer, from humanistic to Gestalt to cognitive, their benighted European counterparts—or so the common wisdom goes—stoically accepted that the best they could hope for from analytic treatment was that, as Freud so memorably put it, their neurotic misery might be transformed into common unhappiness. Further, as Ernst Falzeder reminds us, Freud famously disdained America, adducing among other complaints the greedy materialism and sexual hypocrisy of its inhabitants and, vexed by their insufficient appreciation for political and paternal authority, repeatedly invoking the specter of New World political and gender anarchy—or, as his translator James Strachey so dismissively rendered it, "petticoat government"—in contrast to venerable Old World respect for hierarchy and tradition. Yet, perhaps paradoxically, America is the nation in which, among all others, Freud's science of psychoanalysis has arguably enjoyed the greatest purchase, the most far-reaching cultural influence, the most powerful institutional instantiations—its bleak pessimism and patently un-American severity notwithstanding.

The question of why psychoanalysis so prospered in the United States is still open, despite a good deal of excellent commentary and scholarship addressed to it. It is worth underscoring that the Americanization of Freud is not new. Rather, it is visible from the start, as a hastily sketched history shows. Freud's first American enthusiasts—James Jackson Putnam, L. E. Emerson—translated his stark strictures into a distinctively meliorist American idiom and infused them with moralism notably absent from Freud's own texts and worldview. Cultural radicals in the 1910s and 1920s seamlessly conscripted the Freud who was a critic of civilized sexual morality into their own programs as the prophet of sexual and social liberation. American analysts in the interwar years proffered an improbably effective and upbeat Freudianism, with, for example, the country's psychiatrist-in-chief Karl Menninger suggesting that those submitting to psychotherapy could, as he evocatively put it, "change their spots."[1] And American theoretical eclecticism squared off against a reinvigorated European doctrinal orthodoxy through the 1940s and 1950s, with the prewar and wartime emigration to the United States of a clutch of ego psychologists, many of them Viennese with close ties to Freud—among them Heinz Hartmann, Kurt and Ruth Eissler, Edith Jacobson, and Robert Waelder. Rising quickly to leadership of the analytic establishment in their adopted land, these so-called ego psychologists contributed to the consolidation and hegemony of classical analysis in the United States. Characterized by an austerity and abstinence consonant with Freud's technical recommendations but absent from his actual practice, classicism and the "Freud" who authorized it were produced, as other essayists in this volume have argued, not in late nineteenth-century Vienna but in mid-twentieth-century New York and Chicago.

The Americanization of Freud is, then, less a singular turning point in the long history of Freud in America than constitutive of that history, a constant—and contested—process of appropriation, translation, supplementation, and purification. Freud in America, like any other immigrant to American shores, has always been subjected to the forces of Americanization. The debut of the Americanized Freud of the Viennese-born, Chicago-based psychoanalyst Heinz Kohut—the focus of this essay—is from this perspective but the latest chapter in this century-long saga of cultural and intellectual translation. Indeed, some—focusing especially on Kohut's explorations of narcissism—have seen it as an exemplary chapter, characterizing him as quintessentially American in his optimism and sug-

---

1. Karl Menninger, cited in Nathan G. Hale Jr., *The Rise and Crisis of Psychoanalysis in the United States: Freud and the Americans, 1917–1985* (New York: Oxford University Press, 1995), 83.

gesting that his revisionism reflected, expressed, and, as one formulation puts it, "fit perfectly" with the culture of the postwar United States in which it was articulated.² There is something to this line of argument. Kohut brilliantly situated his interventions at the crossroads where long-simmering dissatisfaction both with Freud's drive-based theories and with the brittle asceticism of the orthodox analytic setting met long-standing concerns about the shape of the modal American self. In a series of analytic papers published in the 1960s, at the height of Freud's influence in the United States, and then in two landmark books that appeared in the 1970s, Kohut challenged the primacy Freud had assigned to the drives in understanding human behavior, brought provision and gratification back into discussions of analytic technique, and outlined a normal narcissism that was the wellspring of human ambition and creativity, values and ideals, empathy and fellow feeling. He burst onto the cultural scene in the 1970s brandishing an appealingly normalized narcissism that, in the estimation of social critics, was symptomatic of the nation's precipitous decline. To them, both Kohut, whom they cast as the analyst of abundance and plentitude, and the figure of this new narcissist—greedy, solipsistic, entitled, grandiose—were *echt* American.

Yet to characterize Kohut's achievement primarily as a reflection of his times is to underestimate it. One of the most striking aspects of Kohut's analytic career is that he managed to attack head-on the fundamentals of Freudianism while escaping both the banishment from the analytic mainstream *and* the marginalization that was the fate of so many of his dissenting forebears, among them Carl Jung, Alfred Adler, and Sándor Ferenczi. Despite the audacity and ferocity of his attacks on Freud and Freudian analysis, Kohut is very much part of, by some accounts at the center of, the analytic mainstream today. He insured the survival of "Freud" both externally, in making psychoanalysis newly relevant to the culture at large, and internally, nourishing, even healing, the analytic field as he laid the groundwork for the re-appropriation in the 1980s and 1990s of the banished and vilified Ferenczi and the largely ignored W. R. D. Fairbairn as well as of the British object-relations perspective more generally. Kohut, that is, managed simultaneously to kill off Freud and to insure his survival in America. In what follows, I first provide an overview of Kohut's career and thought before turning to examine the externalist story, looking at how social critics picked up on his explorations of narcissism, bringing them into a wide-

---

2. Philip Cushman, *Constructing the Self, Constructing America: A Cultural History of Psychotherapy* (Reading, MA: Addison-Wesley, 1995), 211.

ranging conversation about the American self that was already, fortuitously for the public fortunes of psychoanalysis, framed in analytic terms. I then turn to the internalist story, suggesting that among the factors accounting for his singular success was that he fashioned himself a revolutionary while at the same time channeling spectral presences that had long haunted the discipline of psychoanalysis.

Kohut was in many respects the unlikeliest of spokesmen for an Americanized narcissism. Born in 1913 into an assimilated Jewish family, he fled Vienna in March 1939, a mere five months before the outbreak of war, settling temporarily in a refugee camp in England before managing to move to London and, within the year, landing on American shores with barely twenty-five dollars to his name.[3] He made his way to Chicago, where a childhood friend was living, and, a medical degree from the University of Vienna in hand, he quickly secured an internship and then a prestigious residency in neurology in his adopted city. Advancing to the rank of instructor, he switched his appointment to psychiatry and, in 1946, began to train as a psychoanalyst at the Chicago Institute for Psychoanalysis. In analysis with Ruth Eissler, an exemplar of orthodox technique, and methodically plowing through Freud's works,[4] Kohut was situating himself very much in the analytic mainstream. He would brook no criticism of Freud, to whom his idealized devotion was manifestly evident. By the 1950s, he was recognized as a brilliant and creative analyst as well as an adept psychoanalytic politician, friend and correspondent to the stars—among them Anna Freud—in the analytic firmament. He was, he explained, "beloved by everybody and on the right kind of handshaking terms. In every room I entered there were smiles."[5]

Soon enough, everybody would be looking away.[6] The precise moment

---

3. Charles B. Strozier, *Heinz Kohut: The Making of a Psychoanalyst* (New York: Farrar, Straus and Giroux, 2001), 68.
4. Kohut to August Aichorn, 12 October 1946, in Heinz Kohut, *The Curve of Life: Correspondence of Heinz Kohut, 1923–1981*, ed. Geoffrey Cocks (Chicago: University of Chicago Press, 1994), 53–55.
5. Strozier, *Kohut*, 135.
6. Kohut in Susan Quinn, "Oedipus vs. Narcissus," *New York Times*, 9 November 1980. Bernard Brickman, "The Curve of Life: Correspondence of Heinz Kohut, 1923–1981," *Journal of the American Psychoanalytic Association* 45 (1997): 591–92, refers to the analysts who "reviled and shunned him at meetings," many of them "former friends and admirers." Kohut was well-enough known among American analysts to be ranked fifth in a list of those named as influential and important in a survey of 188 analysts conducted in 1969; narcissism was ranked fourth in a list of "important discoveries in psychoanalysis during the past 30 years": Charles K.

at which Kohut's apostasy became evident is a matter of some dispute. Some see it as early as his 1959 paper on introspection and empathy as modes of observation in psychoanalysis, which occasioned responses that Kohut remembered as ranging from the almost violent to the warmly accepting when he first shared it with his colleagues.[7] Others see him struggling, with varying degrees of success, to negotiate between Freud and his own evolving new perspective through the period that eventuated in *The Analysis of the Self*, published in 1971. Most agree that with the publication, in 1977, of *The Restoration of the Self*, the break with Freud's drive-based metapsychology was complete and irreversible. The once-fierce guardian of orthodoxy, the latter-day psychoanalytic paladin who would "wipe the floor" with anyone daring to dishonor Freud's genius,[8] had launched a successful assault on the very foundations of Freudianism, formulating a patently optimistic alternative to its bleak pessimism in language his detractors dismissed as sentimental, mawkish, and—echoing as it did the themes of growth and possibility that fueled the earlier stabs at analytic revisionism that had flourished on native grounds—*echt* American.[9] In the space of three decades, Kohut—the self-appointed "Mr. Psychoanalysis"—moved from high priest to excommunicated heretic to founder of the new church of "self psychology," from president of the resolutely classical American Psychoanalytic Association in the early 1960s to banished "deviant" to widely celebrated spokesman for what many deemed the field's "new scientific paradigm" in the late 1970s.[10]

In making his journey, Kohut broke not only with the American keepers of the Freudian faith—among them his training analyst and important mentors—but also with what he called the archaic Freud who lived on in the analyst's breast as a constraining and curbing force. The death of this idealized Freud—and, more important, the deaths of those analysts who were charismatically tied to him by virtue of having known him

---

Hofling and Robert W. Meyers, "Recent Discoveries in Psychoanalysis: A Study of Opinion," *Archives of General Psychiatry* 26 (1972): 518–23.

7. Heinz Kohut, "Introspection, Empathy, and Psychoanalysis: An Examination of the Relationship between Mode of Observation and Theory," *Journal of the American Psychoanalytic Association* 7 (1959): 459–83. For Kohut's memories of the paper's reception, see Kohut, "Introspection, Empathy, and the Semi-Circle of Mental Health," *International Journal of Psychoanalysis* 63 (1982): 395–407.

8. According to the testimony of a Chicago colleague, who claimed Kohut had "wiped the floor with me": Strozier, *Kohut*, 132.

9. Mawkish: Janet Malcolm, *Psychoanalysis: The Impossible Profession* (New York: Knopf, 1981), 119.

10. See, for example, Robert Stolorow, "Kohut's *Restoration of the Self*: A Symposium," *Psychoanalytic Review* 65 (1978): 622–24.

personally—was to Kohut an opportunity, an open door portending "a surge of independent initiative," explorations that would take the intrepid into the vast territories of the psyche left uncharted by the founding generation of analysts.[11] Admitting that his need of the Freud within had lessened over the years, Kohut gradually consigned his Freud to the status of admired historical figure, respected but no longer idealized. Where Freud was in Kohut's estimation clearly a man of the nineteenth century, Kohut fashioned himself a child of the twentieth, looking to the future, not fixated on the past, however comfortable and familiar it might have been.[12]

Freed of his inner need of Freud, "the symbol of the father," of his need to lean on him for "self-confirmation or support,"[13] Kohut was able to spell out what was at stake in his abandonment of classicism. In papers published and in interviews granted before his death, Kohut spiritedly took on, among other targets, orthodoxy's closed-system thinking, its covert moralism, and its developmental telos, maintaining that "values of independence are phony, really. There is no such thing. . . . It is nonsense to try to give up symbiosis and become an independent self."[14] He challenged Freud's cherished personal mythology, suggesting that the latter's well-known comparison of himself with Copernicus and Darwin as one who had delivered a wounding blow to man's megalomania and had in so offending humanity's narcissism brought down upon himself "the most evil spirits of criticism,"[15] was misguided. Kohut suggested that Freud's "fancy idea that there was an unconscious," among other great discoveries in the history of science, might have occasioned heightened self-esteem as much as wounded pride among those familiar with them.[16] And he combatively closed a posthumously delivered address by suggesting that psychoanalysis needed to grow up, to internalize Freud in the way a growing child would internalize a parent, and to "turn from the study of Freud to the study of man."[17]

A good part of Kohut's achievement consisted in recasting narcissism

11. Heinz Kohut, "The Future of Psychoanalysis," *Annual of Psychoanalysis* 3 (1975): 325–40, at 328.
12. Kohut to Henry D. von Witzleben, 7 April 1977, in Kohut, *Curve*, 344–46.
13. Kohut, "Future of Psychoanalysis," 327; Kohut to Henry D. von Witzleben, 7 April 1977, in Kohut, *Curve*, 345.
14. Kohut interviewed by Strozier, 6 June 1981, in Kohut, *Self Psychology and the Humanities: Reflections on a New Psychoanalytic Approach*, ed. Charles B. Strozier (New York: Norton, 1985), 262.
15. Sigmund Freud, *Introductory Lectures on Psycho-Analysis* (1916–17), S.E. 17:284.
16. Kohut interviewed by Strozier, 12 March 1981, in Kohut, *Self Psychology and the Humanities*, 250; Heinz Kohut, *How Does Analysis Cure?* (Chicago: University of Chicago Press, 1984), 58.
17. Kohut, "Introspection, Empathy, and the Semi-Circle," 405.

as a desirable, even necessary, dimension of personhood. Freud had conceived of narcissism as an early stage in a developmental sequence that originated in infantile solipsism and culminated, ideally, in the sovereign self. Within this framework, narcissism, once abandoned, was a fallback position to which one might revert under threat—think here of Freud's striking imagery of the amoeba with its pseudopodia, the false feet thrust outwards and pulled back when in danger. Recall as well that in his essay "On Narcissism" Freud had outlined an opposition between love of oneself, termed "narcissistic," and object love, love of another.[18] He and his followers generally argued that narcissistic investment in the self was optimally displaced by mature object love. Kohut objected not only to Freud's closed-system thinking but also to a pejorative stance toward narcissism that he held was manifest in analysts' preference for object love over self-love—however much they might maintain that their stance on narcissism was morally neutral, "psychoanalytic locker-room chitchat" assigned it a negative valence.[19] Kohut argued that object love, as well as "any other intense experience," strengthened the self, which in turn could then experience love more intensely.[20] He maintained that Freud's closed-system thinking could not account for the fact that reciprocated passionate love did not diminish but rather enhanced self-esteem—an observation that Freud's amoeba imagery was inadequate to explain.[21] Where Freud had seen childish narcissism superseded by mature object love, Kohut argued it was instead *transformed*—that archaic forms of it, such as grandiosity, were "remobilized and reintegrated" in the service of ideals, self-esteem, creativity, and other useful attributes of a healthy personality. Object love did not replace narcissism, as Freud had argued; rather, narcissism followed its own line of development "from the primitive to the complex and advanced,"[22] assuming different forms at different points in the curve of life. Complex forms provided the very basis for civilized life.

To start with the most primitive, infantile forms: Kohut admired Ferenczi's portrayal of infantile grandiosity, and his infant was as much a fantasist as was Ferenczi's. Both were cared for, in ideal circumstances, by an empathic maternal figure who accepted the child's idealization of her as

18. Freud, "On Narcissism: An Introduction" (1914), S.E. 14:67–102.
19. Heinz Kohut, "Value Judgments Surrounding Narcissism," in *The Kohut Seminars on Self Psychology and Psychotherapy with Adolescents and Young Adults*, ed. Miriam Elson (New York: Norton, 1987), 6.
20. Kohut, *How Does Analysis Cure?*, 53.
21. Kohut, "Thoughts on Narcissism and Narcissistic Rage," *Psychoanalytic Study of the Child* 27 (1972): 360–400, esp. 364.
22. Kohut to Robert Sussman, 8 April 1967, in Kohut, *Curve*, 165–66.

perfect and all-powerful—acting as what Kohut called the "idealized parental imago"—while mirroring the child's grandiosity, enabling it to delight in its own feelings of omnipotence and to revel in its exhibitionism. This empathic figure smoothed the child's confrontation with the inevitable frustrations of reality, allowing it to maintain pleasurably narcissistic feelings of power and fullness where it might otherwise, absent her actual and internalized presence, feel powerless and empty. Kohut maintained that the child experienced this figure as part of itself, as a sustaining "selfobject"—part self, part internalized other. As the child grew, it gradually took on more of the self-esteem-regulating and tension-reducing functions that the internalized selfobject had performed, and a sense of self, cohesive and not fragmented, was achieved.

Kohut's writings on narcissism entered a cultural field already focused—quite critically—on narcissism. Through the 1970s, commentators were arguing that American culture was increasingly narcissistic. In a 1973 essay prophesying that the 1970s would "come to be known as the Me Decade," Tom Wolfe skewered the newly emergent penchant for unceasing "analysis of the self," terming the impulse to do so narcissistic and linking it to the postwar prosperity that was endowing so many with the leisure to dwell on themselves.[23] Wolfe's indictment was followed two years later by Peter Marin's widely cited, plangent analysis of the beleaguered, solipsistic retreat into the self that, he argued, portended the rise of a "new narcissism."[24] Others chimed in, branding the United States a nation of narcissists and seeing its young deformed by a media-fueled collective narcissism that emptied the self while mandating reverence for "the image."[25] The stunning, and almost instantaneous, visibility of Christopher Lasch's *Culture of Narcissism*, published in 1978, positioned psychoanalysis at the center of a long-running conversation about the failings of the modal American. Lasch skillfully—if promiscuously—mined the discipline, fashioning a contradictory theoretical hodgepodge of Kohut, Otto Kernberg, and Melanie Klein, among other analysts, into a manifestly convincing and rhetorically persuasive account of precipitous national decline. It was the "Age of Narcissism," proclaimed the *New York Times*,[26] and the term of-

---

23. Tom Wolfe, "The 'Me' Decade and the Third Great Awakening," *New York Magazine*, 23 August 1976, 26–40.

24. Peter Marin, "The New Narcissism," *Harper's*, October 1975, 45–56.

25. Jim Hougan, *Decadence: Radical Nostalgia, Narcissism, and Decline in the Seventies* (New York: William Morrow, 1975), esp. 151–55. Christopher Lasch, in his "The Narcissist Society," *New York Review of Books*, 30 September 1976, 15, stakes out his particular take on narcissism as "the key to the consciousness movement and to the moral climate of contemporary society."

26. Eugene Kennedy Franklin, "The Looming 80's," *New York Times*, 2 December 1979.

fered a range of critics a beguiling new language in which to voice venerable complaints. In their hands, narcissism usefully brought together under one snappy rubric the rampant individualism, the spiritual questing, the preoccupation with self, and the flight from commitment they argued was newly prevalent. Throughout the 1970s and 1980s, Cassandras of cultural decline issued dire assessments of the nation's fall in tandem with narcissism's rise.

Kohut was centrally part of this conversation, but he, in contrast to the critics, highlighted the positive aspects of narcissism, arguing, for example, that childhood grandiosity—anathema to the critics—was gradually tamed but not wholly expunged, transformed, and available to the adult, acting as "instinctual fuel" for ambitions and self-esteem.[27] The point as he saw it was not to deny or to eradicate the child's narcissistic grandiosity and pleasurable exhibitionism but, rather, to see them at once frustrated and lovingly supported. Narcissism transformed provided critical support to the adult personality, in particular to its creative capacities but also to its humor and even wisdom. Kohut held that it was when the child's strivings were not supported that problems arose—the feelings of emptiness, aimlessness, and fragmentation that together constituted the social critics' indictment of the modal modern American.

Almost from the start of his musings on narcissism and a full decade before social commentators homed in on the diagnosis, Kohut was situating it sociologically as "the social pathology of our age."[28] Disorders of the self were not new but newly prevalent,[29] he maintained, explaining that the bustling Victorian households in which Freud's patients had been reared offered children too much sexual and other stimulation, whether from servants or members of extended families living together, and that by contrast the modern household offered them too little. In Freud's time, children had been over-involved with their parents. Now, isolated in homes superintended by one or two parents, children were far too under-involved with their elders.[30] Children reared by loving parents, empathically attuned to

---

27. Heinz Kohut, "The Psychoanalytic Treatment of Narcissistic Personality Disorders: Outline of a Systematic Approach," *Psychoanalytic Study of the Child* 23 (1968): 86–113, at 87.
28. Kohut to Alexander Mitscherlich, 22 February 1965, in Kohut, *Curve*, 111–12.
29. Kohut to Margrit Hengaertner, 22 March 1977, in ibid., 342–43.
30. Kohut in Quinn, "Oedipus vs. Narcissus"; Kohut to Evan Brahm, 7 February 1977, in Kohut, *Curve*, 335. In *The Restoration of the Self* (Chicago: University of Chicago Press, 1977), Kohut expanded on this, speculating that the damage inflicted on the young by "narcissistically disturbed parents" in Freud's time may have been less than in the present, due to the presence of extended family members and servants, many of them "young, healthy unmarried country-girls who, without ties in the big city, became deeply involved with the families for whom they

their needs, grew into adults secure in their self-worth and capable of mobilizing their narcissism to embrace life exuberantly, to love themselves and others too. Those reared by preoccupied or cold and unempathic parents could grow up to be pathological narcissists, fated to seek desperately from others the admiration—the mirroring and feeding of their grandiosity—that their upbringing had failed to provide. Narcissism was rooted in deprivation.

Kohut, explaining that Freud was "not exuberant enough" for his tastes,[31] crafted a psychoanalysis that was organized around the development of a cohesive self capable of articulating its ideals, pursing its ambitions, and relating to others around it. By his own telling no ascetic, Kohut celebrated the preoccupation with the self that social critics found intellectually bankrupt and morally suspect. In the context of a Western culture that extolled activity and disparaged "concern for one's self," critics might contend that looking inward "to contemplate one's navel" was the province of a few eccentrics, but, he maintained, it was precisely in man's interiority that the sources of gratification that would make life worth living would in the future be found.[32] Gesturing toward a grand history of the passions, Kohut suggested that mankind had formerly found some relief from civilization's demands that lust and aggression be contained in performing manual labor, in roaming about freely, and in the pleasures of parenthood—all realms of activity that, as machines replaced muscles and as the human population grew at an unsustainable rate, would of necessity be further curtailed. He applauded the rising generation's search for intensification of inner experience, whether abetted by surrender to the intoxications of drugs and music or by immersion in the teachings of Eastern philosophy, maintaining that the countercultural young better than their parents grasped that the path to psychic health lay in responding "with a full range of emotions" to the challenges presented by a rapidly changing world.[33] Turning humanity from the battles and war that had long engaged its energies toward harmony and peace necessitated a culturally supported shift inward. Only when persuaded of what Kohut called "the enriching potentialities of the inner life" would mankind have strength enough to

---

worked." Their presence counteracted the "emotional isolation" of the children under their care: 276, and n. 4.

31. Kohut to Roger Petti, 24 March 1981, in Kohut, *Curve*, 426–27.
32. Heinz Kohut, "Psychoanalysis in a Troubled World," *Annual of Psychoanalysis* 1 (1973): 3–25, at 22.
33. Ibid., 23.

temper their dangerously aggressive drives, and only then would world peace prevail.[34] The path to restraint, that is, was paved with what looked to critics like self-indulgence.

Kohut was confronting the cultural Cassandras head-on here, proposing that external scarcity called not, as they contended, for a psychological stance of asceticism but rather for a compensatory internal plentitude, not for a refusal but instead for an embrace of gratifications and satisfactions. In proposing that what could easily be construed as solipsistic self-absorption would enhance rather than imperil the public good, Kohut was scrambling the critics' categories. If they would mourn the demise of the nineteenth century's purportedly unified culture, in which disciplined restraint governed society and shaped social character, he would contend, in a unifying spirit, that the social environment had changed since then, calling forth new characterological constellations more suited to it than to "the world of yesterday."[35] If they would condemn the newly ubiquitous narcissism of the present as pathological, he would contend that, in "his groping toward the enlargement and intensification of his inner life," the narcissist might be seen as responding more creatively and courageously to the possibilities offered by the world around him than the purportedly normal person. The new psychic forms that drew the censure of both professionals and laity alike were best conceptualized not within the framework of disease and illness but rather "as a way station on the road of man's search for a new psychological equilibrium."[36] New times called for new psychic forms. Kohut charged the cultural arbiters who would wish narcissism out of existence with hypocrisy akin to that of the Victorians on the question of sex—denying the existence of what was everywhere evident, if in disguised and distorted form.[37] History—specifically, two thousand years of Christianity—had shown that suppression of human drives, "the meek acceptance of an ascetic existence," was neither possible nor advisable.[38]

Kohut's brief for the prerogatives of the newly expansive self patently smacked of what the social critic Daniel Bell would call "the debasement of modernity,"[39] and it might easily be construed as exemplary of what Lasch

---

34. Kohut, "Future," 338.
35. Kohut, "Troubled World," 23; Kohut, "Future," 336.
36. Kohut, "Troubled World," 22, 21.
37. Kohut, "Narcissistic Rage," 365.
38. Kohut, "Troubled World," 21.
39. Daniel Bell, *The Cultural Contradictions of Capitalism* (New York: Basic Books, 1978 [1976]), xv.

saw as the defining self-absorption of contemporary culture.[40] But Kohut was no simple-minded prophet of liberation. To the end, he was enough the Freudian to hold that humanity's abandoning itself to lust and aggression would lead only to disaster. Further, the self untrammeled by any and all convention that was to Bell a specter of modernity at its worst was to Kohut an impossibility, so ubiquitous were the forces of cultural control that tempered this self's yearnings at every turn. As Kohut saw it, the point was to acknowledge what lay within, not to deny it in the name of an impossible-to-honor ascetic ideal. Like Bell and his fellow critics, Kohut saw humanity at a critical cultural turning point, in Bell's words "a watershed in Western society," that would herald the end of the bourgeois character type. Yet where Bell saw the end of creativity, Kohut saw its renaissance, and while Bell denounced modernism's "idolatry of the self," Kohut embraced it.[41]

Kohut conceived of narcissism as a necessary component of a self robustly engaged with its environment, holding it was to be not suppressed but transformed into something culturally useful. In his hands narcissism was not the antithesis of ambition but the condition of its flourishing. It was not, that is, an impediment to worldly efficacy. This dimension of narcissism would, by the 1970s, be commonly referred to as "healthy narcissism." The term, coined by the Viennese analyst Paul Federn in a little-known paper on the difference between healthy and pathological narcissism published in 1936, was absent from Freud's oeuvre.[42] Federn and the few other analysts who invoked the concept before its popularization used it in reference to the self's needs for growth and mastery, with its "feelings of triumph over difficulties"[43] and, more capaciously, with the "capacity to enjoy life."[44]

From the start, healthy narcissism fit uneasily with Freud's metapsychology, with his emphasis on the pathological nature of narcissism and its

---

40. Christopher Lasch, *The Culture of Narcissism: American Life in an Age of Diminishing Expectations* (New York: Norton, 1978), 25.

41. Bell, *Cultural Contradictions*, 16, 7, 19. See Edward Jones, "Critique of Empathic Science: On Kohut and Narcissism," *Psychology and Social Theory* 2 (1981): 29–42, for a different perspective than mine on Kohut and the critics.

42. Paul Federn, "Zur Unterscheidung des gesunden und krankhaften Narzissmus," *Imago* 22 (1936), 5–39.

43. Henry Harper Hart, "Narcissistic Equilibrium," *International Journal of Psychoanalysis* 28 (1947): 106–14, at 108.

44. Martin S. Bergmann, "The Place of Paul Federn's Ego Psychology in Psychoanalytic Metapsychology," *Journal of the American Psychoanalytic Association* 11 (1963): 97–116, at 103.

infantile roots, referring as it did to an altogether different dimension of personhood, whether it was an experiential orientation[45] or a capacity—for exuberance, for liveliness and resourcefulness,[46] for "inner freedom and vitality,"[47] issues on which orthodox psychoanalysis was largely silent. These were but minor points, however. It fell to Kohut to bring healthy narcissism from the periphery of the analytic conversation to the center, to celebrate what defenders of Freud's orthodoxy—*plus royaliste que le roi*—imagined would have occasioned squeamish "theoretical embarrassment" in the master.[48] Kohut used the term "healthy narcissism" early in his career to refer to the pleasure enjoyed by the musical virtuoso, pleasure that enhanced self-esteem.[49] Later, proclaiming that "we should not deny our ambitions, our wish to dominate, our wish to shine," he branded as legitimate aspirations conventionally associated with an unseemly grandiosity. The point, he argued, was not to deny hypocritically that narcissistic forces lay within but rather to see them transformed into realistic self-esteem and "the socially useful, adaptive and joyful capacity to be enthusiastic."[50]

By the early 1980s, psychoanalysts and popular writers alike were touting healthy narcissism as "vital for satisfaction and survival," as a "bank account of self-esteem" on which one could draw to bolster oneself against the many insults and small traumas of everyday life.[51] Challenged at work, the patently self-assured but in fact deeply vulnerable pathological narcissist might react with rage, devaluing those who would question his perfection and withdrawing into a brooding depression. The healthy narcissist, in contrast, would better be able to maintain his equilibrium—by drawing on his banked self-esteem—and to get on with living life to its rough-and-tumble full. Given that the price of worldly success was high, "you have got to have a bit of narcissism to succeed," as a leading New York analyst put it in 1984. Pride in oneself and one's achievements, even "the urge to be

45. Paula Heimann, "Notes on the Anal Stage," *International Journal of Psychoanalysis* 43 (1962): 406–14, esp. 413.

46. Joseph D. Lichtenberg, "The Development of the Sense of Self," *Journal of the American Psychoanalytic Association* 23 (1975): 459–84, at 477.

47. Alice Miller, "Depression and Grandiosity as Related Forms of Narcissistic Disturbance," *International Review of Psycho-Analysis* 6 (1979): 61–76, at 62.

48. C. Hanly and J. Masson, "A Critical Examination of the New Narcissism," *International Journal of Psychoanalysis* 51 (1976): 49–66, at 50.

49. Kohut, "Observations on the Psychological Functions of Music," *Journal of the American Psychoanalytic Association* 5 (1957): 389–407, at 391.

50. Kohut, "Narcissistic Rage," 365.

51. James Masterson and Paul Ornstein, quoted in Daniel Goleman, "Narcissism Looming Larger as Root of Personality Woes," *New York Times*, 1 November 1988.

great," were now conceived of as within the compass of a healthy narcissism.[52] Modern life insistently called on everyone's reserves of healthy narcissism, whether in the service of realistic appreciation of one's strengths coupled with loving acceptance of one's limitations[53] or, more grandly, in sustaining the pain and sacrifice, the delayed gratifications, that were prelude to mastery and success.

Lasch marshaled the Kohut who was theorist of the empty self's fragmentation in support of his own dour prophecies of immanent cultural disaster while all but ignoring the Kohut who was celebrant of the self's rich potentialities. Lasch's is thus a curiously tendentious reading of Kohut. It is not clear he even realized that Kohut—avatar of a transformed healthy narcissism, harsh critic of the West's "heritage of altruism that condemned anything that tended to enhance the self"[54]—was not his ideological ally but rather antagonist. Harkening back to an imagined past of fullness and plentitude, Lasch bemoaned the displacement of "the imperial self of yesteryear" by the minimal self he argued was decreed viable by times of impending austerity.[55] Kohut, by contrast, welcomed the debut of the imperial self, and he celebrated the expressiveness and liveliness Lasch condemned. There is no underestimating the extent to which Kohut's writings, with their invocations of joy, creativity, affection, growth, and adjustment, and their focus on the self's potentials instead of its pathologies, marked a break with the austerity of analytic orthodoxy and a reorientation of the analytic field.

Where others saw a world in decline, Kohut saw a different world. His questioning of whether the world of the present was really worse than the one in which he'd grown up set him apart from the critics who were disposed to see decline everywhere. He played with the notion that the world of his adulthood was not worse but decisively different from the world of his youth, demanding of those who would evaluate and comprehend it "new values, new yardsticks, new viewpoints."[56] Along these lines, Kohut

---

52. Robert Michels and Arnold Cooper, quoted in Goleman, "Analyzing the New York Syndrome," *New York Times*, 4 November 1984.

53. Susan Prince, quoted in Alexandra Penney, "Showing Some New Muscle," *New York Times*, 15 June 1980.

54. Kohut, in Nathan P. Segel, "Narcissistic Resistance," *Journal of the American Psychoanalytic Association* 17 (1969): 941–54, at 953.

55. Christopher Lasch, *The Minimal Self: Psychic Survival in Troubled Times* (New York: Norton, 1984), 15.

56. Kohut, as paraphrased by Richard Chessick, "Perspectivism, Constructivism, and Empathy in Psychoanalysis: Nietzsche and Kohut," *Journal of the American Academy of Psychoanalysis* 25 (1997): 373–98, at 388.

historicized the conflicts between man and civilization that Freud had cast as timeless. For all their professed disdain for the therapeutic ethos and psychological man, social critics were insistently drawn to the Freudian notion that civilization was built on the repression of human drives and was, as such, antithetical to the fulfillment of human desire. In *Das Unbehagen in der Kultur*—which was translated by Freud himself as "Man's Discomfort in Civilization" but famously rendered in English as *Civilization and Its Discontents*—Freud had argued that the demands of society were antagonistic to the individual's claim to personal gratifications, in particular to sexuality but also to the expression of aggression. Civilization imposed sacrifices on man such that it was difficult for him to find happiness in it. In fact, Freud suggested, though "primitive man" enjoyed little security, he "was better off in knowing no restrictions of instinct."[57] Adopting Freud's rough economic calculus, critics would maintain renunciation was an imperative, inhibition "the price of entry into every real satisfaction." In the words of Philip Rieff, there were no "pleasures unpaid for in parallel pains." Culture ruled over man by means not of sublimation but of a more draconian repression.[58] If Western civilization was premised on what Philip Slater called the "control release dialectic," then liberation was at best only apparent, at worst a means to more efficient manipulation of the populace,[59] a line of argument developed by Frankfurt school theorists and adopted by Marcuse and Lasch, among others. From this perspective, increased liberties in the sexual and other spheres were procured at the price of intensified societal domination and bureaucratic control.

Through the 1970s, social critics brandished the sociological Freud both to excoriate student radicals for their utopianism and to discredit the meliorism of the neo-Freudian psychologists, holding that to bridle against limits was to protest the very essence of humanity.[60] Kohut would have none of this. "Where is the *Unbehagen*?" he asked.[61] Maintaining that culture had to be thought of as more than drive-taming, he argued that dis-

57. Freud, *Civilization and Its Discontents* (1930 [1929]), S.E. 21:59–145, at 115.
58. Philip Rieff, *Freud: The Mind of the Moralist* (Chicago: University of Chicago Press, 1979 [1959]), 372; see also Fred Siegel, "The Agony of Christopher Lasch," *Reviews in American History* 8 (1980): 285–95.
59. Philip Slater, *The Pursuit of Loneliness: American Culture at the Breaking Point* (Boston: Beacon Press, 1980), 92; see also Abram de Swaan, "The Politics of Agoraphobia: On Changes in Emotional and Relational Management," *Theory and Society* 10 (1981): 359–85, esp. 380.
60. Siegel, "Christopher Lasch," 292.
61. Kohut interviewed by Strozier, 7 May 1981, in Kohut, *Self Psychology and the Humanities*, 254. Kohut, "Troubled World," 21 n. 2, wrote: "The English rendition of the title of Freud's great essay *Das Unbehagen in der Kultur* is *Civilization and Its Discontents*. Actually neither the words 'discomfort' nor 'discontent' do full justice to the meaning of *Unbehagen*, although 'dis-

comfort resulted not from civilization itself, but came when persons were not *supported* in civilization, for example, when one was bereft of the sustaining comforts provided by one's language, music, and art, by familiar voices and by the endearing habits of friends and acquaintances. Freud's model of *Homo natura* at war with his surroundings, if marvelously consistent and lovely to behold, "an esthetic pleasure," was at bottom mechanistic: "There is a certain tension, and when the tension rises you put the lid on." Kohut argued that the murderous, drive-fueled man of Freud's theorizing—"man wants to kill, man wants to fuck, man wants to eat ravenously," and then he has restrictions slapped on him—was not the norm but the exception, explaining that Freud had seen the essence of man in what was in fact the breakdown of civilized relations. Only when the self was not supported did the lust and hate that Freud took as foundational come to the fore. Consider the Native Americans subjected to the civilizing mission of their colonizers, Kohut asked. Were they depressed, as Freud's *Unbehagen* would suggest, because they could no longer kill each other, or was it that the continuity of their culture had been disrupted? As he put it, "don't they drink because their all-sustaining culture, their own traditional self, has become valueless?" Murderousness only resulted when man's assertive strivings were stymied. Likewise, Oedipal conflicts were not universal, but arose when the child's caretakers failed to meet his exhibitionism and assertiveness with pride and joyful acceptance and his gropings for affection with sexual stimulation.[62]

Psychoanalysts may have bristled at critics' plundering of their discipline to level wholesale indictments of their fellow citizens, but at least some of them reveled in the possibilities this heady moment presented. Kohut was featured in popular publications on the diminishing quality of modern family life and interviewed in pages of *People* magazine, and Otto Kernberg similarly enjoyed a remarkable public visibility. There is no question that psychoanalysis as a discipline benefited from its newfound visibility, even as any sense of theoretical consistency and purity—defense of which looms large in the discipline's history—was sacrificed on the altar of celebrity. Narcissism's transformation—which escaped critical notice—from a clinical concept associated with emotional impoverishment into a cultural indictment of an unseemly plentitude was central to its appeal; a protean category, it could signify all things to all people.

---

comfort,' with its milder connotation of suffering and without the implication of resentment, is the closer equivalent."

62. Kohut interviewed by Strozier, 7 May 1981, in Kohut, *Self Psychology and the Humanities*, 254–57.

Analysts had been discussing the emergence of the "new type of patient" for decades before Kohut and his explorations of narcissism were conscripted into a wider vernacular conversation about the American character. Among the effects of this conversation was the extraordinary visibility of psychoanalysis in 1970s and 1980s American culture, much of it focused on the appeal of narcissism—for or against, it mattered little. Think, for example, of the buzz that attended the publication of Janet Malcolm's 1981 book, *Psychoanalysis: The Impossible Profession,* in which orthodoxy and revisionism, austerity and gratification, neurosis and narcissism dramatically and satisfyingly squared off.

Psychoanalysis: The Impossible Profession now reads as a brilliant ethnography of a tribe of healers—the orthodox New York–based Freudian establishment—fitfully attempting to comprehend, and parry, the threat to their sovereignty posed by "a fervid cult in Chicago." Arrivistes worshipping the new god Kohut and proffering a new species of magical healing, the Chicagoans elicited a scathing contempt, leavened with tidbits of grudging respect, from the New Yorkers, who saw them as but the latest in a long line of pretenders whom they had faced down—"savagely fought," in Malcolm's words—and successfully defeated in the defense of their founding god's science (indeed, one of Malcolm's more colorful informants boasted of having at a conference done "a hatchet job on Kernberg"—a New Yorker but like the Chicagoans a revisionist—and having thereby proved his bona fides: "I had done my homework, and I crushed him, and everyone knew I had. . . . People started noticing me, inviting me to parties"). This time would be no different. Adler and Jung in the 1920s, Alexander in the 1940s—psychoanalysis, Malcolm's chief informant, the pseudonymous Aaron Green, maintained, "has waves of this kind of thing, and it serenely lets them wash over itself, because eventually they all subside"[63]—occasional recourse to the hatchet notwithstanding.

We, with the benefit of historical hindsight, know better than Malcolm and her informants could have how the story would unfold; in the decade-long subsiding, Kohut was assimilated into—not like his forebear Ferenczi, banished from—the analytic mainstream, and the high orthodoxy of the New York Freudians was more washed out than washed over. It is clear now that Malcolm swooped down on the orthodox at the point when their commitment to an uncompromising austerity of technique had become untenable, attacked from without but also, more interestingly, eroded from

---

63. Malcolm, *Psychoanalysis,* 104, 4, 88, 118.

within. Freud, as is well known, famously wrote that analytic treatment "must be carried out in abstinence." It was, he added, "a fundamental principle that the patient's need and longing should be allowed to persist in her," for only in such a state of suspended satisfaction would she be impelled to do the work analysis demanded. No surrogate satisfactions were to be offered her, for her frustration was critical to the progress of the treatment.[64] "Cruel though it may sound," he later told his colleagues, it was the analyst's task to insure that the patient's suffering was not prematurely foreclosed and, if it was, to "re-instate it elsewhere in the form of some appreciable privation."[65]

The cruelty that Freud admitted was the necessary corollary of abstinence has long shadowed it. For example, among the objectives of its observance as enumerated by one mid-century proponent was that of keeping "the intensity of psychic conflict at its optimal level,"[66] while allowing, *contra* orthodox precepts, that "maximal frustration is not always the most favourable condition for analytical work."[67] Green, a paragon of analytic orthodoxy, in the process of extolling the virtues of adopting a "fanatically pure" technique—namely, the greater freedom it, as "the more libertarian perspective," allowed the patient—could not help but highlight the same gratuitous cruelty. "No one likes to hurt people," Green told Malcolm, unwittingly caricaturing classical technique in terms of causing pain, standing silently by in the face of suffering, and withholding help from patients "when they plead for it," as he expounded on this insight. Green maintained that tempering the rigors of orthodox technique with "judicious doses of kindliness and friendliness" deprived the patient—all pleading aside—of her freedom to decide what was best for her. Green characterized the difficulties abstinence imposed on the analyst as "the real wear and tear of analysis," invoking the "chronic struggle to keep oneself from doing the things that decent people naturally and spontaneously do."[68]

It would be hard to overestimate the centrality of abstinence to psychoanalytic practice—especially in the mid-twentieth-century heyday of ego-

---

64. Freud, "Observations on Transference-Love (Further Recommendations on the Technique of Psycho-Analysis III)" (1915 [1914]), S.E. 12:159–71, at 165.

65. Freud, "Lines of Advance in Psycho-Analytic Therapy" (1919 [1918]), S.E. 17:163. Freud worried the question of analytic cruelty in "Analysis Terminable and Interminable" (1937), S.E. 23, part 4, pp. 230–34.

66. Rudolf Lowenstein, transcript of presentation in Poul M. Faergeman, "Meetings of the New York Psychoanalytic Society," *Psychoanalytic Quarterly* 27 (1958): 622–24, at 622.

67. Rudolph M. Loewenstein, "Remarks on Some Variations in Psycho-Analytic Technique," *International Journal of Psychoanalysis* 39 (1958): 202–10, at 204.

68. Malcolm, *Psychoanalysis*, 77.

psychology in the United States. Although frequently invoked before then, it was only in the 1950s that it was enshrined as a rule, the so-called "rule of abstinence."[69] Freud had, it should be noted, good reasons for issuing his prohibition on analyst-patient sexual relations. Such relations, now called boundary violations, were rife in—even, one might argue, in their ubiquity constitutive of—early analytic practice, and it appears that Freud was concerned about his disciples' promiscuous mixing of sexual and analytic relations.[70] Carl Jung and his analysand and later co-worker and fellow analyst Sabina Spielrein had an affair four years after her two-month-long analysis that ended violently; Ernest Jones met Loë Kann, with whom he lived for years, when she was in treatment with him; and an especially messy thicket of analysis and sex ended in Ferenczi's marrying Gizella Palos—not her daughter Elma, with whom he was also in love—a patient of his and Freud's alike. Freud involved himself in managing a number of such relationships at a distance, and though he was disconcerted by Ferenczi's messy triangle and chided Jones for his sexual impulsiveness, Freud's stance was not one of moral condemnation. He was less concerned with the sexual transgressions in themselves than with the ignominy he feared these relationships would bring analysis.[71] As important, abstinence was consonant with Freud's closed-system, energic thinking more generally. The transference as he conceived of it was entitled to monopolize the patient's libido, and all of her desires and demands were to be refused gratification such that, in a state of frustration, she would be propelled toward a cure.

But Freud was never so ascetic in his actual practice as his own recommendations prescribed, and neither was he so ascetic as these recommendations would become in the hands of those who followed him. Mid-twentieth-century American analysts expanded the compass of Freud's recommended abstinence to proscribe any words, gestures, actions, or behaviors on the part of the analyst that might interfere with the purity of the analytic process. Kurt Eissler, for example, introduced the concept of parameter as a way of bringing into analysis deviations from orthodox technique; for example, a phobic might be commanded "to expose himself to

---

69. Otto Fenichel, "Problems of Psychoanalytic Technique," *Psychoanalytic Quarterly* 8 (1939): 57–87, esp. 63, was the first to use the term, but references to it are sparse before the 1950s.

70. Glen O. Gabbard, "The Early History of Boundary Violations in Psychoanalysis," *Journal of the American Psychoanalytic Association* 43 (1995): 1115–36. See also Lisa Appignanesi and John Forrester, *Freud's Women* (New York: Basic Books, 1992), esp. chap. 7, and Forrester, "Casualties of Truth," in *Proof and Persuasion: Essays on Authority, Objectivity and Evidence*, ed. Suzanne Marchand and Elizabeth Lunbeck ([Turnhout,] Belgium: Brepols, 1996): 219–62.

71. Appignanesi and Forrester, *Freud's Women*.

the dreaded situation despite his fear of it and regardless of any anxiety which might develop during that exposure," and it might be necessary to threaten to break off treatment if he refused to do so.[72] Others delineated modes of relationship—the working alliance, the therapeutic relationship, the real relationship—that might supplement but not replace the ascetic and authoritarian transference. In so doing they attempted to preserve the latter's purity while bringing a measure of simple humanity into the orthodox consulting room. Both the parameter and these extra-transferential relationships testify to just how impoverished the analytic relationship had become in the hands of the orthodox. Dissidents pointed to the "superfluous deprivations" exacted by "overzealous and indiscriminate" adherence to the rule of abstinence and chastised their colleagues for the austerity, aloofness, and authoritarianism that characterized their interactions with patients.[73] The literature is peppered with accounts of analysts so under the sway of orthodoxy they cannot express any compassion over the fate of a patient's seriously ill infant or, conversely, congratulate a patient for a major achievement for fear that in doing so they might harm the patient.

Malcolm, an insightful ethnographer, was more interested in how her informants talked about what they actually did—how they conceived of the analytic setting—than in any of their theoretical speculations and commitments, with the result that her story unfolds most compellingly at the level of technique. And it is in Green's ambivalence on this score—which Malcolm masterfully evokes—that we can glimpse something of the magnitude of Kohut's achievement. Malcolm's Freudians are ascetics to the core, disdainful of the laxness and sloppiness of the upstarts, the faddishness and mawkish sentimentality of their therapeutic ambitions. Yet Green—for all of his commitment to a "fanatically pure" technique, his disdain for Kohut's misguided theorizing, his "hate" for self psychology—cannot help but be drawn to Kohut's recommendations on technique, almost as if in spite of his better self. This is perhaps not surprising, given the terms in which he conceptualized the constraints imposed by adherence to orthodoxy. Green grudgingly admitted to respecting Kohut's technique with dif-

---

72. K. R. Eissler, "The Effect of the Structure of the Ego on Psychoanalytic Technique," *Journal of the American Psychoanalytic Association* 1 (1953): 104–43, at 110.

73. Leo Stone, *The Psychoanalytic Situation: An Examination of Its Development and Essential Nature* (New York: International Universities Press, 1961), is the *locus classicus* of this line of critique; at 21. See also Stone, "The Psychoanalytic Situation and Transference: Postscript to an Earlier Communication," *Journal of the American Psychoanalytic Association* 15 (1967): 3–58, at 3.

ficult, widening-scope patients: "Whenever I read his clinical discussions, my therapeutic technique improves. It's true. . . . He reminds me of my obligation to the patient, which is to think analytically about everything he says and does."[74]

Green's ambivalence towards Kohut is fully on display in his impassioned recounting of his reading "with utter amazement" of Kohut's controversial 1979 paper, "The Two Analyses of Mr. Z." In the paper, Kohut contrasted the dead end of a by-the-book classical analysis characterized by its many "empathic failures" with the hopefulness and joy generated by a re-analysis conducted along self-psychological lines.[75] The paper came under withering criticism—even before it was revealed after Kohut's death that it was autobiographical, that Mr. Z. was Kohut himself.[76] Skeptics from the orthodox camp argued that the first analysis was wrongly carried out,[77] that it presented a distorted picture of classical technique. Green objected that the first analysis "just didn't make sense," adding that "in the second, 'Kohutian' analysis, he finally did what any one of us 'classical' analysts would have done in the first place. His description of the first analysis reads like a caricature of analysis, while the second analysis is made to seem rich and profound, subtle and empathic, humanistic and humane."[78] That is, self psychology was just orthodoxy by another name. Or, was it the reverse, that orthodoxy at its best had "succeeded because it was using self-psychological methods without knowing it was doing so"?[79]

Other critics similarly charged Kohut in general with having served up old wine in new bottles, of repackaging what "everyone always knew" in an attractive new form.[80] From an object-relations perspective, the charge

---

74. Malcolm, *Psychoanalysis*, 117–19.

75. Heinz Kohut, "The Two Analyses of Mr. Z," *International Journal of Psychoanalysis* 60 (1979): 3–27.

76. Cocks, in his introduction to Kohut, *Curve*, was the first to assert that the work was autobiographical: 4–6.

77. Randolf Alnoes, "Treatment of Narcissistic Personality Disturbances: The Kernberg-Kohut Divergence," *Scandinavian Psychoanalytic Review* 6 (1983): 97–110.

78. Malcolm, *Psychoanalysis*, 118.

79. Arnold M. Cooper, review of *How Does Analysis Cure?* by Heinz Kohut, ed. Arnold Goldberg with collaboration of Paul Stepansky (Chicago: University of Chicago Press, 1984), *Journal of the American Psychoanalytic Association* 36 (1988): 175–79, at 178.

80. Martin James, review of *The Analysis of the Self: A Systematic Approach to the Psychological Treatment of Narcissistic Personality Disorders*, *International Journal of Psychoanalysis* 54 (1973): 363–68, at 363. This was a common critique; see also, for example, Roman N. Anshin, review of *Progress in Self-Psychology*, vol. 1, edited by Arnold Goldberg, *Journal of the American Academy of Psychoanalysis* 15 (1978): 415–18. Arnold Goldberg, "One Theory or More," *Contemporary*

was that Kohut's new perspective could be found in the works of Ferenczi, Michael Balint, Harry Guntrip, and Donald Winnicott.[81] From an American interpersonal perspective, it was the pioneering work of Harry Stack Sullivan to which critics pointed. It is worth emphasizing how remarkable are these nothing-new-under-the-sun reactions to Kohut's work in light of the decades-long furor that attended his deviations from Freudian orthodoxy. Critics of Kohut leveled another sort of charge that highlights the same issue from a different angle, namely, that he borrowed and appropriated without acknowledgment—or, more seriously, plagiarized—from his disciplinary forebears, chiefly Ferenczi and Fairbairn. The charge of intellectual theft insistently arises around Kohut. He was charged with plagiarism upon the publication of his first book[82] and, on the appearance of the second, with being "strangely unable to acknowledge" his debts[83] and with failing to situate his findings in the discipline's rich heritage.[84] He vigorously defended himself whenever the charge arose, even pointing out that a similar charge of borrowing from forebears had been leveled against Freud. On numerous occasions he pointed out that, whatever his analytic predecessors had written, none of them had pulled their contributions on the self into a systematic and comprehensive whole, as he had, and, more to the point, once he'd knitted the medley of their isolated observations together, he'd made it easy for critics retrospectively to locate his ideas in others.[85]

Psychoanalysis 17 (1981): 626–38, provides a friendly overview of the controversy Kohut's work occasioned.

81. See, for example, Howard A. Bacal, "British Object-Relations Theorists and Self Psychology: Some Critical Reflections," *International Journal of Psychoanalysis* 68 (1987): 81–98.

82. See Kohut to Martin James, 18 June 1973, in Kohut, *Curve*, 278–80; written upon receiving an advance copy of James's review of *The Analysis of the Self*, in which the charge—subsequently excised, before publication in the *International Journal of Psychoanalysis*—of "unconscious plagiarism" is leveled against Kohut, with the qualification that such was "an endemic force in psychoanalysis." James was here recycling a charge he'd earlier made, that "plagiarism is endemic in the world of ideas, and in psycho-analysis priorities are especially hard to place": James, review of *The First Year of Life*, by René A. Spitz, *International Journal of Psychoanalysis* 48 (1967): 118–21, at 118.

83. Gerald J. Gargiulo, "Kohut's *Restoration of the Self*: A Symposium," *Psychoanalytic Review* 65 (1978): 616–17, at 616.

84. Saul Tuttman, "Kohut's *Restoration of the Self*: A Symposium," *Psychoanalytic Review* 65 (1978): 624–29. Criticism of Kohut for the inadequacies of attribution may also be found in, among others, Ruth R. Imber, "Reflections on Kohut and Sullivan," *Contemporary Psychoanalysis* 20 (1984): 363–80; Chessick, "Perspectivism, Constructivism, and Empathy"; and Neil McLaughlin, "Revision from the Margins: Fromm's Contributions to Psychoanalysis," *International Forum of Psychoanalysis* 9 (2000): 241–47.

85. Heinz Kohut, *The Search for the Self: Selected Writings of Heinz Kohut*, ed. Paul H. Ornstein (New York: International Universities Press, 1990), 3:227. Kohut here cited Heinz Hart-

Visionary or shameless plagiarist? For our purposes what is most interesting in all this is analysts' assertion of a fundamental continuity in their discipline, a continuity that calls into question characterizations of Kohut as non-analytic, outside of the mainstream, a dangerous revolutionary. The furor around the question of Kohut's authorship and originality—premised as it was on analysts' facility with the works of Ferenczi, Fairbairn, and Winnicott, among others—highlights the fact that the hegemony of classicism was less complete than chroniclers of the fortunes of psychoanalysis have assumed.

This is a complex issue; what is relevant here is that, evaluative judgments aside, both sorts of charges may be seen as evidence of the degree to which Kohut's theorizing—for all if its jargon, coining of awkward neologisms, and lack of writerly grace—was received by analysts as deeply and comfortingly familiar. We might even go further and suggest that the so-called "Ferenczi renaissance" of the last ten to fifteen years is enabled by and indebted to Kohut, who brought the long-banished Ferenczi, a troubling spectral presence in the history of psychoanalysis, back into the mainstream.[86] Aaron Green scoffed at the idea that his version of analysis would "have to assimilate" Kohut's renegade systematizing, but in his—and his colleagues'—sniffing claim that there was nothing new in self psychology, we can see enacted the incorporating, assimilating impulse that was among the conditions of Kohut's eventual absorption into—and reshaping of—the mainstream of psychoanalysis in United States.

---

mann, "The Development of the Ego Concept in Freud's Work," *International Journal of Psycho-Analysis* 37 (1956): 425–38, at 426: "Her [M. Dorer's] statement that Freud's psychology was in the main derived from earlier sources is quite obviously wrong, and Jones's objection to it is indisputable. What happened to that historian of pre-analysis has happened to other historians before: looking at even the greatest work from the angle of 'precursors' only, one cannot help finding similar ideas in the history of human thought."

86. See, for example, Carlo Bonomi, "Editorial: Ferenczi and Contemporary Psychoanalysis," *International Forum of Psychoanalysis* 7 (1998): 181–85.

NINE

The Walking Man and the Talking Cure

JEAN-CHRISTOPHE AGNEW

Sigmund Freud may have sailed only once to the United States, but Freudian*ism* has been a frequent flyer. Not so surprising when one recalls that even at those moments when Freudian orthodoxy has had to steer its way through the stiff headwinds of American popular culture, the early touchdowns on this side of the ocean were remarkably smooth. For several generations of American writers and critics, Freudianism had stamped its own passport to the New World by offering a brilliant, interpretive *passe-partout*—a master-key—to modernity's discontents. And as American intellectuals opened the gate to a variety of Freudianisms "after Freud left," so the theoretical rigors and narrative power of psychoanalytic theory opened the higher reaches of the nation's intellectual and cultural life to writers and thinkers—many of them second-generation immigrants—who might otherwise have despaired of entering for lack of adequate documentation. For these reasons among others, Part II of this book has shifted our focus to high culture, where the evidence of Freudianism's impact is richest and where the personal, political, and professional stakes were most intense.

By the time of Freud's own death, Dorothy Ross's chapter reminds us, the intellectual ground had been well prepared for his ideas by literary modernism. And upon that soil stood that wartime structure of feeling that Louis Menand calls the "discourse of anxiety"—a temporary construction, to be sure, but one that turned out to be surprisingly hospitable to the darker, transferential struggles that have for so long marked the accounts we have of psychoanalytic theory and practice.

Totalitarianism furnished one of the principal objects of this Cold War discourse of anxiety, as Menand rightly notes, but so too did the global experience of total war and the postwar threat of nuclear annihilation. Still, what is at stake in these chapters is the intellectual and cultural history that identifies how that threat was "handled," which is to say the specific forms of thought through which the "anxiety about anxiety" was worked up, if not worked through, by America's mid-century intelligentsia. Dorothy Ross, Louis Menand, and Elizabeth Lunbeck each offer us a different angle into a historical problem, and perhaps the easiest way to think these three approaches together would be to treat them as nesting inside one another. Dorothy Ross treats the broad arc of Freudianism in America after 1940 as a forty-year-long chapter in the epic journey of modernism from Europe to America and in the more prosaic though no less significant journey of second-generation Jewish thinkers into the American mainstream. The introspective and interpretive rigors of Freudian theory, she argues, credentialed a generation of public intellectuals as experts on the modern condition at the very moment when that condition was becoming the common currency of academic and middlebrow exchange, with college bookstore shelves displaying stacks of Camus's *The Stranger*, Freud's *Civilization and Its Discontents*, and Lionel Trilling's *The Liberal Imagination*.

Louis Menand looks to the war itself as the propulsive force behind the culture's postwar romance with Freud, existentialism, and tranquilizers. The mix may seem an odd one at first glance—Merseault and Miltown—and Menand does see this unstable "amalgam" of prescriptive thought and prescription drugs imploding by the mid-1960s. But, he adds, that implosion had as much to do with the culture's own romance with personal psychology, whether understood in a Freudian, modernist, or pharmacological framework. "Once the political has been made personal," he concludes, "the personal can become political," as of course it did with the politics of authenticity, identity, and consciousness embraced by the New Left, the counterculture, black power, feminism, and gay liberation.[1]

That sixties moment of implosion—or explosion—marks the beginning of the story that Elizabeth Lunbeck tells of Heinz Kohut's Americanization of Freud; the Dionysian Freudianism and modernism that Trilling had deplored as an "adversary culture" in 1965 became, ten years later, a national debate over American decline as the result of its "culture of narcissism," a debate in which Kohut's work was used or, as Lunbeck shows, misused in order to bring what was seen as a "renegade" modernism and Freudianism to heel. Lunbeck identifies Kohut as a pivotal or hinge figure between the bleak, drive-based theories of Freudian orthodoxy and the more gener-

---

1. For a more detailed history of the war, the rise of psychology and psychologism, and their impact on second-wave feminism, see Ellen Herman, *The Romance of American Psychology: Political Culture in the Age of Experts* (Berkeley: University of California Press, 1995).

ous, more hybrid, more plenitude-based therapies on offer today—in other words, precisely the kind of self-serving therapeutic vision that Christopher Lasch deployed Kohut's theory to diagnose. Ironies abound throughout all three accounts, we see, with ideas sabotaged by their success and enemies misread or mistaken as allies. But this is as one might expect of the history of Freudianism and modernism, where time and again we have been told that *we* are our own worst enemies.

Yet why were Americans told such things (and told them so often) at midcentury? Why, at the moment of the U.S.'s wartime triumph, did its highbrow culture cleave to a tragic sense of itself—a sense infused with equal measures of Freudianism and existentialism—only to lament the loss of that same sensibility some thirty years later, at a moment of national crisis, decline, and "malaise"? The pages that follow venture a tentative answer to those questions; they do so by scaling postwar Freudianism and modernism to the expansive geopolitical and institutional history of America's intelligentsia in those years and to the forms of intellectual muscularity that that history modeled. If Freudianism was the medicine that modernists prescribed for themselves at mid-century, it was an emphatically heroic medicine they had in mind.

The years spanned by the papers of Ross, Menand, and Lunbeck, with background from Makari and Usak-Sahin, which is to say the 1940s through the 1970s, have often been called (following Henry Luce) the "American Century," and even though thirty to forty years makes for a very short century, it is still worth thinking about this extended, triumphalist moment when mapping the specifically *American* trajectory of modernist and Freudian orthodoxies, and thinking, too, about what it meant to "domesticate" Freud during those years. Let us not forget, for example, that Luce's famous call to Americans to fulfill their geopolitical destiny was steeped in the imagery of paralysis and anxiety. "We Americans are unhappy," his landmark editorial of February 1941 began. "We are not happy about America. We are not happy about ourselves in relation to America. We are nervous—or gloomy—or apathetic." There is "no peace in our hearts," he insisted, because "we have not been honest with ourselves.... [W]e have been at various times false to ourselves, false to each other, false to the facts of history and false to the future."[2] Nothing could have been more political than this

2. Henry R. Luce, "The American Century" [February 1941], reprinted in *Diplomatic History* 23 (1999): 160–61.

openly personal and subjective appeal to his readers' apprehensions about the war; Luce effectively renamed these fears as anxieties specific to a collective state of indecision and inauthenticity.

Luce's secular sermon was scarcely Freudian or Sartrean in its inspiration. Still, the rhetorical strategies animating "The American Century" suggest how labile was the language of the Jeremiad in which Luce, a missionary's son, had been steeped, and how easily that language could be translated into the modernist lexicon of existentialism, even without the aid of Walter Lowrie and Reinhold Niebuhr. Fittingly, it was with Luce, and not Freud (or Kohut), that Christopher Lasch chose to open his best-selling *The Culture of Narcissism* (1978). "Hardly more than a quarter-century after Henry Luce proclaimed 'the American century,'" Lasch reminded his readers, "American confidence has fallen to a low ebb. Those who recently dreamed of world power now despair of governing the city of New York. Defeat in Vietnam, economic stagnation, and the impending exhaustion of natural resources have produced a mood of pessimism in higher circles, which spreads through the rest of society as people lose faith in their leaders."[3] And, as if to signal the hollow or "minimal self" hiding behind the mask of American consumerism, Lasch subtitled *The Culture of Narcissism* "American Life in an Age of Diminished Expectations." This was not the language of abundance.

For that reason alone, Lunbeck points out, one could hardly imagine a more inappropriate Freudian companion for Lasch in his 400-page journey through the morally and emotionally impoverished world of work, politics, and consumption than the apostle of internal plenitude, Heinz Kohut; nor could one imagine a broader, more extra-transferential context or canvas for Lasch's call to return to the discipline of a classic, if not a modernist, Freudianism. Forget metapsychology, Lasch advised. "Psychoanalysis best clarifies the connection between society and the individual, culture and personality, precisely when it confines itself to careful examination of individuals. It tells us most about society when it is least determined to do so."[4] A case history was a document, not a parable. *"It tells us most about society when it is least determined to do so."* Lasch was taking his cues—or clues—less from what Kohut's cases said about American culture than what they unwittingly *betrayed*. This, perhaps more than any of the numberless

---

3. Christopher Lasch, *The Culture of Narcissism: American Life in an Age of Diminishing Expectations* (New York: Norton, 1979).

4. Ibid., 76–77.

references to Freudian and neo-Freudian theory in Lasch's text, strikes me as itself a sign or symptom of how the *modernist* Freud had become an intuitive interpretive style for historians—and especially cultural historians—over the forty years or so spanned by the American Century.

The Culture of Narcissism was the last great exemplar—a self-liquidating exemplar—in the tradition of inquiry about the American character or what Lunbeck refers to as "the shape of the modal American self." We could, if we wished, track that inquiry all the way to Hector de St. John Crevecoeur's iconic question about the identity of "the American, this new man." But in the modern or modernist context, we need only reach as far back as the 1930s, to Karen Horney's *The Neurotic Personality of Our Time* (1937) and, before that, to anthropologist Ruth Benedict's *Patterns of Culture* (1934). For Benedict, the Apollonian and the Dionysian figured as ordering psychological principles for arranging the cultures of the Pueblo, the Dobu, and the Kwakiutl—and by collective refraction, the United States. When Margaret Mead summarized Benedict's approach to culture as "personality writ large," it was 1958, the high-water mark of the so-called "culture and personality" school associated with international area studies.[5] Dorothy Ross reminds us that it was also high noon for modernist Freudianism in literary studies and cultural criticism.

By 1958, though, the peculiarly American form of metapsychology that was the culture-and-personality school had become indissolubly associated with the modernization (as opposed to modernism) component of American foreign policy. Modernization theory is a missing fragment in the puzzle of the American Freud that Ross, Menand, and Lunbeck piece together in this volume—missing, perhaps, because modernization was at once cognate with and anathema to high modernists. By modernization theory, I mean that five-foot shelf of social-scientific work that both formulated and licensed the projection of American models of economic, social, and political development into Europe after World War II and into the so-called "third world" during the first decades of the Cold War; work associated with names like Talcott Parsons, Walt Rostow, Lucian Pye, and the like.[6]

---

5. Karen Horney, *The Neurotic Personality of Our Time* (New York: Norton, 1937); Margaret Mead, introduction, Ruth Benedict, *Patterns of Culture* (Boston: Houghton Mifflin, 1959 [1934]).

6. The best account of the relation between modernism and modernization theory is Nils Gilman's *Mandarins of the Future: Modernization Theory in Cold War America* (Baltimore: Johns Hopkins University Press, 2003).

Closest to this cohort of modernization theorists, perhaps, was Arthur M. Schlesinger Jr., whose influential *Vital Center* (1949) set the characteristically "tough-minded" course and tone of Cold War liberalism and whose *A Thousand Days* (1971) further personalized (and canonized) the twilight struggle against totalitarianism by distilling it down to the story of "John F. Kennedy in the White House." Menand thus highlights a critical dimension of Cold War liberalism in its modernist *and* modernizationist dimensions when he quotes Schlesinger's embrace of anxiety as the "official emotion of our time." Here was Henry Luce again, but a Luce rewritten in the psychological registers of Erich Fromm and Niebuhr. Menand accents the emotional balancing act of *The Vital Center*—the modulation of anxiety to its ideal, centrist, and centering level—but it is also worth underscoring Schlesinger's almost Bergsonian intimations of life force. What made anxiety the "official" emotion of the age was its role or "office" as the regenerative reminder that choice was inescapable in the face of totalitarianism.[7]

Curiously, though, that face was deceptively warm. As K. A. Cuordileone has pointed out, totalitarianism was for Schlesinger a markedly infantilizing and feminizing force that appealed to men's willingness to surrender their selfhood and retreat to the "womb-dark sea" or "broad maternal expanse of the masses." Should American democracy fail to "produce the large resolute breed of men capable of the climactic effort" of resistance against this temptation, Schlesinger warned, it would "founder."[8] If we hear the echoes of 1940s Momism (not to mention anticipations of the 1980s Nanny State) in Schlesinger's womb and apron-string imagery, we should not be entirely surprised. Anxiety was for him a politically bracing stimulant, not in the evolutionary sense of an adaptive instinct but in the intellectual sense of an unsettled state of mind—a state of mind to be confronted, plumbed, interpreted, debated, and, finally, decided. The complexity of this exercise was not to be underestimated, but neither was its emotional strenuousness: the agony and the ecstasy of what was, after all, a "climactic effort." Schlesinger's *Vital Center* implicitly vindicated—it could even be said to have rehearsed—the global heroism of the talking cure over against the domestic surrender to the pharmaceutical one. It was thus one thing to be "in analysis," another to be in therapy. The psycho-

---

7. Arthur M. Schlesinger Jr., *The Vital Center: The Politics of Freedom* (New Brunswick, NJ: Transaction Press, 1998 [1949]).

8. K. A. Cuordileone, *Manhood and American Political Culture in the Cold War* (New York: Routledge, 2005), chap. 1.

analytic couch was an intellectual and political crucible; to lie down was to man up.

As Schlesinger's book reminds us, modernizationists sprang from the same Enlightenment ground as modernists, and for all the suspicion they may have felt toward one another, the public fate of one party was quietly bound to the public fate of the other. Modernism, like romanticism before it, was dependent, if not parasitic, on an advanced technological context—material and ideological. Freud the scientist was also Freud the moralist, and the century-long "modernization of sex" about which cultural historians like Paul Robinson and Jane Gerhard have written was always in intimate, if vexed, conversation with the sexual "modernism" of Freudians.[9]

By and large, modernization *theorists* built on (and within) what the sociologist Max Weber had earlier prophesied about a thoroughly rationalized modernity, whereas modernist *critics* excavated the ambivalence, if not the outright dread, that Weber had felt about the "iron cage" of bureaucratic instrumentalism—a dread that, to paraphrase Lunbeck's concise formulation, was appropriated, translated , supplemented, and purified into a mid-century neo-Freudian mix of crisis humanism and existential psychology. Menand remarks that 1958 was also the year that *echt*–New York school modernist William Barrett published his *Irrational Man*, the pocket guide to the existential condition that instantaneously appeared in every college bookstore. Anchor Books created a startlingly aqua cover as background to Alberto Giacometti's sculpture of "Walking Man," gaunt, stiffly erect yet slightly hunched, stepping forward into the void.[10]

The memory of Giacometti's overwrought-iron figure was brought back to me as I read through the chapters of Ross, Menand, and Lunbeck and again and again came across the same portrait—the same self-portrait—of

---

9. See Paul Robinson, *The Modernization of Sex: Havelock Ellis, Alfred Kinsey, William Masters and Virginia Johnson* (New York: Harper & Row, 1976); Jane F. Gerhard, *Desiring Revolution: Second-Wave Feminism and the Rewriting of American Sexual Thought, 1920–1982* (New York: Columbia University Press, 2001).

10. William Barrett, *Irrational Man: A Study in Existential Philosophy* (Garden City, NY: Doubleday, 1958); two years earlier, an equally austere portrait of Freud had appeared on the cover of the April 23 issue of *Time* to honor the centenary of the birth of the "Explorer of the Unconscious"; the cover, drawn by Ben Shahn, was a perfect example of the Cold War transition from a popular-front heroism (e.g., Shahn's famous portrait of Sacco and Vanzetti) to more universal themes of the human condition; cf. Frances K. Pohl, *Ben Shahn: New Deal Artist in a Cold War Climate, 1947–1954* (Austin: University of Texas Press, 1989); and Mark Greif, *The Age of the Crisis of Man* (Princeton, NJ: Princeton University Press, forthcoming).

9.1. William Barrett's *Irrational Man*, a widely read American book of 1958 symbolizing the symbiotic relationship between existentialism and psychoanalysis. Courtesy of the Athenaeum of Ohio.

the modernist/Freudian hero: austere, abstinent, stoic, aloof, Apollonian—a figure of discipline, a figure *for* a discipline. "Everything that Freudian man gains," Ross quotes Lionel Trilling, "he pays for in more than equal coin." Whether Trilling drew his wisdom in this instance from Vienna or Queens mattered not; his diction and his imagery were pure Henry James. "No themes are so human," James once wrote, "as those that reflect for us out of the confusion of life, the close connection of bliss and bale, of things that help with things that hurt, so dangling before us forever that bright, hard metal, of so strange an alloy, one face of which is somebody's right and ease and the other somebody's pain and wrong."[11] Here then, in miniature, we have a splendid example of the rhetorical resources that modernism afforded an outsider like Trilling to translate both a European orthodoxy—Freudianism—and himself into an American academy (especially an Ivy League English department) indifferent or hostile to both.

Like Freud in his way before him, Trilling had had to acquire "ritual competence" in the Protestant ethic, etiquette, and aesthetic of the mid-century university, had to endure what John Murray Cuddihy once called the "ordeal of civility."[12] Freudian modernism enabled Trilling to practice a version of the close reading that New Criticism demanded without at the same time sacrificing himself to its textualist or formalist insularities. Inside the psychoanalytic establishment the patterns of social and intellectual courtship do not appear to have been that much different; Heinz Kohut's account of Protestants and Jews on the "analytic scene" echoes Dorothy Ross's and David Hollinger's account of the rapprochement between disaffected Protestants and assimilated Jews in the university.[13] At Harvard, Puritanism itself was rehabilitated—resurrected—as a recognizably modernist intellectual vocation by Perry Miller; his 1949 biography of Jonathan Edwards may have avoided the psychoanalytic lexicon, but it was in every other respect a modernist psychological and existential portrait of Walking Man: a Conradian "errand in the wilderness."[14]

So modernism was itself the coin, the currency—what we would now

---

11. Henry James, preface to *What Maisie Knew* (1909 "New York" edition; New York: Penguin Books, 1966), 7.

12. John Murray Cuddihy, *The Ordeal of Civility: Freud, Marx, Levi-Strauss and the Jewish Struggle with Modernity* (New York: Basic Books, 1974).

13. David A. Hollinger, *Science, Jews, and Secular Culture: Studies in Mid-Twentieth Century American Intellectual History* (Princeton, NJ: Princeton University Press, 1996).

14. Perry Miller, *Jonathan Edwards* (New York: W. Sloane, 1949); David Hackett Fisher later took Miller to task for making Edwards a "living anachronism . . . a contemporary of Paul Tillich or Marcel Proust," *Historians' Fallacies: Toward a Logic of Historical Thought* (New York: Harper & Row, 1970), 199.

call the cultural capital—in which a New York intellectual could gain access to the university chairs and highbrow press of which Ross speaks. In fact, thanks to the war, New York *was*, in the 1950s, a cultural capital; an international capital of modern art, cultural criticism, and, of course, psychoanalysis. And it is that same double intimation of high-priced knowledge and highbrow access or entrée that one detects in Frederick Crews's claim that he was "first drawn to Freud by his promise of a Faustian key to knowledge." Ross is properly skeptical that scientific objectivity was Crews's goal, but I'm as dubious that it was some broader quest for certainty. To me Crews's image is of an occulted, buried, hidden, even illicit knowledge that the Devil may promise but that the analytic key unlocks.

And in that respect, Crews's figure of speech strikes me as itself quite "Freudian"—as if he were discreetly referring his readers to Freud's famously failed analysis of Dora and to its complex metaphorical apparatus of keys and jewel boxes. If so, perhaps the metaphor of a Faustian key was Crews's sly way of alluding to Freud's obliviousness to the counter-transference infusing his treatment and the account he gave of it. No matter. As John Forrester once observed, Freud's frank confession of failure in the Dora case was for Freud the mark of his commitment to the rigors of science as opposed to the easy pleasures of a *roman à clef*. But for us, it is just this confession of failure (think Henry Adams or Marcel Proust) that marks Freud as a modernist. What he has learned from Dora, Freud assures us, *he* has paid for in more than equal coin. And it is as modernist, scientist, and Viennese Jew, Forrester adds, that Freud "writes up" his case in a way that assures his readers that the knowledge he seeks in the consulting room is not to be confused with the gossip—the female sex talk—into which he has been so assiduously inquiring.[15] Not for Freud (or Trilling) the vulgar pleasures of a novel that so seductively—or hospitably—offers its key to the reader.

As Christopher Lasch might have said at this point, psychoanalysis *"tells us most about society when it is least determined to do so."* And what Freud's and Crews's talk of keys reminds us here is that Freudian orthodoxy has consistently rejected any taint of the domestic—the homely, the sentimental, the feminine—so that when we speak of the domestication of Freud in America, whether by James Jackson Putnam, Erik Erikson, or Heinz Kohut, we are (as Dorothy Ross notes) talking about something more than the meliorist colorings given to the chapter and verse of Freud's thought. We

---

15. John Forrester, "The Untold Pleasures of Psychoanalysis: Freud, Dora, and the Madonna," in *The Seductions of Psychoanalysis: Freud, Lacan, Derrida* (New York: Cambridge University Press, 1991).

are talking about the consulting room, the transferential space, as a masculine operating theater. And we are talking, too, of the space of countertransference, where, as Lunbeck quotes Heinz Kohut, "psychoanalytic locker-room chitchat" sloughed off its public neutrality toward his revisionist views and assigned narcissistic investment in the self a "negative valence." The locker room of the 1960s was still very much a man's world, a place where one let one's guard—not one's hair—down.

The social geography of modernism—the analytic "scene," the university chair, the highbrow journal—is as good a place as any to close these remarks, for we can see how much that geography had changed at the moment of modernism's collapse and of Christopher Lasch's postmortem analysis in the 1970s. It was not just that the American Century had failed in Vietnam and in New York—capital of the Luce Empire as of modern art and psychoanalysis. The demographics of modernism had changed as well. Thanks to the Cold War infusion of resources, the 1965 immigration act, and the cumulative impact of the civil rights and women's movements, the modern multiversity, for all its managerialism, was now open to a wider mix of students and especially to women. The vital center had shifted, and with it had gone the whole metaphorical apparatus that had once so seamlessly mixed the Calvinist, the Apollonian, and the Freudian into a single, masculinist vision of intellectual engagement. The old-boy rituals, the old-boy civilities, the old-boy *system* that had for so long operated as the means by which modernism reproduced itself, syndicated itself, were now giving way to something else.

What that something else was remains a matter of debate, but Elizabeth Lunbeck's account makes clear that the collapse was *extra*-transferential—outside the analytic scene of the consulting room and outside the shoptalk of the psychoanalytic locker room, too. The Dionysian impulses of the counterculture may have had something to do with this shift, Dorothy Ross suggests, as well as the modernist recoil against the unrestrained libidization of culture itself. As the spaces of therapy proliferated, the singularity of the psychoanalytic setting as a theater of battle lost its practical and symbolic hold on the American imagination. Not surprisingly, President Jimmy Carter's Laschian moment—the infamous "malaise" speech of 1979—helped lose him reelection.[16] The Jeremiad had not lost its teeth,

---

16. For a shrewd analysis of Christopher Lasch's, Robert Bellah's, and Daniel Bell's misadventures as emergency advisors to Carter, see Daniel Horowitz, *The Anxieties of Affluence: Cri-*

only its bearings. Cynics even mused that Americans had made *The Culture of Narcissism* a best seller under the illusion that it was a how-to book, wanting to think of themselves not as their worst enemies but as their best friends.[17]

Was this the fate of the talking cure? Happy talk and happy pills? I don't think so. Trauma theory's resurgence in the 1980s and 1990s is grounds alone for skepticism.[18] What had changed by the turn of the new century, though, were the gender politics organizing and warranting psychoanalytic authority in the broader culture and, conversely, the capacity of psychoanalytic orthodoxy to sustain its own, deeply gendered model of intellectual and introspective heroism. "Today," Mark Micale has written, "medicine no longer plays a commanding role in producing the dominant fictions of masculinity."[19]

Could the same be said for the authority of modernism? For what it's worth, Giacometti's haunting, existentialist icon—*Walking Man*—recently sold at auction for a record-breaking $104 million.[20] Should we take that figure as expressing a collective emotional investment—a nostalgic cultural cathexis upon high modernism's masculine rigors? Or was it merely a financial investment, a hedge against the irrational exuberance of other markets? An artifact of the Collectible Unconscious, if you will, modernism's and Freudianism's cultural and psychosexual archaeology reduced to the dimensions of a Sotheby's catalogue or an *Antiques Roadshow*. It's hard to know which scale or metric to use when weighing the sunk costs of modernism and Freudianism for those who tried to live by their exacting strictures. Art historians and intellectual historians rarely treat human suffering as more than the idea or image of it, even if they refuse to put a price on it. So Elizabeth Lunbeck's allusion to the emotional pain in Aaron Green's consulting room is a timely reminder to all of us about who was still paying *that* coin after Freud left.

---

tiques of American Consumer Culture, 1939–1979 (Amherst: University of Massachusetts Press, 2004), chaps. 7 and 8.

17. See Mildred Newman and Bernard Berkowitz, with Jean Owen, *How to Be Your Own Best Friend* (New York: Harper, 1971).

18. Here, it is tempting to treat the turbulent controversies over incest, satanic ritual abuse, and recovered memory in this period as, among other things, a belated cultural rebuke to the eroticization of the father-daughter bond in mid-century popular culture, psychoanalytic theory, and the modernist novel; cf. Rachel Devlin, *Relative Intimacy: Fathers, Adolescent Daughters, and Postwar American Culture* (Chapel Hill: University of North Carolina Press, 2005).

19. Mark S. Micale, *Hysterical Men: The Hidden History of Male Nervous Disease* (Cambridge, MA: Harvard University Press, 2008), 284.

20. Carol Vogel, "At London, a Giacometti Sets a Record," *New York Times*, 3 February 2010.

That being said, postmodernism—and especially poststructuralism—can be nearly as severe in its attitude as the modernism and humanism it supersedes. True, we now see modernism's and Freudianism's notion of depth psychology dismissed as if it were all a textual effect read through 3-D glasses. Mock heroism, so to speak. Yet for all that condescension, Freud's hermeneutics of suspicion persists in poststructuralism's abiding textual interest in the "defenses, concealments, and counter-stories" that modernism (and Freudianism) deployed in the middle years of the twentieth century.[21] Or, to come back again to Christopher Lasch's words, psychoanalysis *tells us most about society when it is least determined to do so.* Psychoanalysis betrays itself because it cannot help doing so and because we cannot help reading it in this way, thanks in no small part to Freud. As a structure of thought and a structure of feeling, modernism may have fallen in upon itself and with it, Freudianism, too; but if so, we still hold fast to their interpretive keys.

Acknowledgments

I hope it is clear that this essay is deeply indebted to the contributions of Dorothy Ross, Louis Menand, and Elizabeth Lunbeck; I am grateful as well for John Burnham's gracious and insightful editorial encouragement and suggestions.

---

21. For example, see Joel Pfister, *Staging Depth: Eugene O'Neill and the Politics of Psychological Discourse* (Chapel Hill: University of North Carolina Press, 1995).

Conclusion

In the last part of the twentieth century, as our Part II authors indicate, a fundamental shift took place in the venues in which psychoanalytic thinking functioned among the intellectual and well-educated groups in the United States. Freudian psychotherapists and clinical theorists were no longer playing the part of major instigators of exciting insight and rebelliousness, as their predecessors had. Even the age of narcissism brought from the self psychologists adaptation and conformity, not insurrection. Freud's legacy remained a major component in the available modernist intellectual heritage. While many postmodern contrivers of innovative and unsettling ideas tried to avoid or reject Freudian thinking, others still struggled with it. These later disturbers of tranquility remained anchored in the attention to subjectivity found in psychoanalysis and in modernism more generally.

By the late twentieth century, it had become customary, if not required, to quote the poet W. H. Auden, who upon Freud's death in 1939 wrote: "To us he is no more a person / Now but a whole climate of opinion."[1] Louis Menand does not include this now-clichéd profundity in his discussion of Auden. Yet he, Dorothy Ross, Elizabeth Lunbeck, and Jean-Christophe Agnew go a long way toward turning this familiar bon mot into a sum-

---

1. W. H. Auden, *Another Time: Poems* (New York: Random House, 1940), 104: "In Memory of Sigmund Freud (d. Sept. 1939)." John Forrester, "'A Whole Climate of Opinion': Rewriting the History of Psychoanalysis," in *Discovering the History of Psychiatry*, ed. Mark S. Micale and Roy Porter (New York: Oxford University Press, 1994), 174, noted: "If Auden's diagnosis is accurate, writing the history of psychoanalysis is rather like writing the history of twentieth-century cultural weather: Its presence is so constant and pervasive that escaping its influence is out of the question. And precisely because of its inescapable character, it cannot be isolated from the myriad striking events that can more straightforwardly be singled out as part of the histories of science, of medicalization, of great ideas, of cultural movements, of modernization, of all the other movements to which it might apparently belong."

mary of at least the 1940s–1970s decades of U.S. history. An astonishing number of American mainstream intellectuals testified that their familiarity with Freud's ideas brought them a radically shifted perspective on humankind and the world. Like a Gestalt switch, Freudian viewpoints made all of the old rationalism and romanticism and formalism look quaint and outdated. With insights from Freud, thinking people could actually experience modernism, particularly in the ways that Ross identifies.[2] For our consideration of what happened after Freud left, these four final chapters bring us to an end point that is also a point of departure. Tracing the interplay of psychoanalytic ideas with high and even middlebrow culture is a powerful reminder that the subject of American intellectual history of the middle and late twentieth century consisted of much more than politics—even as politics of many varieties framed intellectual productions.

Agnew implicitly uses the metaphor of the Russian matryoshka dolls nested inside each other to evoke the complexity and layers of thinking that surrounded the trajectory of Freudian ideas from the 1930s on. There were Freudians and neo-Freudians. There was the culture and personality school. There was the darkness of totalitarianism and Freud's own dark thoughts, along with American optimism, meliorism, and Kohut's "therapeutic vision." And the framework of two-sided modernism operated alongside ideas of up-to-date modernization and technologization. Picking up on Menand's insights, Agnew casts the story begun by early twentieth-century intellectuals and intensified by Ross, Menand, and Lunbeck as an existentialist tragedy, in which deep knowledge about human beings that Americans took from psychoanalytic thinking exacted the price that any wisdom does. Altogether, if one reads the record, for a century intellectuals did provide the best measure and indicator of the impact of Freud.

By concluding with these explorations, our authors implicitly ask collectively, how could Americans have interacted with a novel psychotherapeutic technology and revolutionary intellectual structure? How could that multilayered complexity leave so many intellectual and social leaders and even ordinary citizens so marked that when communicating they would use Freudian terms—such as "I am being anal" or "Freudian slip"—as a shorthand for concepts, knowing that a surprisingly large audience would understand? How could major intellectuals have learned about the self—their own and others'—and human nature in general from a Viennese

---

2. Benjamin Nelson, preface to *Freud and the Twentieth Century*, ed. Benjamin Nelson (New York: Meridian Books, 1957), 10.

medical man? And how could it happen in America, of all places? As Elizabeth Lunbeck has pointed out, the phenomenon was historically implausible. But so was the combination of Protestant, conscience-driven thinkers with upwardly mobile Jewish intellectuals that our authors have identified as the crucial carrying population.

Students of American culture, regardless of orientation, have for generations commented on how many people were interested in improving themselves, whether in spiritual areas or in social or economic effectiveness. Psychoanalytic treatment and psychoanalytic thinking both offered attractive opportunities to improve oneself in one sense or another. For any number of people, this was transparently a major mechanism by which, constantly over the years, Freud's legacy spread in the United States.

If self-improvement had deep roots in American culture, we are invited to raise the question of American exceptionalism. Is the history of the society and culture that developed in the United States special or distinctive? With the history of psychoanalysis, the question is particularly acute, because the dominant historical narrative has been Eurocentric. Following much the same perspective within which Freud himself operated, most historians have centered their inquiries around the intellectuals of the great European cities, not least Vienna, Berlin, and London. In their accounts, events in the United States were either pale reflections or in other ways subordinate to the main European narrative. These general histories of psychoanalysis have often been compelling and richly insightful.[3] At the same time, many scholars have assumed the special popularity of psychoanalysis in the United States without really studying it.

The authors in this book have worked within a different framework. The framework starts with a demystifying examination of how specific figures carried Freudian ideas transnationally, meaning that people in the receiving culture were active receiving agents and that their reactions were often reciprocal as well as selective, as we see from G. Stanley Hall to Usak-Sahin's main characters. Second, our authors start with the existing dynamics of a changing American culture. This cultural orientation and sense of transnationalization substantially liberates our writers from the older, conventional accounts.

The authors in this book have therefore collectively offered the beginnings of a fresh narrative of the Americans' encounter with Freud's ideas.

---

3. A recent very broad example is Eli Zaretsky, *Secrets of the Soul: A Social and Cultural History of Psychoanalysis* (New York: Alfred A. Knopf, 2004).

Sonu Shamdasani shows clearly that, worldwide, Freud in 1909 did not stand out from the crowd of advocates of various kinds of psychotherapy. Shamdasani underlines that it was by chance, as Richard Skues tells us, that 1909 came to appear as a turning point. G. Stanley Hall, who knew Freud's work on sexuality and childhood, decided to make Freud a celebrity figure in psychology at the Clark conference. Then two things happened. First, Freud for the first time made a clear statement that psychoanalysis embodied a coherent body of beliefs. Second, Freud on his return responded to events in European psychotherapy and founded an international organization to foster the psychoanalytic movement. Quite independently, the appearance of Freud's clear lectures as an American publication, accompanied by translations of other of Freud's works and Ernest Jones's noisy crusading, caused some important Americans within the next few years to "discover" Freud and psychoanalysis.

In the three decades after 1909, psychoanalysis and "the new psychology" became fashionable in parts of medicine and in the highbrow media in the United States. Intellectual and cultural rebels and modernizers found dynamic thinking useful. As Ernst Falzeder emphasizes in his essay, Freud's personal aloofness did not significantly affect the activities of American enthusiasts.

Then in the 1930s, and especially just as World War II approached, the United States moved to center stage in the formal psychoanalytic movement and also in both intellectual and popular psychoanalytic discourse. Ironically but typically, as George Makari points out, the same committee that was asserting American independence of the international movement on the issue of lay analysts suddenly had to mobilize support to move and welcome leadership figures of Viennese psychoanalysis to the New World, and especially New York.

By the end of World War II, orthodox analysts advocating ego psychology and strict standards dominated organized psychoanalysis. Their standpoint had great intellectual power and appeal, not only within psychoanalysis but among social scientists and other American thinkers. It is perhaps classic tragedy that the domination of the ego psychologists came slowly to an end not just because of attacks on the rigidity of their technical standards but also because of problems with theory. The problems did not come from technical philosophers, who never did understand the appeal of psychoanalysis, however much they respected Freud's power as a thinker. As Charles Hanly has commented, "For the most part, philosophers have greeted psychoanalysis with indifference, they have criticized it, or they have made it over into something Freud had not intended it to be."[4] Instead, it was psychoanalytic theorists themselves who developed doubts. It was they who came to believe that the elegant intellectual structures of the ego psychologists were wanting.[5]

Kohut, who started out marching with the orthodox, played off the changing culture of late twentieth-century America and ended as an exemplar of the late twentieth-century diversity in psychoanalysis, a psychoanalysis in part still within psychoanalytic organizations, in part a psychoanalysis spread throughout a variety of types of mental healing and even more importantly the highbrow and popular cultures. Once again, as in 1909, so in the second half of the twentieth century, psychologists like Rollo May were playing an important role in propagating psychoanalytic thinking.

At the end, our authors have concluded that the story of Freud and American culture becomes completely intertwined with almost all of the major intellectual and cultural changes that occurred from the 1920s and 1930s to the 1970s and 1980s and after. To become mainstream at any time was a remarkable achievement for propagators of psychoanalytic thinking, as our Part II authors in particular point out. But since psychoanalytic thinking was so integrally a part of modernism, how could it be otherwise?

In the process of taking soundings along this chronicle of psychoanalysis, our authors identify not just 1909 as a landmark date. There was also 1939, when Vienna moved to New York. And finally, as Menand and others conclude, 1980 is a third landmark, the year when *DSM-III* destroyed the commanding position of psychoanalysis in psychiatry, the cultural area in which Freud's ideas had taken hold with such authority as to pass over to the rest of high culture and thence to American culture in general.

The final bookend to the story that began in 1909, then, is 2009. By that time, workers in clinical psychology and some fields in the humanities had appropriated much of psychoanalytic thinking to further and shape their own agendas. Moreover, proponents of various types of postmodern-

---

4. *Freud: A Collection of Critical Essays*, ed. Richard Wollheim (New York: Anchor Books, 1974); Charles Hanly, "Materialism, Humanism, and Psychoanalysis," in *Psychoanalysis and Culture at the Millennium*, ed. Nancy Ginsburg and Roy Ginsburg (New Haven, CT: Yale University Press, 1999), 298.

5. In his nuanced examination of postwar American psychoanalysis, Paul E. Stepansky, *Psychoanalysis at the Margins* (New York: Other Press, 2009), characterizes the late twentieth-century fate of organized psychoanalysis as "fractionation" rather than "pluralism," a term that tends to have positive overtones. It is striking that scholars writing the general cultural history of the United States in the late twentieth century have found that American society in general was fragmenting or fracturing. See, for example, Daniel T. Rodgers, *Age of Fracture* (Cambridge, MA: Harvard University Press, 2011).

252 / Conclusion

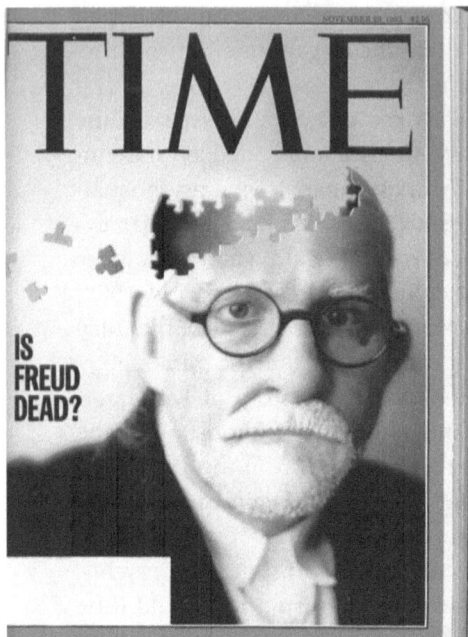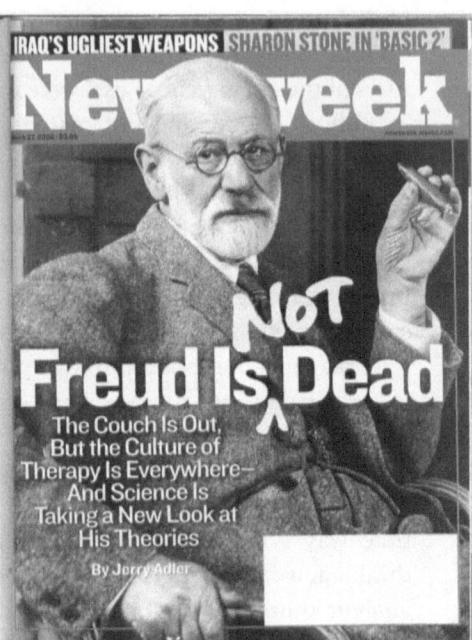

C.1. Freud on the covers of *Time* in 1993 and *Newsweek* in 2006: psychoanalysis as past history but still persistently present in American culture at the turn of the twenty-first century. Courtesy of Upper Arlington Public Library.

ist thinking found justification for their subjectivism in the uniqueness of each psychoanalytic case history even as they tried to reject the universalism in the Freudian schema.[6] Remarkably, some students of the late twentieth-century neurosciences underlying psychiatry and ideas of human nature were still finding resonance in Freud's ideas.[7] Freudian ideas have become

---

6. Robert S. Wallerstein, "Freud and Culture in Our Fin de Siècle Revisited," in *Psychoanalysis and Culture at the Millennium*, ed. Ginsburg and Ginsburg, 355–79.

7. T. M. Luhrman, *Of Two Minds: The Growing Disorder in American Psychiatry* (New York: Alfred A. Knopf, 2000), observed psychiatrists at the end of the twentieth century who were utilizing psychotherapy alongside psychopharmaceutical therapies, in part in reaction against too exclusive a dependence upon chemical treatments. Later, in the period of the centennial of Freud's visit, American psychiatrists had started meeting in committees to prepare *DSM-V*, and their online reports and correspondence made it clear that many specific and general psychoanalytic ideas and procedures—not least transference and countertransference—were still deeply influencing clinical treatment of mental patients and would continue to do so even among organically oriented psychiatrists and in an age of remarkable advances in understanding neurocircuitry in the brain and evidence-based medicine, a conclusion also reached in Jonathan Engel, *American Therapy: The Rise of Psychotherapy in the United States* (New York: Gotham Books, 2008), 257–61.

part of the ever-relevant intellectual heritage on which thinkers continue to draw as they face the constantly contemporary challenges of modernity.

In his 1990 Edith Weigert Lecture, one of the great American theorists, Roy Schafer, pointed out that psychoanalysis originally was a dialogue between doctor and patient, a point that underlay the dialogical nature of postmodernism of the late twentieth century, in which communication, "the linguistic turn," came to constitute reality for many thinkers. In that postmodern vein, Schafer, calling on self-awareness, or reflexivity, then came to the same conclusion that is inherent in the papers in this book and proposed that, for Freud,

> we give up the idea that there is just one legacy to sum up. For in a [psychoanalytic] world forever constituted anew through continuing dialogue, there can never be only one theoretical or technical legacy. There can only be legacies, linguistic legacies, legacies that are theoretical through and through. Freud's texts will remain open forever to alternative readings and writings: scientific, literary, and cultural. The absolutist writings and readings on theory and technique, with which we are so familiar and which still are published in official analytic journals, will with time become a thing of the past; already they come across to some of us as narrowly doctrinaire if not old-fashioned bravura performances. In the perspective of the modern Enlightenment, it will be Freud's readers and Freudian writers who will continuously co-create Freud's legacy. This they will do by how they read his texts and by how and what they write. As the readers and writers change—and they do change—Freudian psychoanalysis changes.[8]

The authors in this book have exemplified this insight, and to it they have added in each chapter a number of suggestive glimpses of the American culture with which Freud's legacies have been in dialogue for a century. These specific glimpses cover an enormous range of types of events over the century after 1909. Yet as just a moment in the universe of historical change, each glimpse can by itself add much to understanding. Together, however, they offer every one of us the opportunity to connect those moments in different ways as we reflect on American encounters with psychoanalytic thinking in the eventful ten decades after Freud left.

8. Roy Schafer, "Reading Freud's Legacies," in *Telling Facts: History and Narration in Psychoanalysis*, ed. Joseph H. Smith and Humphrey Morris (Baltimore: Johns Hopkins University Press, 1992), 1-20, quotation from 6-7. On p. 9, he added, "This pluralistic view of Freud's legacy, this view that there can only be legacies that are forever subject to change, is itself one of Freud's legacies."

ACKNOWLEDGMENTS

Beyond the generous concern for the collaborative effort of all of the authors of the essays printed above, important intellectual support for the content of this book came at an early stage from James William Anderson, Patricia R. Everett, Raymond E. Fancher, James Gilbert, Leon Hoffman, Lila Kalinich, Martin Rauchbauer, Inge Scholz-Strasser, and Andreas Stadler. Special mention should also be made of the contributions of two anonymous referees of the University of Chicago Press.

Basic financial support was provided by the Rosenzweig Foundation for Personality Dynamics and Creativity of St. Louis, with additional funding from the Austrian Cultural Forum of New York, and the New York Academy of Medicine. Other institutional benefactors included the American Psychological Association Division 26, the Association for Psychoanalytic Medicine, and the Sigmund Freud Museum and Sigmund Freud Foundation of Vienna, along with these individuals: Jules Bohnn, George S. Goldman, Sheila Hafter Gray, and Nathan G. Hale Jr.

Individual donors included Bernard W. Bail, Helen Beiser, Donald L. Burnham, Lawrence Friedman, Irving B. Harrison, Leonard Horwitz, Deborah Johnson, Lila Kalinich, Nathaniel P. Karush, Anton O. Kris, Margaret Morgan Lawrence, Jerome M. Levine, Peter Loewenberg, Marvin Nierenberg, Paoli Psychiatric Associates, Dorothy Ross, Harvey D. Strassman, Landrum Tucker Jr., Herbert M. Wyman, and Abraham Zaleznik.

Additional special thanks are due to Eric Nuetzel, Arlene Shaner, and Christian Warren.

CHRONOLOGICAL GUIDE TO EVENTS

1909 Sixth International Congress of Experimental Psychology (Geneva)
1909 Münsterberg publishes *Psychotherapy*
1909 Forel founds International Society for Medical Psychology and Psychotherapy
1909 American Therapeutic Society meeting in New Haven discusses psychotherapy
1909 Freud and Jung speak at Clark University
1909 Works by Jung and Freud appear in translation in the United States
1910 Freud's Clark lectures, summarizing and synthesizing psychoanalysis for the first time, published in English in the *American Journal of Psychology*
1910 Founding of the International Psychoanalytical Association and the beginning of exclusion of those diverging substantially
1913 Founding of the *Psychoanalytic Review* (eclectic, but the first American and the first English-language psychoanalytic professional journal)
1914 Freud, "On Narcissism"
1914–17 Freud moves into a new phase—theory and metapsychology, loosening personal control of the psychoanalytic movement so that it becomes psychoanalysis, not Freudianism
1920s Psychoanalysis centered in Vienna, Berlin, London, and Budapest
Late 1920s Frankfurt school applying psychoanalysis to sociology/Marxism
1931 New York Psychoanalytic Institute institutes orthodox training pattern
1932 Founding of the *Psychoanalytic Quarterly* (orthodox second-generation American analysts)
ca. 1933 Destruction of the Berlin Psychoanalytic Society and movement of significant leadership figures to the United States
1936 Anna Freud, *The Ego and the Mechanisms of Defense* (basic new departure for psychoanalytic theory)
1937 Re-founding of the *Partisan Review*

1938 American analysts break with the International Psychoanalytical Association over the issue of lay analysis
1938 Second wave of refugee analysts, most notably leaders from Austria
1939 Karen Horney, *New Ways in Psychoanalysis*
1939 Death of Sigmund Freud, in London
1940 Lionel Trilling, "Freud and Literature"
1941 First splitting off of neo-Freudians in New York and Washington, D.C.
1941 Erich Fromm, *Escape from Freedom*
1941–45 U.S. participation in World War II leads to major professional and popular validation of psychoanalysis
1943 (republished 1945) Roy Grinker and John Spiegel, *War Neuroses*
1945 Otto Fenichel, *The Psychoanalytic Theory of Neurosis*
1946 "Orthodox" Freudians and ego psychologists in control of the American Psychoanalytic Association, emphasizing adaptation and abstemious, detached style of treatment
1947 W. H. Auden, *The Age of Anxiety*
1948 Sartre, *Existentialism* (English translation)
1950 Lionel Trilling, *The Liberal Imagination*
1950 Rollo May, *The Meaning of Anxiety*
1950 Erik Erikson, *Childhood and Society*
1953–74 *Standard Edition of the Complete Psychological Works of Sigmund Freud*
1955 Herbert Marcuse, *Eros and Civilization*
1956 Celebrations of the centennial of Freud's birth, including *Freud and the Twentieth Century*, edited by Benjamin Nelson
1958 H. Stuart Hughes, *Consciousness and Society*
1959 Philip Rieff, *Freud: The Mind of the Moralist*
1959 Norman O. Brown, *Life Against Death*
1963 Betty Friedan, *The Feminine Mystique*
1966 Philip Rieff, *The Triumph of the Therapeutic*
1971 Heinz Kohut, *The Analysis of the Self*
1977 Heinz Kohut, *The Restoration of the Self*
1978 Christopher Lasch, *The Culture of Narcissism*
1980 *DSM-III* removes dynamic psychological language from psychiatric diagnoses
1980 Janet Malcolm, *Psychoanalysis: The Impossible Profession*
1980 Frederick Crews, "Analysis Terminable," anchors the Freud wars in the culture wars
1993 Freud appears on the cover of *Time*
1995 Nathan G. Hale Jr., *The Rise and Crisis of Psychoanalysis in the United States*
1995–98 "Freud wars" culminate in a controversy over a Freud exhibit at the Library of Congress

2006 Freud appears on the cover of *Newsweek*
2006 "New Freud Studies" recognized and named
2008 George Makari, *Revolution in Mind: The Creation of Psychoanalysis*
2009 The centennial of Freud's visit to the United States stimulates new reflections on a century of the relationship of American culture to psychoanalysis

CONTRIBUTORS

Jean-Christophe Agnew
American Studies Program and Department of History
Yale University
New Haven, CT 06520-8236
USA

John Burnham
Department of History
Ohio State University
Columbus, OH 43220-1367
USA

Ernst Falzeder
Alberto Susat-Strasse 4
A-5026 Salzburg
Austria

Elizabeth Lunbeck
Department of History
Vanderbilt University
Nashville, TN 37235-1802
USA

George Makari
DeWitt Wallace Institute for the History of Psychiatry
Weill Medical College of Cornell University
New York, NY 10065
USA

Louis Menand
Department of English
Harvard University
Cambridge, MA 02138
USA

Dorothy Ross
Department of History
Johns Hopkins University
Baltimore, MD 21218
USA

Sonu Shamdasani
Wellcome Trust Centre for the History of Medicine
University College London
London NW1 2BE
UK

Richard Skues
Faculty of Social Sciences and Humanities
London Metropolitan University
London N7 8DB
UK

Hale Usak-Sahin
Sonnenpark Lans
Zentrum für psychosoziale Gesundheit
6072 Lans/Tirol
Austria

INDEX

abreaction: Freud, 76; World War II, 197
abstinence, 225–27. *See also* heroism; orthodoxy
academics. *See* intellectuals
adaptation: as adjustment, 174, 180, 198, 228; ego psychology, 123; late twentieth century, 171
Adler, Alfred, 85–86, 112, 117, 211
Age of Anxiety, The (Auden), 190–94, 256
aggression. *See* death instinct
Albrecht, Adalbert, 55
Alexander, Franz, 113, 115, 117, 118, 120, 122
alienation, 176; compounded, 174; transformed, 165
American century, 18, 20, 243; and anxiety, 235–37; and existentialism, 236
American culture, 1–4, 9, 16–21, 27–30, 47, 80; Freud and, 90–109; hypocrisy, 91, 99; lack of intellectual rigor, 92, 99, 100; money and greed, 91, 92, 93, 97–99, 104–8; national character, 93–94, 99, 100, 102, 237; not a passive receiver of psychoanalysis, 17–20, 28; politics, 91; social equality, 91, 94 (*see also* women). *See also* communication of ideas; sixties
American Institute for Psychoanalysis, 121
American Psychoanalytic Association, 123
American Therapeutic Society, 41–42; meeting in 1909, 41–44, 47, 255
Analysis of the Self, The (Kohut), 213, 256
"Analysis Terminable" (Crews), 184, 256

angst. See anxiety
Anschluss, Austria, 114, 124
anti-Semitism, 17, 99, 108–9, 241; Nazi, 16, 113, 128, 130 (*see also* National Socialism)
anti-utopianism. *See* utopianism
anxiety: and American culture, 18, 194, 199–200; and civilization, 198–99; and Cold War, 115, 160, 189–90, 234; discourse, 189–90, 202–3, 233; and existentialism, 194–95, 198–200; Freud and validation, 190; historicization, 198–99; meaning, 198, 199, 200, 202; and neurosis, 199–202; politics and psychology, 238; and psychoanalysis decline, 206; religious origins, 192–94; and totalitarianism, 18, 203–4
Apollonian modernism, 18, 160, 165, 167, 237; conservative elements, 180–82; decline, 179–81; Eriksonian mutuality, 176; and Freud, 168, 172, 173, 174, 186–87
Arendt, Hannah, 203
art, 180. *See also* humanities; intellectuals
Aschaffenburg, Gustav, 45
Association for the Advancement of Psychoanalysis, 121
association test, 43, 46, 51, 52–53, 62–63, 68, 70, 71, 73. *See also* complex; Jung, C. G.
Atatürk, Mustafa Kemal, 130, 136, 137. *See also* Turkey
atomic bomb fears, 160, 202, 233

Auden, W. H., 190–92, 193, 247, 256
authenticity, 18, 168, 174, 176, 180, 187, 234, 236. *See also* alienation; self
automatic writing, 34
avant-garde, 2, 113, 162, 167. *See also* intellectuals
Avicenna, 132n29

Baldwin, B. T., 63
Balint, Michael, 230
Baltimore, MD, 30, 144–46, 149, 150–51
Barrett, William, 163, 167–68, 194–95, 239–40
Barthes, Roland, 134
Barzun, Jacques, 191
battle fatigue, 10. *See also* trauma; World War II
behaviorism, 35
Bell, Daniel, 163, 181, 219–20
Bellow, Saul, 195
Benedict, Ruth, 237
Bennet, Edward A., 98
Berger, Frank, 201
Berlin, 112, 113, 119–20, 124, 249, 255
Berlin, Isaiah, 203
Berman, Marshall, 187
Bernays, Eli, 104
Bernays, Minna, 85–86, 107
Bernheim, Hippolyte, 39. *See also* Nancy school
Bernstein, Leonard, 191
Berry, C. S., 62
Bettelheim, Bruno, 203
Beyond the Pleasure Principle (Freud), 169, 204
Binswanger, Ludwig, 198
biography, 8
biology, 170–71, 206–7. *See also* human nature
Bleuler, Eugen, 46, 51, 112, 130, 133–34. *See also* Zurich school
Boas, Franz, 59, 69
Bonaparte, Marie, 103
Bornstein, Bertha, 119
Boston, 32; Boston school of psychotherapy, 40, 54; and psychoanalysis, 75, 77
Boston Psychoanalytical Society, 75
bourgeois society: nineteenth century, 160; post–World War II, 175–76; sixties, 180–81. *See also* modernism
Bremen, 27, 28
Breuer, Josef, 46, 76, 102
Brill, A. A., 41, 55–56, 75, 77, 91, 107
Brown, Norman O., 163, 167, 176–77, 178, 179, 200, 256
Burgerstein, Leo, 59, 66, 69, 70
Burghölzli, 51, 130, 152. *See also* Bleuler, Eugen; Forel, August; Jung, C. G.; Zurich
Burnham, W. H., 70, 71
Burrow, Trigant, 47n54

Camelot, 160
Camus, Albert, 195, 234, 256
Cannon, Walter B., 115, 116
Caplan, Eric, 47
Carter, Jimmy, 243
cartoons, 6
catharsis. *See* abreaction
Cattell, J. M., 63
centennial of Freud's visit to the United States, 2, 27, 47, 250, 253, 257
Chambers, Whittaker, 194
Chestnut Lodge, 148, 149
Chicago, IL, 210, 212, 219, 225
Chicago Institute for Psychoanalysis, 212
child development, 12, 54, 175–76
child guidance movement, 26
Childhood and Society (Erikson), 175–76, 256
chlorpromazine, anti-psychotic, 201
Chodorow, Nancy, 187
Christianity: and existentialism, 192–94, 197–98; and self psychology, 219. *See also* religion
Civilization and Its Discontents (Freud), 168–69, 204, 205, 207, 234
Clark conference, 14–15, 25, 46, 49–84, 111, 255; audience, 64–66, 73–74; Freud's aims at, 77–78, 103; Freud's reaction to, 50, 56–57, 78–79; Freud's starring role, 54–55, 70, 71; group photos, 57, 58, 59–64, 66–67, 72, 74, 82–84; iconic event, 1, 2, 14, 28, 32, 46, 49–51, 57, 82, 257; impact, 74–77, 250; insignificance of in 1909, 41, 46, 47, 50–51, 55–56, 74–75, 76–79, 82;

invitations, 55–57, 67–73; Jung at, 51, 52–54, 56, 66–73; psychoanalysis at, 49–51, 66–67, 74–75; structure, 57–58, 65–66
Clark conference lectures by Freud, 65–66, 69, 72, 78, 82, 250, 255; importance of, 76–77, 250; translation, 74–77, 250, 255. *See also The Origin and Development of Psychoanalysis*
Clark University, 1, 14–15, 28; honorary degree to Freud, 49–50. *See also* Clark conference
Cold War, 19, 20, 191; culture of, 160, 166, 169, 171, 172, 195, 198; and death instinct, 205–6; discourse and anxiety about, 206; discourse and culture of, 202; discourse origins of, 190; historiography of, 190
Columbia University, 122, 179
Commentary, 184
communication of ideas, 11–12, 13–14, 16, 20–21, 25, 52–53; cultural differences, 158, 171; European prejudices, 109. *See also* American culture; psychoanalytic communities
complex: Adolf Meyer, 143; before Freud, 51; Morton Prince, 34–35; Walter Dill Scott, 45. *See also* association test
Concept of Dread, The (Kierkegaard), 193–94
conformity, persistent cultural force, 247; fear of, 170–71; Freud as agent, 162
Consciousness and Society (Hughes), 173, 256
conservative reaction, late twentieth century, 169, 180–85; factor in decline of psychoanalysis, 181–82
consumer culture, 11, 171, 181, 236
"conversion" to psychoanalysis, 79–82
Coriat, Isador, 41, 65–66, 73–74, 75
Cotkin, George, 9
counseling, factor in decline of psychoanalysis, 159, 243
counterculture, 179, 183, 243. *See also* sixties
Crews, Frederick, 163, 183–84, 242, 256
crystal gazing, 34
Cuddihy, John Murray, 241

cultural comparison, 90, 94, 95–96, 99–100, 105, 109, 125, 159
cultural radicals, interwar, 210. *See also* avant-garde
culture and personality studies, 26, 237, 248
Culture of Narcissism, The (Lasch), 216, 236, 237, 244, 256
Cuordileone, K. A., 238

Daniels, George, 115, 116, 122
Darwinism. *See* evolution
death instinct, 116, 169, 177, 204–5
Deliorman, Altan, 135
dementia praecox. *See* psychoses
Derrida, Jacques, 184
Dessoir, Max, 32
development theory. *See* modernization theory
dilution. *See* eclecticism
Dionysian modernism, 18, 160, 165, 167, 176–78, 234, 237; denial of, 180–81; in Freud, 173
dissociation, 35, 42–43
domesticated modernism. *See* Erikson, Erik
Don Giovanni, 87–88
Dorsey, John M., 87
drive theory, 12–13, 117, 211, 223–24, 234–35
Drucker, Peter, 194
DSM (*Diagnostic and Statistical Manual of Mental Disorders*), 200, 206, 251, 256
Dubois, Paul, 36, 37, 39, 40
Dufresne, Todd, 4n7
dynamic psychiatry. *See* psychiatry and psychoanalysis

eclecticism in the United States, 29, 80, 81, 122–23, 159, 196, 210; and decline of psychoanalysis, 188
education in psychotherapy, 39, 43
Edith Weigert Lecture, 253
ego psychology, 4, 157, 159, 175, 226–27, 251; and émigrés, 16, 210; and the United States, 122–23, 250. *See also* orthodoxy
Einstein, Albert, 92n33
Eissler, Kurt, 105, 107, 210, 227–28

Eissler, Ruth, 210, 212
Eliot, T. S., 166
elites, 157, 253. *See also* avant-garde; intellectuals
Emergency Committee on Relief and Immigration, 114
Emerson, L. E., 210
emigrant analysts, to U.S., 16–17, 111, 113–26, 157, 158, 196, 233; to Turkey, 130, 135–38
emigration. *See* migration
Emmanuel Movement, 40–41, 45, 80
energy in psychotherapy. *See* James, William
English translations, 14, 39, 46, 52–54. *See also* Freud, translations of works
Enlightenment, 164, 165, 173, 253; source for both modernism and modernization, 239
environmentalism, 6, 12–13, 210, 223; and anxiety, 199; in Kohut, 161, 248; and modernism, 170
Equanil. *See* meprobamate
Erikson, Erik, 18, 163, 167, 175–76, 178, 185, 256
Erkoç, Şahap, 132n28, 135
eros. *See* sexuality
Eros and Civilization (Marcuse), 177, 178, 256
Escape from Freedom (Fromm), 170, 256
ethical imperative, 193–94; anxiety and, 193–95; Knight of Faith and, 193–94
Evans, Rand, 55
evolution, 165
existentialism: academics, 195; and anxiety, 172, 195, 234; atheistic, 194–95; Christian, 191; dread and neurosis, 198; European, 194–95; and feminism, 185; and freedom, 195; French, 195; and humanism, 195; individualism in, 195; and psychoanalysis, 19, 234

failure and modernism, 242. *See also* heroism
Fairbairn, W. R. D., 211, 231
family therapy, 146, 147–48
Federn, Paul, 116–19, 220
feminine mystique, and Freud, 186

Feminine Mystique, The (Friedan), 184–85, 207, 256
feminism: and Erikson, 185; and Freud, 185–86, 187; late twentieth century, 207; and modernism, 185–86. *See also* sixties; women
Fenichel, Otto, 115, 120, 123; and anxiety, 199–200; and *Rundbriefe*, 12
Ferenczi, Sándor: boundary violation, 227; and Clara Thompson, 121; and Clark conference, 27, 57, 61–62, 66; "Ferenczi renaissance," 231; on Freud at Clark, 78, 107; and Kohut, 215; and Riverside Drive incident, 105–7; as schismatic, 211
Finnegans Wake (Joyce), 191
Firestone, Shulamith, 187
Five Lectures. See *The Origin and Development of Psychoanalysis*
Flournoy, Théodore, 32
Ford, Henry, 31
Forel, August, 37–38, 46, 130, 255
Forel, Oscar, 130
Forrester, John, 242
Frankfurt school, 170, 177, 200, 255
Freud, Anna (sister), 88
Freud, Anna (daughter), 123, 212, 255
Freud, Ernst, 97
Freud, Martha, 107
Freud, Martin, 89
Freud, Mathilde, 57, 97
Freud, Sigmund: ambitiousness, 77–79, 98–99, 106–7; ambivalence toward the United States, 89–90, 94, 95–96, 108–9; and American accents, 95–96; and American journalists, 100; and American psychoanalysts, 100–102; and American publishers, 100; and American toilet facilities, 96, 106; and American wealth, 95–96, 103, 108–9; antipathy toward Americans, 15–16, 28–29, 86, 89–90, 94–99, 104, 200; and bicycles and motorcycles, 86; Central European conventionality of attitudes, 15–16, 92, 94, 104–5, 109; and Clark conference, 49–84; criticism turns personal, 187; death of, 256; early reputation, 14–15, 34–35, 40, 43–47, 51–55; emigration to London, 102, 103, 135; gastrointes-

tinal upsets, 96–97; and hairstyles, 86; hater, 85–89, 102; impact of his ideas, 11, 26–27; incontinence, 105–8; as an intellectual, 20, 25, 253; International Society, 38–39, 112, 255; interpretations of antipathies, 104–8; misanthropy of, 90; and music, 86–89; personal impressions of the United States, 94–95; and philosophy, 86–87; reports from the visit to the United States, 78, 95–97; telephones, 86; and tobacco, 90–91; translations of works, 46, 75–77, 196, 255, 256; as a transmitter of ideas, 28–29, 250; travel to the United States, 1, 25, 27–28, 49–84, 233; valued loyalty, 85; and Vienna, 86, 87, 89; and women, 94, 103; worldview, 25

Freud, Sigmund, as a symbol: authority, 112, 116–19; birth centennial celebrated, 5, 12, 172; historiography, 2, 7–10, 12–13; ideas separated from man, 182–83; modernism of, 171–75, 178, 236–37; not charismatic, 213–14; in retreat from modernism, 178–85, 187–88; in textbooks, 1. *See also* Freud, reputation; heroism; modernism

Freud: The Mind of the Moralist (Rieff), 173, 256

"Freud and Literature" (Trilling), 168, 256

Freud and the Twentieth Century (Nelson), 5, 172, 256

Freud Wars, 7–9, 184, 256

Friedan, Betty, 163, 185–86, 207

Frink, Horace W., 101–2

Fromm, Eric, 121–22, 170, 174, 175, 178, 198, 203, 238

Fromm-Reichman, Frieda, 125, 148; modifies technique, 148–50; relationship to Edith Weigert, 150–51; relationship to Ruth Wilmanns Lidz, 148, 149, 150

Gay, Peter, 90, 104–5
Genet, Jean, 186
Geneva conference, 1909, 31–34, 46
George Washington (ship), 27, 98
Gerhard, Jane, 239
German Medical Association for Psychotherapy, 113
Gerrish, Frederick, 42

Giacometti, Alberto, 239–40, 244
Gilbert, Stuart, 195
Goldman, Emma, 65–66n47
"Green, Aaron," 225–26, 228–30, 244
Grinker, Roy, 197, 256
Grossman, Atina, 126, 128–29, 142
Grünbaum, Adolf, 184
guessing device in psychotherapy, 45
Guilbert, Yvette, 88
Guntrip, Harry, 230
Guraba Clinic (Istanbul), 138–42

Habermas, Jürgen, 184
Hale, Nathan G., Jr., 2, 26, 256
Hall, G. Stanley: invitation to Freud, 27, 103; orchestration of Clark conference, 54–56, 74–75; and psychoanalysis at Clark, 66–67, 72; publicity of Freud and Clark, 14, 70, 74–75, 249–50. *See also* Clark conference
Hammerstein Roof Garden (New York), 108
Hanly, Charles, 250–51
Hartmann, Heinz, 16, 119, 122–28, 210
Harvard University, 54, 241; connection to Clark conference, 62
Hawthorne, Nathaniel, 183
healthy narcissism, 220–22. *See also* narcissism
Heidegger, Martin, 184, 194–95
Heidelberg school of psychiatrists, 127
Heller, Erich, 188
heroism: in Americanized Freud, 20, 165, 169, 170–72, 239–41; and modernism, 174, 176, 235; sexism in, 243, 244, 245. *See also* ethical imperative
Herzberg, David, 201–2
hidden motives, 6, 11, 24, 26, 188, 223, 245
Hilger, Wilhelm, 40
Hill, Lewis, 146–147, 149
historians, 2–3, 7–11, 13–14, 25–26, 189–90, 249, 251; and Clark conference, 49–52, 57, 164
Hitler, Adolf, 113, 129, 196
Hoboken, NJ, 27
Hollinger, David, 241
Holocaust, 191–92. *See also* anti-Semitism; National Socialism

Holt, Edwin B., 62
homosexuality theorists and Freud, 186, 187.
Horney, Karen, 113, 117, 118, 119–20, 121–22, 123, 170, 200, 256
Hughes, H. Stuart, 158, 163, 173, 256
humanities and psychoanalysis, 4, 162, 164, 188, 239, 241, 251. *See also* intellectuals
human nature, 3, 4, 6, 11, 169–71, 174, 176, 188, 207, 234, 248, 252. *See also* environmentalism; existentialism; self
hypnoid states, 43–45, 46, 47
hypnotism, 36, 37, 39, 40, 42, 43
hysteria, 35, 42

identity, 175, 185, 234. *See also* self
industrialism, 164
inner life. *See* hidden motives; narcissism
instincts: 116, 169, 171, 181. *See also* drive theory; Freud
insulin shock treatment, 141, 142, 145–46, 150; and psychoanalysis, 150
insurance and psychoanalysis, 7
intellectuals and psychoanalysis: anxiety discourse, 189–95; applying modernism, 172, 235, 240–42; channel for ideas, 3–6, 17–19, 26, 157–59, 160–62, 163–88; continuing regard for Freud, 172, 174–75, 178, 181; cultural authority, 165–66, 169, 189, 234; desertion of Freud, 9, 182–83; existentialism crossover, 195, 198–99; gauge of impact of Freud, 11, 159, 248; Jewish, 166, 167, 233, 234, 241, 249; Marxism and, 167; persistent interest, 188, 248; Protestant, 166, 241, 247, 249; rebelliousness and, 167
international area studies, 239
International Congress of Experimental Psychology, 31–34, 46, 255
International Psychoanalytical Association, 38–39, 112, 114, 250, 255
International Society for Medical Psychology and Psychotherapy, 37–39
Interpretation of Dreams (Freud), 107, 169
Irrational Man (Barrett), 195, 239–41
Islamic beliefs. *See* Turkey
Istanbul University, 125–26, 132, 138

Jacobsen, Edith, 210
Jaffé, Aniela, 68
James, Henry, 241
James, William, 37, 71, 111; and Clark conference, 59, 60–61, 62; in early psychotherapy, 37, 42, 43, 44
Janet, Pierre, 32–33, 35, 44
Jekels, Ludwig, 119
Jennings, Herbert S., 59, 69
Jeremiads, 206–7, 235–36, 243–44
Jones, Ernest: at American Therapeutic Society meeting, 41–43; and boundary violations, 227; and Clark conference, 62, 66; on conversion, 79–80; early publications, 39–40, 45; publicizing psychoanalysis, 77–78; rescue efforts in 1930s, 115
Journal of Abnormal Psychology, 33, 34, 42, 75
Joyce, James, 166
Jung, Carl Gustav: and Auden's *The Age of Anxiety*, 191; boundary violations, 227; Clark conference invitation, 55–56, 67–71, 73; Clark conference role, 54, 66–67, 68–73, 255; early prominence in the United States, 34, 35, 43, 47, 51–53, 74, 111; in early psychotherapy, 44; financial support from Americans, 103; Fordham lectures, 69; Freud traveling companion, 27, 98–99; Riverside Drive story source, 105–6, 107; as schismatic, 112, 117; writings translated, 46, 52–53, 255. *See also* association test; Clark conference

Kafka, Franz, 166
Kardiner, Abram, 117, 118, 119, 120, 122, 123
Karlson, J. K., 64
Katzenellenbogen, E. W., 62–63
Kaye, Howard L. 105
Kazin, Alfred, 173
Kernberg, Otto, 161, 224, 225
Kierkegaard, Søren, 192–94, 197–98; and concept of anxiety, 192–94, 199
Knight of Faith, 193–94, 198
Koelsch, William, 55, 68–69, 73
Koestler, Arthur, 203
Kohut, Heinz, 210–31, 256; and American

culture, 19, 210–11, 230–31, 234, 251; biography, 212–13; challenges Freud's teachings, 211; critics of, 229–30, 243; deviation from orthodoxy, 19, 161, 213, 251; following, 159; historicizes Freud, 213–14; ideas absorbed into psychoanalysis, 225–26, 228–31; personal psychoanalysis, 229; predecessor thinkers, 229–30; preserves psychoanalysis, 211; and social pathology, 217–18, 220–21; transforms narcissism, 214–15, 218, 219–23, 235–36. *See also* Lasch, Christopher; narcissism; self psychology
Kris, Ernst, 119, 122–23
Kris, Marianne, 119
Kroeber, Alfred, 27
Kubie, Lawrence, 114–15, 118–19, 121

Lacan, Jacques, 184
language problems of migrants, 95, 118, 119, 136, 138, 144–45, 145n82
LaPiere, Richard, 5–6
Lasch, Christopher, 187, 216–17, 219–20, 222, 223, 236, 243, 245, 256
Lawrence, D. H., 166, 186
lay analysis, 100, 104, 114, 121, 256
left-wingers: European analysts, 29, 123; U.S. intellectuals, 167, 169, 185. *See also* New Left
Levy, David, 115, 116–17, 118–19, 122
Lévy, Paul Émile, 39
Lewin, Bertram, 115
Liberal Imagination, The (Trilling), 169, 234, 256
Library of Congress, 256
Librium, 201
Liddell, Howard, 200
Lidz, Ruth Wilmanns, 125, 126, 152–53; childhood, 127–28; emigration to Turkey, 138–41, 157; emigration to the United States, 142, 144–46; escape from Nazis, 129–30; learns and practices insulin shock therapy, 142, 145–46; and psychoanalytic family therapy, 147–48; relationship to Edith Weigert, 150; relationship to Frieda Fromm-Reichman, 148–50; and Turkish culture, 138–42, 157; undergoes psychoanalytic treatment and training, 146–47, 149–50

Lidz, Theodore, 146, 147–48
Lidz, Victor, 138, 146, 149
Life Against Death (Brown), 177, 178
linguistic turn. *See* postmodernism
literature, 5, 6. 163. 166–72, 175, 177, 179–80, 183–84, 188, 190–92, 233, 234, 241
local, importance of, 25–26
London, 89, 112, 123, 249
Lowenstein, Rudolph, 122–23
Lowrie, Walter, 192–93, 198, 236
Luce, Henry, 235–36, 238, 243
Lynd, Helen, 198–99
Lynd, Robert, 198–99

Mahony, Patrick, 90, 105
Mailer, Norman, 186
Malcolm, Janet, 225–26, 228–29, 256
Mann, Thomas, 166
Marcuse, Herbert, 163, 167, 177–78, 179, 200, 223, 256
Marin, Peter, 216
Marxism, 166, 167, 168, 189, 199–200, 204–5. *See also* utopianism
Maslow, Abraham, 186
Masson, Jeffrey, 184
May, Rollo, 198, 202, 203, 204, 256
McCarthyism, 160, 169
McComb, Samuel, 41
Mead, Margaret, 237
Meaning of Anxiety, The (May), 198, 203, 256
"Me Decade," 216
medicine and psychoanalysis, 3–14, 201–2; 1930s, 113, 122; post–World War II, 159, 164; and sexism, 244
Menninger, Karl, 210
mephenesin, 201
meprobamate, 201
Meyer, Adolf: attitude toward psychoanalysis, 64, 69, 71, 81, 143–44, 152–53; career in the United States, 125, 143–44; at Clark conference, 30, 59, 64, 69, 71, 125, 143; emphasizes adaptation, 43, 143; hires Ruth Wilmanns Lidz, 141, 142–43; and schismatics, 121, 122
Middletown studies and anxiety, 198–99
migration of psychoanalysts: difficulties of migrants, 114–15, 120–31, 151–52;

migration of psychoanalysts (*continued*)
  impact on New York, 115-23; interwar movement, 3-4, 25, 29-30, 104, 111, 113-15, 118-19, 123-24, 136-52, 157-58, 210; via Middle East, 151-52, 157
Miller, Perry, 241
Millett, Kate, 163, 186
Miltown. *See* meprobamate
modernism, 14-15, 17-18, 20, 157, 234; carrier of psychoanalysis, 160, 165-67, 172, 178, 180-81, 233, 234, 235, 240-41, 247-48, 251; decline of, 179-85, 188, 234, 243-44, 245; definition of, 164-65, 167; and feminism, 185; high point of, 163; Kohut and, 220; and modernization, 239; and politics, 166-67; social geography of, 243; and technology, 239; and varieties of psychoanalysis, 175, 235; *See also* Apollonian modernism; Dionysian modernism; intellectuals
modernity, 20, 26; and anxiety, 198-99; and psychoanalysis, 219-20, 233, 252-53
modernization, 157; and death instinct, 157; and modernism, 239; theory, 237
Molnar, Michael, 94
Momism, 238. *See also* sexism
Mowrer, O. Hobart, 158, 197-98, 200
Mozart, Wolfgang Amadeus, 88
Müller, Max, 142
multiple personality. *See* dissociation
Münsterberg, Hugo, 36-37, 41, 62, 255

Nancy school of psychotherapy. *See* hypnotism
narcissism, 18, 19-20, 224; in American culture, 216-17, 234, 247; and civilization, 215, 218-19; Freud's version of, 215; Kohut's version of, 161, 210-11, 214-15, 217-18; and national decline, 211, 216-17; and self, 211-12, 217-18. *See also* healthy narcissism; Lasch, Christopher
national character, 20, 237. *See also* American culture; cultural differences
National Institute of Mental Health, 196

National Socialism, 16, 25, 113, 125-26, 128, 148, 152, 170, 177, 196, 204-5
Nazis. *See* National Socialism
Nelson, Benjamin, 5, 172, 256
neo-Freudians, 6, 122, 158, 164, 170, 172, 175, 178, 200, 239, 248
neurosciences and psychoanalysis, 252
neuroses, 34-35, 39, 43. *See also* psychiatry; psychoanalysis; psychotherapy
Neurotic Personality of Our Times (Horney), 119, 237
New Criticism, 183, 241
New Freud Studies, 8-10, 257
New Haven conference, 1909, 41-44, 46, 47, 74, 255
New Left, 179, 183, 188, 234. *See also* sixties
Newman, Barnett, 194
Newsweek, Freud on cover, 252, 257
New Ways in Psychoanalysis (Horney), 119-20, 256
New York City: as cultural capital, 75, 89, 241-43; in Freud's visit, 27, 95; haven for Viennese refugees, 11, 29, 114-16, 251; symbol of orthodoxy, 122-24, 210, 225, 250
New York Psychoanalytic Society and Institute, 101, 115-23, 171, 255
Niebuhr, Reinhold, 192, 236, 238
Nietzsche, Friedrich, 173, 180, 184
1960s. *See* sixties
Nunberg, Hermann, 119
Nuremburg meetings, 1910, 112. *See also* orthodoxy

Oberndorf, Clarence, 51, 67, 112
object love, 215-16
object relations school, and Kohut, 211, 229-30
Oedipus complex, 173, 199, 225
Ogburn, William Fielding, 27
opera, 88
Origin and Development of Psychoanalysis, The (Freud), 76; translated into Ottoman and Turkish, 132. *See also* Clark conference lectures
orthodoxy in psychoanalysis: and adjustment, 171; diluted but persistent,

225-26, 235; division in the United States, 122, 151, 161, 164, 256; ego psychologists intensify, 210, 253; established in Europe, 10, 112, 189; high point in the United States, 162, 248, 250; Kohut and, 212-14, 221, 229, 234-35
Orwell, George, 203

Pappenheim, Else, 85-86
Parker, W. B., 40
Partisan Review, 147, 163, 168, 194-95, 255
patients, change in, 159, 161, 225
Pavlov, Ivan, 115
People magazine. *See* self psychology
personal becomes political, 18, 19, 162, 206-7, 234. *See also* sixties
personality, 13, 26, 170, 216, 237
persuasion, 36, 37, 39
Pfister, Oskar, 56
Phillips, William, 167
philosophers and psychoanalysis, 250
Phipps Clinic, Johns Hopkins University, 143-46
physiology of emotion, 115
Pinel, Philippe, 39
politics, 9-10, 18, 29, 205-6, 248. *See also* personal becomes political
Popper, Karl, 184
popularization of psychoanalysis, 11-12, 26, 28, 181, 189, 221, 224. *See also* psychoanalysis
postmodernism, 18, 160; Freud and, 181, 183-85, 187, 188, 247; intellectual stage, 160, 165, 184, 251-52, 253
Prince, Morton: and Boston school, 40; at New Haven congress, 42-43; and psychoanalysis, 34-35, 45-46, 75; and psychotherapy movement, 33-35, 38, 44
psychiatry: dominated by psychoanalysts after 1945, 196-97, 251; dynamic, 31, 161, 201-2; expansion after World War II, 196; Jung known for, 52-53; and psychoanalysis, 159, 189, 196, 198; shift to organic basis, 201, 206; and World War II, 196-97. *See also DSM*; neuroses; psychoses

Psychic Treatment of the Nervous Disorders (Dubois), 39
psychoanalysis: becomes distinctive, 76, 250; boundaries uncertain, 44-46, 53; change constant, 111, 253; conservative aspects of, 174-75; decline of, 3, 6-8, 160, 163, 244-45, 188, 247, 250-51; as doctor-patient communication, 253; in early psychotherapy, 14, 31-47, 53; emergence as a system, 14-15, 76; European high culture, 4, 112-13; and existentialism, 197-201, 235; fragmentation in late twentieth century, 248; growth following 1909, 76-77; high point of, 3-6, 157, 159, 160, 163, 164, 178, 188, 189, 211, 237, 250; local aspects of, 25-26, 111-12, 225; in medical schools, 196; psychopathology and, 10-11; and psychotherapy, 43-45, 50, 161, 250; in special academic areas, 162, 188, 251; subject attractive, 1; survival after 2000, 162, 252, 253; theory, 113, 115-16, 119-21, 152, 157, 183, 212-16, 221, 233, 237, 250-51; in Turkey, 132-36, 137-38. *See also* schismatics
psychoanalysis, American: Americanization of, 113, 209-10, 210-11, 249; break from international, 113-14, 250; centralization post-1945 of, 123; cultural incompatibility of, 189, 250; cultural penetration of, 1-6, 10, 17-20, 26, 108, 158-59, 189-90, 209-10, 233, 243, 248, 249, 252-53; and Frink incident, 101-2; how organized, 10, 16, 17, 27, 29, 196; and lack of contribution to world psychoanalysis, 112; pre-1939 style, 170; splits, 16, 19, 121-22; survival in late twentieth century, 211, 251. *See also* Kohut; modernism
Psychoanalysis: The Impossible Profession (Malcolm), 225, 256
psychoanalytic communities: Berlin, 112, 113, 117, 118, 119-22, 123; Budapest, 112; Chicago, 119; London, 112; New York, 111-23, 243; Vienna, 112, 117, 118, 120-22, 123; Zurich, 46-47, 112

psychoanalytic movement, 38–39, 101–2, 103, 111–12, 157, 250; cultural content of, 111–12; international, 38–39, 111–13
Psychoanalytic Quarterly, 255
Psychoanalytic Review, 255
Psychoanalytic Theory of Neurosis (Fenichel), 199–200, 256
psychological man, 1, 174, 181–82
psychological mechanisms, 11, 248
psychologization of the United States, 1, 174–75, 181, 182, 206–7. *See also* American culture; psychological man
psychology and psychologists: and Clark conference, 58–64, 72–73; clinical, 159; and ego psychology, 123; and psychoanalysis, 4–5, 7, 13–14, 172–73, 196, 251; and psychotherapy, 31–32, 37
Psychology of Dementia Praecox (Jung), 46, 52
psychopharmaceuticals, 6, 7, 19, 160, 200–202; compatibility with psychoanalysis, 19, 202; as feminine, 238–39
psychotherapy: as heroic, 238; movement, 13–14, 31–47, 50; optimistic American, 209; popularized, 40–41; and psychoanalysis, 10, 37–39, 43–46. *See also* environmentalism; psychiatry; psychoanalysis
Psychotherapy (Münsterberg), 36–37, 255
Psychotherapy (Parker), 40–41
psychotic patients, 125, 128, 145–46, 147–48, 149, 150, 152; pre-reform Turkey, 131
psychotic syndromes, 17, 34, 46, 125, 128, 152
Putnam, James Jackson: and Clark conference, 74, 77; "conversion" of, 80; and Freud, 74, 75; as pioneer in psychoanalysis, 42, 46, 111, 210

Radó, Sándor, 113, 114, 115–19, 122
Rahv, Phillip, 163, 166, 167
Rank, Otto, 87, 117, 199
Rapaport, David, 123
rationalism (Enlightenment), 40, 168, 181, 198–99, 203, 248
reality principle, 168, 169
recapitulation, 54
reeducation, 39, 43. *See also* education
reflexology, 115
regression, 177–78
Reich, Annie, 119
Reich, Wilhelm, 200, 204
religion, Freud and post–World War II, 172. *See also* existentialism
repression, 177, 219, 223–24
Restoration of the Self, The (Kohut), 213, 256
revisionist history of psychoanalysis, 13. *See also* New Freud Studies
Revolution in Mind (Makari), 257
Ricksher, Charles, 62
Ricoeur, Paul, 184
Rieff, Philip, 163, 167, 173–75, 181–82, 223, 256
Riesman, David, 178
Riklin, Franz, Jr., 102, 103
Riverside Drive incident, 105–8
Roazen, Paul, 85
Robbins, Jerome, 191
Robinson, Paul, 184, 239
romanticism, 160, 164–65, 168, 248. *See also* modernism
Rosenzweig, Saul, 27, 53, 54, 67–68, 72, 105
Rothko, Mark, 194

Sachs, Hanns, 113
Şadan, Izeddin A., 132–36
Sadger, Isidor, 85
Sakel, Manfred, 141
Salinger, J. D., 197
Sanford, E. C., 70, 71
Sartre, Jean-Paul, 195, 256
Schafer, Roy, 253
Schilder, Paul, 115
Schildkraut theory of depression, 206
schismatics in psychoanalysis: American, 116–12, 225, 256; European, 112, 152, 211, 255. *See also* Kohut, Heinz; orthodoxy
Schlesinger, Arthur, Jr., 203–4, 238–39
Schloss Tegel clinic, 126–27, 152
Schopenhauer, 87
science and psychoanalysis, 115–17, 121, 164, 172–73, 184
Scott, Walter Dill, 44–45
self: American, 211–12, 237; conflicted, 204; disorders of, 217–18; and femi-

nism, 185; and modernism, 18, 165, 171, 173–74, 175; and narcissism, 215–22; and objectivity, 184; potential, 19, 209, 222; and society, 19, 181–82, 204. *See also* alienation; identity; narcissism; subjectivity

self-improvement, 20, 222, 249

self psychology, 19–20; and abundance, 219; emotions in, 219; founding, 213; interiority as basis, 218–19; visibility in the 1970s and 1980s, 225. *See also* Kohut, Heinz

Selye, Hans, 197

service industry society, 11

sexism: and anxiety, 238; and modernity, 242–43; and psychoanalysis, 238–39, 242–43

sexuality: aversion to, 56, 142–43; Freud, modernism, and modernization, 239; Hall's interest in, 54; Kohut and, 219; psychoanalysis and, 223, 227; Reich and, 204; social version in Erikson, 175–76

sexual revolutions, 179, 187, 204, 210. *See also* sixties

Sheppard and Enoch Pratt Hospital, 150

Sidis, Boris, 42; at New Haven meetings, 43–44; and psychoanalysis, 44

signal anxiety, 116

Simmel, Ernst, 127

Sixth International Congress of Experimental Psychology. *See* International Congress of Experimental Psychology

sixties: anxiety and Freud in, 19; decline of modernism and psychoanalysis, 6, 160, 162, 179–81, 234; Freud and, 18, 187; Freud blamed, 180–83

Slater, Philip, 223

social sciences, 4–5, 26, 163, 171. *See also* modernization theory

somaticism, 6, 159, 171

Spiegel, John, 197, 256

Spock, Benjamin, 12

Springfield State Hospital, 145–46

stages in life, Erikson, 175–76

Statue of Liberty parodied, 91, 99

Stekel, Wilhelm, 112

Stern, William, 59, 66, 69, 70, 72

Stranger, The (Camus), 195, 234, 256

stress, 197, 201–2. *See also* anxiety; trauma; war neurosis

subconscious, 32–37, 43, 45, 45; definition of, 33–34, 36–37

subjectivism, 164–65, 183, 247, 251–52

suggestion, 36, 39–40, 42, 45

Sullivan, Harry Stack, 118, 121, 148, 170, 198, 230

Sulloway, Frank, 184

suppression of Freud's legacy, 2

Taylor, Edward W., 42, 43

Taylor, Eugene, 40

Thalidomide disaster, 201

theory, 158; social theory, 136–37. *See also* modernization theory; psychoanalytic theory

Thompson, Clara, 121–22, 198

Thorazine. *See* chlorpromazine

Tillich, Paul, 194

Time magazine, Freud on cover, 252, 256

Titchener, Edward B., 59–60, 64–65, 66, 69, 70

Toptaşı Bimarhanesi, 132–34

totalitarianism, 19; and anxiety discourse, 203–6; challenge post–World War II, 162, 170, 206, 233, 238, 248; choice in, 203, 238; Freud and totalitarian discourse, 204–5; psychologization of, 203. *See also* National Socialism; USSR

tragic pessimism: in Freud, 18, 169, 172, 174, 241; post–World War II, 160, 171, 172, 235, 248. *See also* existentialism; heroism

tranquilizers: and anxiety, 19, 160–61, 201–2; and Freud and existentialism, 234; use of psychoanalytic concepts for, 202

transference, 121, 148–49, 227–28, 243

translations. *See* English translations; Turkish translations

transnationalization, 2, 20–21, 25–30, 233, 241

trauma and catharsis, 76, 202; late twentieth century, 244; World War II and anxiety, 196–97

Trilling, Lionel: abandonment of Freud and modernism, 178–79, 179–80, 205–6, 241; as modernist intellectual, 163,

Trilling, Lionel (*continued*)
    167, 174, 175, 234; and psychoanalysis, 168–72, 256
Triumph of the Therapeutic, The (Rieff), 181, 256
Truman Doctrine. *See* Cold War
Tunç, Mustafa Şekip, 132
Turkey: emigrants in, 125–26, 153, 157; modernization of, 157; psychiatry in, 131–34, 152; psychoanalysis in, 17, 131–36; reforms in, 125–26, 130
Turkish translations, 132, 135

unconscious. *See* psychoanalysis; subconscious
University of Basel, 130
USSR, 167, 195, 196. *See also* Cold War; McCarthyism
utopianism, 169, 170, 175–76, 178, 204–6, 223. *See also* Marxism
utopia of genitality, 176

van Renterghem, Albert, 40
Vienna: psychoanalytic center, 9, 46, 112, 249; sentimentalized, 28, 86, 87, 89, 99–100; transfer to New York, 16, 115, 118–19, 122–24, 256
Vietnam War, 243. *See also* sixties
Vital Center, The (Schlesinger), 203–4, 238

Waelder, Robert, 210
Walking Man, 239–41, 244
Wallerstein, Robert, 161
War Neuroses (Grinker and Spiegel), 197, 256
war neurosis, 10, 196–97, 202. *See also* anxiety; trauma
Washington-Baltimore Psychoanalytic Institute, 149, 150, 151
Washington Psychoanalytic Institute, 148
Weber, Max, 173, 239
Weigert, Edith, 125, 126; career in the United States, 150–51; emigration to Turkey, 130–31; emigration to the United States, 138, 150; isolation in Turkey, 135–38, 157; relationship to Frieda Fromm-Reichman, 150, 151; relationship to Ruth Wilmanns Lidz, 150; at Schloss Tegel, 127
Weigert, Oscar, 130
Weisskopf, Walter, 12–13
Wells, F. L., 62–63, 64
White, William Alanson, 121
William Alanson White Institute, 121–22, 198, 203
Wilmanns, Karl, 127–29, 130, 148
Wilson, Colin, 195
Wilson, Woodrow, 104
Winnicott, Donald, 230, 231
Winterstein, Alfred, 85
Wittels, Fritz, 120–21
Wolfe, Tom, 216
women physicians: conservative constraints on, 17, 142–43; emigrant and socially oriented work of, 142; finding new social status, 151–52; in Weimar, 126, 127–28, 129–30, 142, 151. *See also* feminism
Worcester, Elwood, 40–41
word association test. *See* association test
World War I: Hitler's hysteria, 129; and intellectuals, 167, 168; and neurosis, 202; and psychoanalytic movement, 112
World War II: and anxiety, 18–19, 160, 190, 191–92, 233; facilitates psychoanalytic thinking, 196–97, 256; and personal psychology, 234; and pharmaceutical industry, 200–201; and W. H. Auden, 191–92
Wright, Richard, 195

Yale Institute of Human Relations, 26
Yale University French department, and existentialism, 195
Yalta Conference, 190
Yerkes, Robert, 62

Zaretsky, Eli, 8
Zurich school of psychoanalysis, 9, 34, 46, 51, 112. *See also* Jung, C. G.

www.ingramcontent.com/pod-product-compliance
Lightning Source LLC
Chambersburg PA
CBHW021938290426
44108CB00012B/885